DIET NATION

DIET NATION

EXPOSING THE OBESITY CRUSADE

Patrick Basham, Gio Gori and John Luik

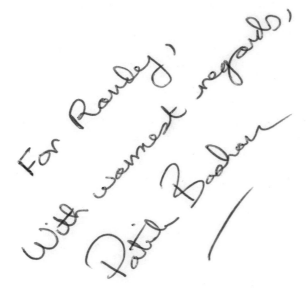

For Rawley,
With warmest regards,
Patrick Basham

British Library Cataloguing in Publication Data
A catalogue record of this book is available from the British Library

Printed and bound in the United Kingdom

ISBN-10: 1-904863-19-1
ISBN-13: 978-1-904863-19-9

Social Affairs Unit
314–322 Regent Street
London W1B 5SA
www.socialaffairsunit.org.uk

CONTENTS

ACKNOWLEDGEMENTS

We would like to thank Michael Mosbacher and the Social Affairs Unit for their willingness to publish this highly contrarian volume, and for the helpful comments of their anonymous reviewers. We are grateful to our editor, Clive Liddiard, for his careful attention to and constructive suggestions about the manuscript.

The central ideas and research for this book began a couple of years ago. The food and beverage industry has had neither input into nor influence upon the planning, research, writing or editing stages of this project.

We are equally critical, where necessary, of some of the positions, policies and actions of the major players in the obesity 'epidemic', including obesity crusaders, governments, organisations such as the World Health Organization, and the weight-loss, pharmaceutical and food and beverage industries.

Patrick Basham
Gio Gori
John Luik

THE AUTHORS

PATRICK BASHAM, a Channel Islander, is the founding director of the Democracy Institute, a new public-policy research organisation. A Cambridge-educated political scientist, he was previously Senior Fellow at the Cato Institute's Center for Representative Government. He is a Cato Institute Adjunct Scholar and a Lecturer at Johns Hopkins University, where he lectures on health care policy. Before joining Cato, he was founding director of the Social Affairs Center at the Fraser Institute, where he led the Institute's research in the areas of consumer choice and social policy regulation. He has authored, co-authored and edited books, studies, reviews and scholarly articles on a variety of policy topics. A highly regarded political commentator, he lectures on both sides of the Atlantic and appears regularly on British and American radio and television.

GIO BATTA GORI, an Italian émigré, first worked in the USA with the late Dr Jonas Salk of polio vaccine fame. In 1968, he joined the National Cancer Institute, where he was deputy director of the Division of Cancer Cause and Prevention. At the Institute, he founded and directed the Diet, Nutrition and Cancer Program, and was instrumental in organising the epochal US Congress hearings that gave life to the first nutritional guidelines for Americans, sparking the huge worldwide interest in nutrition as a public health issue. He has lectured in North America, Europe and elsewhere, and has been an advisor to international organisations. In 1976, he was recognised with the USA Public Health Service

Superior Service Award. Dr Gori holds a doctorate in biology from Italy, a Master of Public Health in epidemiology from Johns Hopkins University, and is a fellow of the Academy of Toxicological Sciences. For a quarter of a century he was the founding editor of *Nutrition and Cancer*, and he is now editor of *Regulatory Toxicology and Pharmacology*, as well as being the author of scientific papers and books.

JOHN LUIK is a leading public-policy analyst with expertise in the regulation of the food and beverage industry. Educated as a Rhodes Scholar at Oxford University, where he obtained a DPhil degree, he has taught at a number of universities. As Senior Associate of the Niagara Institute, he was responsible for its work in public policy, and leadership and organisational change. He has also worked as a director at a management consulting practice, and has served as a consultant to governmental institutions, professional organisations, and corporations in the United States, Europe, Asia, Africa, the Middle East and Latin America. A frequent media commentator and conference speaker, he is the author of several books and numerous scholarly articles. He writes regularly for newspapers and magazines on food and health issues.

INTRODUCTION

It is by now a received truth that the world, or at least a good portion of it, is in the grip of an unprecedented obesity epidemic that threatens a health catastrophe. Speaking at an EU conference on obesity in early 2005, Professor Philip James, chair of the International Obesity Task Force, noted that obesity 'took off in the 1980s and looks as if it was accelerating in the last five to 10 years. It's beginning to look as if we have an exponential rise.'[1]

Professor James is not alone in his worries. The US surgeon general has claimed that obesity, at least for Americans, was a 'greater threat than weapons of mass destruction', a threat that could only be averted by a 'cultural transformation'.[2] This theme was the centrepiece of a March 2004 press conference that featured the heads of the US Department of Health and Human Services (DHHS), the National Institutes of Health (NIH) and the Centers for Disease Control and Prevention (CDC) announcing the results of a CDC study, which claimed that 400,000 Americans died annually from poor diet and physical inactivity, making 'obesity' a killer to rival tobacco.[3]

Indeed, it has become impossible to pick up a newspaper or turn on the television without encountering a new claim about the damage done by fat, the causes of obesity, or what the government should do about it. For example, in the UK in 1985, the word 'obesity' appeared in only ten articles in *The Times*, but in 55 articles in 1995, and 205 from September 2002 to September 2003.[4] A search of the *Guardian* archives by year shows that 'obesity' featured 75 times in 1999 and

727 times in 2004, while 'childhood obesity' was found only twice in 1999, compared with 201 times in 2004.[5] In the US in 1994 there were just 33 newspaper and periodical references to an obesity epidemic, compared with nearly 700 in 2004.[6] Indeed, according to a recently published study, obesity issues now attract far more media attention than tobacco. Based on an analysis of eight years of media coverage from 1995–2003, the authors found that tobacco stories appeared to peak in 1996 to 97, while stories on obesity rose steadily from 1995 onward.[7]

While the sources of this epidemic are variously described as being linked to a growing fondness for sloth, the over-abundance of cheap food, the decline in physical activity, the inevitable corruptions accompanying post-modernity, the absence of manual labour, and the development of technology, particularly the Internet, for the pundit and the political and policymaking class the apparent causes of the epidemic are much more likely to be found in an increasingly fat-friendly environment; an environment engineered by the food and drink industry. Though there is a passing nod to personal responsibility in this tale of growing obesity, since obviously eating is a voluntary act, the major claim in the story is that the primary cause of obesity is to be found in the manufacturing and marketing practices of something increasingly referred to as 'Big Food'.

Not surprisingly, given this diagnosis, the prescription proposed to halt the growth of obesity focuses on government regulation and control: controlling food content and the conditions of selling food, controlling the pricing of food, and, perhaps most significantly, controlling the marketing of food. For instance, the UK's Food Standards Agency is considering warning labels for certain unhealthy foods, and at the same time is pressuring the food industry to change the constituents of some of its most popular foods. In France the French food standards authority, AFSSA, has argued that snacking by children must be discouraged, and new regulations will provide for fines for food makers who advertise 'junk foods' without health warnings. In the UK, in June 2005, the British Medical

Association recommended a total ban on advertising 'unhealthy' food to children.

In November 2005, the UK Department of Health published an advisory document which argued, in a move reminiscent of arguments about cigarette advertising, that celebrities and cartoon characters should be banished from advertisements that promote 'unhealthy' foods to children. Also, Ofcom, the UK's broadcasting regulator, is considering similar restrictions on food advertising. The December 2005 publication of the EU Green Paper, 'Promoting Healthy Diets and Physical Activity', also raises the question of whether involuntary restrictions on food advertising are required. This follows an April 2005 report by the European Heart Network (EHN), which concluded that children require protection from food advertising and recommended a ban on TV advertising of 'unhealthy' food to children.

We call the individuals who have manufactured this story about the obesity epidemic, and who endlessly repeat it, the 'obesity crusaders'. They are a relatively small group of public health officials in the United States, the EU and the World Health Organization, assorted academics (very many with close ties to the weight-loss and pharmaceutical industry), the International Obesity Task Force, a collection of so-called public-interest science groups such as the US Center for Science in the Public Interest, and representatives of the multi-billion-pound weight-loss industry. Their message is that obesity is a disease, not a moral failing; that very many of us are much too fat; that our extra pounds reduce our life expectancy; that our extra pounds are largely the result of a food environment produced by the food industry; that weight loss is necessary, achievable, sustainable and associated with significant reductions in mortality; that the public health community should assume a leadership role in tackling this epidemic through a variety of largely regulatory interventions; and that failure to deal with the obesity epidemic, especially amongst children, portends an unprecedented public health disaster (approaching the Black Death, according to the director of the Centers for Disease Control and Prevention).

This book offers a critical look at the various claims that make up the obesity story. While we are no apologists for obesity, and do believe that it represents a genuine risk for the morbidly obese, we find that the case against it is significantly and, more disturbingly, deliberately flawed. Not only are the claims of an obesity epidemic, particularly an epidemic of childhood obesity, often wildly exaggerated, but the science linking weight to unfavourable mortality outcomes is also frequently nonexistent or distorted. Moreover, not only is the causal account of the sources of obesity an account that roots obesity in an environment shaped by 'Big Food', at odds with the best evidence, but the policy prescriptions for solving the obesity crisis are most likely ineffective and at the same time threaten a fundamental assault on core democratic values.

Our objection to the obesity epidemic story focuses specifically on three areas:

● the absence of scientific evidence to support the main components of the story, namely that childhood obesity is increasing at an alarming rate, that overweight and obesity increase one's mortality risks, that the current body mass index (BMI) recommendations represent population ideals, that the overweight and moderately obese should be encouraged to lose weight because such loss will improve their health, and that one of the major causes of obesity is the consumption of inappropriate foods fostered by the marketing activities of the food industry;

● the lack of substantial evidence to suggest that the significant government interventions urged in the effort to stem obesity will actually work, and the considerable evidence to suggest that many policies advanced will be counterproductive;

● the significant risk that many of the policy proposals to prevent obesity will erode further individual liberty by enhancing the State's exclusive power to define what constitutes a good life.

AETIOLOGY AND EVIDENCE

It is a basic requirement of good public policy that the scientific basis for disease interventions be clear and compelling. The assumptions about obesity, diet, disease and mortality, as well as the evidence, are, however, unable to support the obesity epidemic story. For instance, it is now clear that overweight and even modest obesity are not associated with increased mortality risks, and that the claims that obesity represents a threat to health comparable to tobacco are unsupported by the scientific data.[8] To take but one example, the 2004 CDC study, which claimed that annually there are nearly 400,000 deaths in the US that are attributable to diet and physical inactivity, was discredited in April 2005 by a new study from researchers at the CDC and the NIH that put the annual figure for deaths from overweight and obesity at just 25,814.[9]

It is also clear that the claims about rising childhood obesity, whether in the UK or North America, are very much exaggerated and certainly do not reach epidemic proportions, and that childhood obesity does not lead to a greater health risk in adulthood.[10] For instance, as the Social Issues Research Centre pointed out, the Health Survey for England, published by the Department of Health in December 2004, found that the average weight of boys (aged 3–15) in 2003 was 31.9 kg, compared with 32 kg in 1995. The average weight of girls was 32.4 kg in 2003 and 32 kg in 1995. In 2003 the average 15-year-old boy weighed 60.7 kg, compared with 58.8 kg in 1995. Again, from 1995–2003 there was an increase in average BMIs for boys of 0.5 and 0.6 for girls. Clearly, these changes in the BMI of UK children fail to support Professor James's alarmist claim of an exponential increase in obesity, as the Health Survey data do not suggest an accelerating rate of increase.

A similar sense of unsubstantiated alarmism is to be found in claims of an epidemic of paediatric obesity in, for example, Canada. Sheela Basrur, chief medical health officer for the province of Ontario, for instance, in her 2004 report claimed that an 'epidemic of overweight and obesity is threatening

Ontario's health'.[11] Yet the evidence adduced in her report contradicts this claim. For instance, the report notes that 'The proportion of children who are overweight or obese remained relatively stable through the 1990s', a fact that renders absurd the idea of an epidemic of childhood obesity (which requires an *accelerating* rate of increase in overweight and obesity). In fact, Basrur's own data, which compare the percentage of overweight and obese children aged 12–18 between 1990 and 2000, refutes the claim of a paediatric obesity epidemic. For example, in 1990, 19.3 per cent of boys were overweight, compared to 19.1 per cent in 2000. In 1990, 10.8 per cent of girls were overweight, compared with 11.1 per cent in 2000 – a statistically non-significant increase. In 2000, 3.3 per cent of girls were obese, compared with 3.4 per cent in 1990, a non-significant decrease.

Similar data are found in the United States. According to the most recent data, the prevalence of overweight and obesity in US children showed no statistically significant increase from 1999 to 2002.[12] In fact, caloric intake for US children and young people has not changed significantly in recent years.[13] Similarly, in the UK, the latest National Diet and Nutrition Survey found that, since the last survey in 1983, energy intake in both boys and girls aged 4–18 had declined.[14]

Equally unsupported is the claim of an epidemic of adult obesity. While there has been significant weight gain amongst the very heaviest segment of the population,[15] this has not been true of most of the individuals who are labelled overweight and obese, whose weights are only slightly increased. According to Hedley *et al.*, for instance, there was no statistically significant increase in adult weight in the US from 1999 to 2002. Indeed, the abrupt change in the BMI classification of overweight, from 27 to 25, resulted in millions of Americans who had been classified as normal weight suddenly being described as overweight.[16]

Even more crucially, the critical claim that there is a link between excessive food intake and childhood obesity is highly controversial. As Muecke *et al.* have noted, 'Though some studies support the contention that overweight children over-consume food, others contradicted this widely-accepted notion. Comparisons of obese adolescents to normal peers have demonstrated comparable energy intake and nutrient distribution.'[17] More recently, Hanley observed that the 'notion that obesity is caused by excess energy intake is not generally supported in the scientific literature'.[18]

A cross-cultural review of obesity in children and adolescents in the US, France, Australia, Britain and Spain found little evidence to support the claim that overweight and obese children and adolescents consume more calories than others.[19] Indeed, the authors note that some studies find that these children may, in fact, consume less energy than their thinner peers.

Then, too, the entire idea of 'good' food and 'bad' food, and the link between a particular diet and reduced morbidity, is very much open to question. A recently published series of studies, for instance, has found that a low-fat diet has little effect on reducing the risk of breast cancer, colorectal cancer or cardiovascular disease in postmenopausal women.[20] Comparative studies looking at the fat and blood cholesterol levels across different cultures have failed to sustain the claims of a cause-and-effect connection between life expectancies and diets. Crete, for instance, with its 'healthy' Mediterranean diet, has one of the lowest incidences of heart disease, yet has a fat intake of 40 per cent, which is close to that of the UK. The Netherlands, which has one of the highest life expectancies in Europe, has a fat intake of 48 per cent. This compares to the Masai of East Africa, who have very low levels of blood cholesterol, yet derive some 66 per cent of their calories from fat. About all that might be said with reasonable certainty about the obesity–diet–mortality connection is that, as the late epidemiologist Petr Skrabanek observed, 'people who eat, die'.[21]

Equally unsupported are the recommendations for population-wide weight loss that are based on the assumed connections between overweight and modest obesity and premature mortality. For example, the US National Heart, Lung and Blood Institute advises overweight individuals, regardless of their current weight, to lose 10 per cent of their weight.[22] These recommendations not only fail to take into account the extensive evidence that sustained weight loss is extraordinarily difficult for very many people, but also ignore the evidence of an association between weight loss and increased mortality.[23] They effectively counsel a weight-loss programme for the entire population that not only has no scientifically established benefit, but that also carries substantial risks for many individuals. Indeed, it might be argued that such unfounded and reckless health advice constitutes malpractice.

The evidence supporting the claim that advertising is the cause of fat children and adults also looks highly suspect. UK ad-spend on food and drink has actually been falling in real terms for the past five years. It now constitutes 18 per cent of all TV advertisements, as compared to 34 per cent in 1982. Across the Atlantic, advertising during children's TV programming, according to the Federal Trade Commission, has declined by 34 per cent in recent years. Indeed, despite claims about the influence of TV food advertising aimed at children, UK children watch less television daily than any other group in the population.[24]

Again, there appears to be no compelling evidence that even heavily advertised foods like breakfast cereals and fizzy drinks are making children obese. Epidemiological studies fail to support the claim that dietary fat causes obesity in kids.[25] Nor are there any clinical trials that validate the theory that an increase in carbohydrate consumption, through things like breakfast cereals, sweets and fizzy drinks, leads to overeating and obesity.[26]

Equally importantly, the scientific literature contains numerous studies that count *against* the claim that such heavily advertised carbohydrates as fast foods and fizzy drinks lead to fatter kids. A 2004 Harvard study, for instance, looked at 14,000 schoolchildren and found that, however junk food was defined, with or without fizzy drinks, it did not lead to obesity in children.[27]

Then, too, there are extensive and significant econometric studies that have examined the connection between food advertising and the size of the food market, both in Europe and in the United States.[28] For the most part, these studies have found that, while food advertising may influence the consumption of food brands, it does not increase either total food consumption or food category consumption. These findings constitute a near fatal flaw in the claims that advertising causes childhood obesity, for, to have advertising held responsible for obesity, they would need to show convincingly that it influences not simply brands, but either entire diets or at least parts of diets.

Finally, the suggestion that advertising restrictions or bans, voluntary or involuntary, might reduce childhood obesity is contradicted by some real-world evidence. Since 1980 the Canadian province of Quebec has banned all food advertising to children, yet childhood obesity rates and consumption of so-called unhealthy foods are not substantially different there from other parts of Canada. Then, too, for the last decade Sweden has also had a food advertising ban for children, but this has resulted neither in significant reductions in childhood obesity, nor in marked differences in obesity rates compared with other European countries.[29] As even the World Health Organization's (WHO) review of food advertising to children conceded, there is a 'lack of objective research into the effects of regulation on dietary patterns and longer term health'.[30]

EFFICACY

A further problem with the obesity epidemic story centres on the question of efficacy: namely, will the measures being suggested actually work? Or, just as crucially, will they work without unforeseen counterproductive effects? One of the more unfortunate consequences of the exaggerated claims of an obesity epidemic is that such talk, both in the media and amongst politicians and policymakers, has produced an unwarranted sense of alarm and urgency that works against the careful consideration not only of what evidence of harm there really is, but also where that evidence actually points in terms of solutions. Interventions to 'solve' the obesity epidemic are increasingly accorded the privileged position of self-evident truth, rather than being subjected to a rigorous process of examination that asks whether there is a fit between the problem and the proposed remedy, and that leads to the misguided, the ineffective, the wasteful and the positively harmful being winnowed out.

For instance, will the solutions to obesity really change the eating habits not only of individuals but of entire populations, so that they will be, if not thin, then at least less fat? The numbers do not look promising, given that, out of every 100 people who diet, only four are able to maintain their post-diet weight.[31] As the authors of one study concluded, 'Obesity must be recognized as a chronic condition for which no cure can reasonably be expected.'[32] Several studies that have looked, for instance, at dieting (whether through commercial programmes or self-help), at diet types (low carbohydrate, high protein, high fat vs. low calorie, high carbohydrate and low fat) and at weight-loss counselling have concluded that attempts at weight loss are largely unsuccessful, even in highly controlled situations.[33] Describing the results of one study that compared low-carbohydrate and low-fat diets, the researchers concluded that 'Adherence was poor and attrition was high in both groups.'[34] Another study, which compared self-help and commercial diet plans, found that, after two years, the differences in biological parameters between the two groups were statistically non-significant.[35]

More worrisome yet are the health risks that accompany dieting. Several studies have reported that weight loss is associated with increased mortality.[36] The connection between weight loss and increased mortality is particularly evident in two large studies that controlled for smoking – the Iowa Women's Health study and the American Cancer Society (ACS) study – which showed that weight loss was associated with higher rates of mortality. In the follow-up to the ACS study, researchers found that healthy obese women were, in fact, better off *not* losing weight. Healthy women who lost weight had increased mortality risks from cancer, cardio-vascular disease (CVD) and all other diseases when compared to healthy women who did not diet.[37] A subsequent study discovered the same results for men.[38]

Similar questions of efficacy surround the policies advanced to counter childhood obesity, including changing school food, removing vending machines with 'bad' food, and increasing physical education. For instance, in a very large school-based obesity prevention programme – Child Adolescent Trial for Cardiovascular Health (CATCH) – run in the United States and involving 50 schools in four states, there were no statistically significant changes in the children's blood pressure, BMI or cholesterol levels.[39] Such policy failures are hardly surprising, given that several recent studies have shown that adult attempts to control children's eating patterns result not only in children eating more, but in an increased likelihood of body-image problems and eating disorders.[40]

Then, too, there is the substantial worry about unintended outcomes, as some experts suggest that the most significant cause of eating disorders is a food- and diet-obsessed environment. As nutritionist Francis Berg has observed of rising rates of eating disorders, 'Many specialists ... are convinced that the current high rates of eating disorders in the U.S. are the inevitable result of 60–80 million adults dieting, losing weight, rebounding, and learning to be chronic dieters.'[41] Though reliable estimates of the extent of eating disorders are difficult to come by, most experts suggest that in the US eight million people, mostly women, suffer from them, including about 10 per cent of high-school students.[42] Then, too, given the self-esteem problems associated with overweight and obesity in children and adolescents,[43] there may well be a credible risk that the continued talk of childhood obesity, as well as the actual interventions to supposedly remedy it, could, in fact, impair rather than enhance the health of the very people it is designed to help. Warning of these dangers, particularly those associated with screening for overweight and obese children, Ned Calonge, writing in *Pediatrics*, noted that:

A final and pervasive problem is that we have little information about the potential harms of screening, such as labelling, reduced self-esteem, poor eating habits, eating disorders, adverse family relations, or the effects of continuing to lose and regain weight (yo-yo dieting). The first principle of medicine is well known: *primum non nocere*. If we forge ahead with an intervention (whether therapeutic, preventive, or even diagnostic) without knowing whether it is beneficial, we run the risk of causing unintentional harm.[44]

In fact, when one takes into account the revised figures for the relatively few lives lost prematurely through obesity, and weighs these against the very significant health costs associated with both dieting and eating disorders, then a compelling case can be made that damage to health from attempting to lose weight is far greater than the health consequences of overweight and obesity. As Paul Campos has noted:

> The prevalence of and the devastating health effects that sometimes follow from yo-yo dieting, along with the high mortality rates found among people who are just a few pounds under what the government and the health establishment have mischaracterized as an 'ideal weight', along with the fact that there is virtually no compelling epidemiological evidence that significant long-term weight loss is either practical or confirms a health benefit all provide powerful evidence for the proposition that attempting to lose weight causes far more damage to our health than maintaining even very high weight levels.[45]

Indeed, rather than a campaign against obesity, what is required is a war on thinness.

INDIVIDUAL AUTONOMY AND DEFINING A GOOD LIFE

Scientific evidence and efficacy are but quibbles, however, beside the third problem with the war on obesity: namely its enormous potential for eroding individual liberty through employing the engine of the State, particularly its propaganda and regulatory powers, once again to define and enforce a single vision of what constitutes a good life.

At the core of democratic society lies considerable unease with the idea that the government has a role in structuring a citizen's soul through telling him what to think, believe or be. This is because there is a fundamental conflict between the core democratic values of autonomy and respect (values that imply that the government is a creation of its citizens) and any form of social engineering (with its counter-assumption that the State's citizens are legitimately the creation of the government). The war on obesity, however, proposes to ignore, indeed to erase, this unease, since its key assumption is that the State has both the right and the scientific expertise to define what constitutes healthy living. It proposes that the State's judgement is inherently superior to the individual's judgement that fat is, if not good, at least personally tolerable. And it contends that the individual has an obligation to order his life according to the State's judgement about health, and that the State might justifiably force him to conform if he demurs.

This claim of State-enforced healthy living as scientifically mandated is both fundamentally fraudulent and morally illegitimate. Consider the typical argument against, say, eating large amounts of fast food. The champion of the campaign against obesity will claim that it is a scientific fact that if you stop eating large amounts of fast food you will live longer. Therefore, he will say, you should stop eating so much fast food. But this will only work if another premise is added to the argument: namely *if* you value living longer more than you value eating fast food, then you should stop eating so much fast food.

But as soon as this premise is added, the scientific character of the war on fat is exposed for what it is: a semantic trick that attempts to conceal the value-laden and ideological (as opposed to the scientific) nature of the undertaking. Although it might well be science that suggests one could live longer if one ate less fast food (though the evidence on this is very meagre), it is not science (but rather someone's values) that tells me I ought to value living longer more than eating fast food.

This does not make the fat opponent's injunctions about obesity unworthy of attention: it merely suggests that they are not the pronouncements of science, so much as views about the merits of a particular way of living. And this means that they (as every other bit of moral philosophy about the good life) must be justified not by dogmatic faux-scientific pronouncements and the force of law, but by careful argument.

At best, then, the scientific foundations of the war on fat extend only to its claims about the causes of disease, and these, we argue, are highly contradictory. When those in favour of getting the State involved in the obesity business begin to talk about what to do with this information, they cease to speak as scientists. This, in turn, has enormous implications for public policy on obesity. When the critics of obesity tell us that we must all be thinner, even if this involves using the regulatory powers of the State, they must tell us (and this they have never done) not only why a life of, say, 70 years packed full of the self-chosen pleasures of fast food and chocolate, for instance, is in some sense inferior to a life of 73 years lived without those pleasures, but also why the State is justified in intervening to amend the individual's choice of the former over the latter.

This does not mean, of course, that a life of 70 years crammed with fast food and chocolate is necessarily better than 73 abstemious years. What it does suggest is that these are not scientific choices that the promoters of the war on obesity can make for the rest of us, but are individual moral choices about the kind of life we want, and are core instances of what it means to act autonomously in a democratic society. What the war on obesity proposes to do, all under the guise of 'scientific decision-making' or 'evidence-based medicine', is to replace my decision about the tradeoffs between fast food and chocolate and the risk of a possibly shorter life with the government's calculus of what is good for me. Rather than allowing individuals to make their own health decisions about fat and obesity, we are being told to put our faith in a health establishment and bureaucracy that consistently misrepresents scientific findings, issues dietary guidelines that are sloppy and, in many instances, purely arbitrary, and proposes solutions that are without intellectual, moral or practical rigour. At its core the war on obesity presumes a nursery nation full not of rational and self-governing adults, but of docile infants too uncertain of their own values and how best to realise them to be left to make their own way in the world.

The excessive preoccupation with the values of health and longevity over the last decades of the twentieth century appears to have deadened many to the fact that there are other values that are equally important to a full and good life. So taken are we with the new religion of health that we seem prepared to submit to any regimen, surrender virtually any pleasure and compromise any liberty so long as it gains us a deferral of death. In this sense, the war on obesity is about far more than fat: it is about the relentless attempt by both the health establishment and the State to order what we are under the benign idea of health. Stripped to its essentials, the war against obesity is really a war on what the health establishment conceives to be illegitimate pleasure. A proposal to impose, for instance, a 'sin tax' on certain books, plays, ideas or associations in order to change people's behaviour and improve their mental health would not survive a moment of serious consideration. Yet the same policy applied to food appears to many to be uncontroversial precisely because it is 'only' about health.

The lasting legacy of a war on obesity will be both a much fatter government and a much thinner citizenry. The government will be fatter through its expanded power to shape inappropriately the lives of its citizens, and the citizenry will be thinner in its capacity for choice, self-government and personal responsibility. We should prefer a society of the fat and the free to one of the lean who have surrendered to the government the right to decide what constitutes a good life.

A NOT SO MODEST PRESCRIPTION

The last thing that a work of this nature should do is substitute another set of dogmatic pronouncements about obesity for those promulgated by the obesity crusaders. Our main role is critically to examine both the case for an epidemic of obesity and the policies proposed to address it, rather than to explore at length an alternative account of what, if anything, can or should be done. Even though this book is centred far more on diagnosis than prescription, we nevertheless believe that there are six ways, particularly through focusing on the root causes, in which the 'obesity epidemic' might be legitimately addressed.

First, and without doubt the most difficult task, is to address one of the root causes of the 'obesity epidemic', which is neither gluttony nor sloth, neither excessive food consumption nor insufficient energy expenditure, but rather the way in which science and its findings are both misrepresented and used by the obesity crusaders to distort the policy and the regulatory process. To do this requires a new understanding about the significant limitations of observational epidemiology as a basis both for really understanding issues like population-wide obesity and for crafting policy responses to them. Integral to such an understanding will be a real commitment, as opposed to the current mere lip service, to making evidence-based science the basis on which to decide whether there is a public health problem and what the appropriate response to that problem might be. Such an understanding will dramatically reduce the opportunities available for individuals like the obesity crusaders to pass off as genuine science that which is, in reality, a corrupted reading of the scientific process and its results that is intended both to manufacture 'epidemics' and to hijack the policy and political processes to fix these faux events. While this task is both the most fundamental and the most urgent, it is also the most daunting and uncertain of success.

Second, significant attention must be devoted to the public health establishment's uncritical attachment to the tenets of health promotion, most especially its beliefs, none of which is credible, that many illnesses are the result of lifestyle; that there is a scientific consensus about the one 'healthy' way to live one's life; that a major function of the public health establishment is to convince individuals to accept this consensus definition of 'healthy'; and that coercion is justified to prevent unhealthy living. While corrupted science provides the raw materials for the obesity crusaders' claims, it is a health establishment in thrall to health promotion that provides both the environment and the institutions for launching and sustaining a war on obesity. More importantly, it is health promotion's simplistic commitment to health – and indeed public health over individual autonomy and respect – that provides the basis for so many of the more offensive policies proposed by the obesity crusaders. If the extent of obesity is to be properly understood and, once understood, then intelligently and effectively engaged, obesity must be divorced from any association with the scientifically compromised, ineffective and offensively paternalistic practices of health promotion.

Third, focusing on another root cause of the obesity crusade, there needs to be a reversal of the process of medicalising obesity – a demedicalisation of obesity, or at least moderate obesity, if you will; for it is this process that has both allowed the obesity story to become a public 'fact', endorsed by governments at all levels, and permitted the obesity crusaders to dominate and use for their own purposes the national and international public health organisations. Like the reform of science proposed above, the success of this process is extraordinarily hard and will require two things:

a) the unrelenting, patient and systematic exposure of the unscientific character of virtually all parts of the obesity epidemic story, but especially its claims about the extent of obesity, the connection between obesity and mortality and disease, the role of the food industry in 'creating' obesity, the advisability and possibility of significant and sustained population-wide weight loss, and the viability of government regulation as a solution to the 'obesity' problem;

b) a sustained effort to make the public aware of the web of conflicted and self-interested relationships that exists between certain obesity crusaders, with their assertions about obesity and science, and the weight-loss and pharmaceutical industry, certain government panels and task forces, and the wider public health community.

A *fourth* way in which the 'obesity epidemic' might be addressed is through a renewed personal and social commitment to the importance of physical activity, coupled with a candid recognition that a variety of factors, many the natural product of increased affluence, will continue to conspire against it.

Though the evidence about the connections between physical activity and weight gain is not conclusive, it is nonetheless substantial enough to have physical activity recommended for those at risk from obesity. For instance, Lee and Paffenbarger note that 'Almost 60 percent of all US adults today engage in no physical activity or only irregular physical activity.'[46] The same problem is found in the UK, as the House of Commons Health Committee observed in its 2004 obesity report that only around 37 per cent of men and 25 per cent of women currently achieve the Department of Health's activity targets. Again, as Troiano *et al.* note in their study of adolescent weight gain, 'The lack of evidence of a general increase in energy intake among youths despite an increase in the prevalence of overweight suggests that physical inactivity is a major public health challenge in this group.'[47] As Kimm *et al.* observed in the *Lancet* in 2005, 'These results suggest that habitual activity plays an important role in weight gain, with no parallel evidence that energy intake had a similar role.'[48]

Fifth, in addition to changes in levels of physical activity, there are various other approaches to population-wide weight gain that do not depend on government coercion. These include changes in diet and eating patterns, an increase in consumer knowledge about food and nutrition, improved levels of parenting, and even consideration of the use of discrimination. For instance, a recently released survey by the International Food Information Council (IFIC) on consumer knowledge about calorie consumption, dietary fats, sugars and carbohydrates shows that many consumers are confused about dietary issues and advice. Commenting on the survey,[49] IFIC President Susan Borra noted that 'while consumers are getting the message that they need to make positive dietary and lifestyle changes, putting that advice into practice has been challenging and confusing for many of them'.[50]

For example, few consumers were clear about which of the basic food components such as dietary fat, carbohydrates and protein cause weight gain, with only 29 per cent understanding that calories are the source of weight gain and that all calories are the same. Again, the survey found that nearly 90 per cent of respondents did not know the number of calories they should consume in a day. What this suggests is, first, that a major part of the weight-gain problem is rooted in a lack of consumer knowledge, and, second, that rather than coercive regulatory interventions, what might well prove effective is providing consumers with accurate, relevant and easily understood information.

Finally, if there is any scientific justification for concern about obesity, it is generally not with children or with the vast majority of the population (85.7 per cent of the US population) that falls within the categories of overweight or even obese, but rather with the morbidly obese – those with BMIs in excess of 40. For instance, as Wright *et al.* showed, plump children should not excite concern about an 'obesity epidemic' that is threatening paediatric health, since being an overweight or obese child does not carry a greater health risk, and 'whole population interventions in childhood directed at reducing body mass index in childhood may not benefit adult health'.[51]

Moreover, Gronniger's recent analysis of the relationship of BMI to mortality found that mortality rates were essentially the same for individuals with BMIs from 20 to 35 – 'Normal weight individuals of both genders did not appear to be relatively more long-lived than mildly obese individuals (BMIs of 30–35).' This suggests that the only scientific justification for obesity interventions is among a small section of the population with BMIs over 40 (3.3 per cent of US adults in 2002).[52] As Gronniger writes, 'The present results highlight previous findings indicating that mild obesity and overweight are not strongly related to mortality. It would be more reasonable to focus on the smaller group of people in the severely obese category (BMIs of 40 and over) which has a clear relationship to mortality.'

This relatively small group might well benefit from medical and pharmaceutical interventions of various kinds – interventions that will depend on a better biological and medical understanding of obesity. Whatever the nature of these interventions for the extremely obese might be, the important point is that they, and not the merely overweight and obese, should be the focus of any obesity crusade.

CHAPTER 1

COOKING UP A SCARE: HOW FAT BECAME *THE* HEALTH CATASTROPHE

'But wait a bit', the Oysters cried,
'Before we have our chat;
For some of us are out of breath,
And all of us are fat!'

Lewis Carroll,
Through the Looking Glass

INTRODUCTION

Most of the people who have lived in the past would find the current European and North American obsession with fat puzzling. That is because most of them, along with those who today live in traditional societies, saw fat as something that signified both wealth and health. Indeed, in about 85 per cent of the societies for which evidence exists, being comfortably plump was considered highly desirable.[1] Rather than being deviant, being fat for these people suggested someone who had triumphed in mankind's perennial struggle against famine and disease.

But this view of fat, however true for most of human history, has been under attack for at least the last century. From about the 1880s, under the influence of the ideas of the New Nutrition, changing views of feminine beauty and fashion, a growing athleticism, and an increased interest in weight control, members of the middle class on both sides of the Atlantic increasingly came to believe that fat was bad. Writing about this changing perception of fat, food historian Levenstein notes:

As for the middle classes, for almost fifty years they had been bombarded with warnings against the perils of overindulging in this abundance. Since the 1880s the scientists, home economists, cookery writers, advertisers, and faddists to whom they turned for dietary wisdom had been propagating the ideas of the New Nutrition. These taught that all foods could be broken down into proteins, carbohydrates, and fats, and that one should eat only as much of each of them as the body required. The idea that the body's energy needs could be measured in calories took hold, along with the notion that one would gain weight if one ingested more of these than the body burned.[2]

One can see this changing attitude to obesity in, for instance, language. Several new expressions for those of ample size, all of them unfavourable, entered the language during the latter half of the nineteenth century, including porky, jumbo and slob; this last in reference to a Lord Mayor of London who was described as a 'fat slob'. This growing dislike of the fat, and the belief that being overweight was an issue of personal responsibility, is also evident in the increasing number of jokes and cartoons that were steadily directed against the now unfashionably plump. For instance, a popular American play in 1907 was titled *Nobody Loves a Fat Man*. In Edith Wharton's 1913 *The Custom of the Country*, Undine Spragg, musing about her appearance, notes that 'She was tall enough to carry off a little extra weight, but excessive slimness was the fashion, and she shuddered at the thought that she might some day deviate from the perpendicular.'

Spragg's worry about deviating from the perpendicular was supported by a growing medical literature on the weight problem. While there was early work in the middle of the nineteenth century in the UK on corpulence, the major findings on food, diet and weight came from Germany, particularly the work of the German doctor Max Rubner, who discovered the role of carbohydrates, proteins and fat. Part of what drove this nineteenth-century interest in weight was the desire to define scientifically what constituted health and wellness, as well as deviancy. By the middle of the 1880s, British medical journals were regularly carrying articles about obesity and its treatment, and by the early 1900s American medical journals had also begun to include articles on diet and weight reduction. Though this medical research confirmed the growing social prejudice against fat, it appears, unlike the situation today, to have been a product rather than a cause of that prejudice.

While this worry about fat would suffer the occasional and temporary setback, most notably during the Great Depression and World War II, for the most part it has dominated the social, cultural, medical and, most recently, the political and policy landscape so completely that, in most Western societies (and despite the best efforts of the size activists and the anti-diet movement), overweight and obesity are almost invariably seen as deviant, even though they supposedly affect up to 60 per cent of some populations.

In this sense, the century-long European and American preoccupation with thinness and the rejection of fat is very much a social construct in which obesity is increasingly associated with the morally unacceptable. Fat was not naturally bad: rather it became bad, in the sense that fat people were often portrayed and seen as lazy, stupid and weak-willed individuals who were unwilling, rather than unable, to deal with their weight. As Susan Bordo points out, fat became 'indicative of laziness, lack of discipline, unwillingness to conform' and, most importantly in a society focused on mobility, the 'absence of all of those managerial abilities that confer upward mobility'.[3]

It is not, however, the deviant status of fat that has prompted the incessant talk of an obesity epidemic – or the wide-ranging calls for government action to combat it that have dominated the media and the public consciousness in the early years of the new century. This focus – perhaps even obsession – with obesity is due to a carefully orchestrated campaign on the part of a group of researchers, physicians, public health officials, activists and, more recently, the plaintiff bar, many with significant financial interests in the obesity issue, who have managed to use Europe's and America's moral aversion to fat as the foundation for a war by the public health establishment and the government on obesity. This is not to say that there has been no increase in the weight of European and North American adults and children over the last decade. It is rather to say that these increases, particularly for children, have been greatly exaggerated, that the determination of what constitutes being overweight and obese is a wholly arbitrary, rather than a scientifically justified, standard, and that there is little evidence to support the claim that being overweight or modestly obese leads to premature death.

MEDICALISING OBESITY: THE ARCHITECTS OF THE WAR ON OBESITY

Unlike the last century's disapproval of obesity, the new war on fat, while building on society's notion of fat as morally bad, is premised rather on a different sort of claim: namely, that fat is medically bad since it leads to a variety of health problems and early death. The story, in all of its stark simplicity, is that fat equates to disease and early death. In effect, obesity is no longer a moral failing of bad fat people, but a sickness, acquired in large measure from a 'toxic food environment', that requires medical treatment. Instead of getting fat being something that individuals choose to do, or at least allow to happen, getting fat is now something that *happens* to them. In this sense, the architects of the war on obesity learned an important lesson from the war on tobacco, which early on decided that smokers were not the problem, so much as the tobacco industry. This does not mean that there is no moral component in the war on fat; it simply means, as we shall see, that, as with tobacco, the moral story has moved from the individual to the corporate level, from personal responsibility to corporate responsibility. While there are no longer any bad (fat) individuals in the obesity drama, there are now plenty of bad institutions (in the form of, for instance, Big Food), which are indifferent to the ways in which their actions can bring disease and death to individuals.

The medicalisation of obesity, where something that was

previously seen as a moral problem is transformed into an illness to be defined, managed and treated exclusively by the medical profession, began in both Europe and the United States as early as the 1950s, with the medical profession's claims that obesity was a medical problem that required medical treatment.[4]

In addition to these claims about treating obesity, the move to medicalise fat can be seen in the profession's use of professionally neutral terms like obese, adipose and over-weight, in preference to plump, corpulent and paunchy, to describe people, as well as more value-free descriptions to characterise the issues associated with eating problems. For instance, overeating was no longer gluttony but hyperorexia or acoria, and sloth gave way to chronic fatigue syndrome or lethargy.[5] As Chang and Christakis note in their study of the entries on obesity in a widely used medical textbook from 1927 to 2000, while the text consistently attributes the cause of obesity to consuming more calories than are expended, 'Despite the unwavering nature of this basic model, an evolving set of causal factors is superimposed. Early models invoke aberrant individual activities, such as habitual overeating, while later editions drop these factors in favour of genetic and, paradoxically, environmental effects.'[6]

The process of medicalising obesity can also be seen in the move to have obesity officially recognised as a disease (it is listed in the *International Classifications of Diseases* as ICD-9-CM 1990), and in the increasing use of the language of risk factors in discussion of obesity. Obesity, for instance, is now routinely described as a risk factor for cardiovascular disease and type 2 diabetes. Equally important to obesity's 'disease' status has been the development of a recognised medical speciality, in this case the American Society of Bariatric Physicians (based on the Greek root *baros*, weight), with its own publications such as *Bariatric Medicine*, *Obesity Research* and the *International Journal of Obesity*, as well as the development of specific medical treatments for obesity, such as surgery, drug therapy for weight loss, medically devised and supervised dieting regimes, and psychiatric interventions.

Despite the appearance of scientific justification, we wish to argue that the description of obesity as a disease, and of obesity as an epidemic, is unjustified, not simply by the evidence (which is examined in considerable detail in Chapter 2) but as a matter of logic and definition. Epidemics, properly defined, are communicable diseases that increase at an exponential rate. Yet obesity is not communicable: people do not catch obesity from others. At the very most, obesity might be a non-communicable disease. But, of course, there cannot be epidemics of non-communicable diseases.

LOUIS DUBLIN AND THE FIRST WAR ON OBESITY

Despite the fact that the claims of an 'obesity epidemic' (or, more accurately, pandemic, since it is claimed that obesity is now a worldwide problem) have been gradually developed over the last two decades, the foundation for the current obesity problem was laid in the 1950s through the work of the biologist Dr Louis Dublin of the Metropolitan Life Insurance Company (MLIC) of the United States. Indeed, if there were two obesity epidemics in the twentieth century (1950 to 1960 and 1985 to 2006), the first owed its origin more to Dublin than anyone else. Dublin's career lasted almost 60 years, and his prodigious published output (over 600 articles, pamphlets and speeches) was responsible for the core claim that sustains talk of an 'obesity epidemic': the belief that obesity is the major source of illness and premature death. Though Dublin's role in creating the first obesity crisis is now forgotten, his techniques, his claims – particularly their unscientific foundation – and his capacity to convince and galvanise the medical community of the 1950s are all strikingly similar to the elements of today's 'obesity epidemic'.

In some senses, the 1950s were an odd time in American history for a moral panic about obesity. Life expectancies had risen sharply since 1900 (when the average for males was 47), largely as a result of the decline of mortality from infectious diseases. Moreover, after the relative austerity brought by the Depression and the war years, most people were caught up in rebuilding their lives in the midst of a steadily increasing affluence. Then, too, Dublin's message that Americans were digging their graves with their teeth was hardly new, as he had been making similar claims for years. What was new, however, was the urgency he now attached to the weight problem and the way in which he sold his claims about weight as the source of premature death to the medical community.

In June 1951, Dublin was invited to present the results of his newest actuarial studies on weight and mortality to an American Medical Association (AMA) symposium. Dublin's studies were based on 25,998 men and 24,901 women who took out insurance policies from 1925 to 1934 and whose policy anniversary was in 1950. What Dublin found, and what shocked the AMA, was that men with what Dublin called 'marked obesity' had a mortality rate that was 70 per cent higher than average-weight men. Women with marked obesity had a mortality rate 61 per cent greater, while those who were 'moderately obese' in both sexes had an increased mortality rate of 42 per cent over those of average weight.[7]

What caught the attention of Dublin's audience was that weight-related mortality appeared to be causing more deaths than previously, since 'death rates from diseases like pneumonia and tuberculosis, which were high among underweights, have declined sharply in recent decades'.

What was equally striking, according to Dublin, was that the benefits from overweight that he and others had previously found for younger age groups had disappeared. For instance, Dublin had previously suggested that, until age 30, those who were underweight had higher rates of mortality beginning from age 20. Effectively, being overweight now, according to Dublin, had no protective effect. Moreover, while morbid obesity had always been considered a danger to health, Dublin's figures suggested that the problem was also associated with overweight and moderate obesity, effectively bringing millions of people within the danger zone.

The problem, of course, was that Dublin's work rested on a widespread confusion, which he did little to alleviate. His mortality figures were based on average weights – which were themselves problematic – but his recommendations for optimal health and longevity (and those adopted by the medical profession) were based on what Dublin considered to be ideal weights. Whereas the insurance industry had, since 1923, used the notion of ideal weight to represent the weight that was correlated with optimum life expectancy based on the data for average weights, from 1942 Dublin had instead begun to talk about 'ideal weights' that were not statistically connected with mortality outcomes, but represented weights that the population should strive to maintain. As Dublin wrote, these weights were designed to 'help people aim for a weight below the average for their height'.[8] Dublin's ideal weight, in fact, bore no relation to what the average American actually weighed. Thus, Dublin arbitrarily defined overweight as 10 per cent in excess of the ideal, while obesity was 20 to 30 per cent above ideal. Thus, both overweight and obesity were substantially above an ideal that itself was below average weights.

Dublin, of course, claimed that his notion of ideal was, in fact, scientifically based. He pointed to a sample of 2,300 Metropolitan policyholders who had originally been forced to pay more for their insurance because they were overweight and who had subsequently lost enough weight to reduce their premiums. According to Dublin, these policyholders' life expectancy returned to the same level as those whose weights were ideal. Indeed, for the women who lost weight, life expectancy actually exceeded those with ideal weights. For many of his life insurance associates, and several in the medical profession, Dublin's figures provided scientific confirmation that weight was connected to an increased risk of death, and that weight loss could improve health and longevity.

The confusion between ideal and average weights, and Dublin's arbitrary definition of what constituted ideal, overweight and obese, constituted only one problem with his work.[9] The other, and more damning, problem was the self-selected nature of his life insurance cohort. For the most part, those buying life insurance from 1925 to 1934 were not representative of the American population. They tended to be dominated by relatively affluent northern Europeans, and also tended to exclude the overweight because the company actively discouraged them through higher premiums. Women were also discouraged from purchasing policies, so that Metropolitan policyholders were more than likely to be atypical. Dublin's ideal population weights did not, for the most part, include Americans from eastern or southern Europe. Indeed, even as late as the 1960s, Metropolitan policyholders weighed on average nine to ten pounds less than the sample used by the National Health and Nutrition Examination Survey (NHANES).

Equally problematic were the methods of data collection. Policy applicants were weighed fully clothed, with subjective determinations as to the weight of their clothing. In many instances, family doctors were allowed to submit weights, with some no doubt willing to help a patient avoid the extra premium charges for the overweight and obese by providing a 'normal' reading. At least 20 per cent of applicants submitted their own weights – with a systematic bias to underreporting by an average of ten pounds for those overweight or obese. And once they had obtained their policy, policyholders were never reweighed – so that the inevitable weight gain that accompanies ageing was never picked up. The result was that many of the overweight and obese may well have found their way into the 'normal' category, a fact that would have biased Dublin's results in favour of the underweight and normal.

Despite these flaws, Dublin's statistics caught both the public's and the medical profession's attention. Even though infectious diseases like TB had been largely eliminated, there was a worrying increase in cardiovascular disease, with almost 60 per cent of deaths over the age of 45 being associated with it in 1950. Dublin's link between obesity and mortality appeared to provide a ready explanation for this fact – Americans were simply too fat. In response to Dublin's figures, the insurance industry launched a large lose-weight campaign. As Roberta Seid writes:

> By December 1952, *Business Week* reported that the public had been besieged with advertisements warning about the ill-effects of overweight, such as the picture of

a stoutish, middle-aged man, his buttons popping from his spreading girth, gleefully bringing a full fork to his mouth. The caption above the picture read: 'Lengthening His Waistline ... Shortening His Lifeline'. This and similar ads appeared throughout the media and were reinforced by feature articles, many of them written by Dublin himself. A *Reader's Digest* piece in July, 1952, was catchily titled, 'Stop Killing your Husband' (by overfeeding him). *Business Week* explained that 'overweights aren't left alone for a minute', and attributed the sudden and surprising upsurge in sales of dietetic foods to the effectiveness of this campaign.[10]

Dublin worked tirelessly in the campaign to convince Americans that obesity was soon to kill them. Despite his 'scientific' claims about the association between overweight and mortality, there was always a bit of the late-nineteenth and early-twentieth century prejudice about fat that animated Dublin's work. For instance, in August 1952, in the Metropolitan's *Statistical Bulletin*, Dublin authored a piece about the 'Handicaps of Overweight'. Although acknowledging the mortality risks of obesity, Dublin's 'handicaps' were much more a laundry list of popular prejudices about the fat, rather than a scientific critique of obesity. According to Dublin, children made fun of the fat, fat girls had greatly diminished marriage prospects, and employers often preferred normal-weight employees.

Whatever the effects of the insurance industry campaign, what provided the ultimate validation of the obesity epidemic was the imprimatur of the medical profession, the public health community and, ultimately, the government. By 1951, as Dublin noted, not only the AMA but also the US Public Health Service had joined the insurance industry in proclaiming obesity to be America's No. 1 health problem and calling for across-the-board weight reductions. The medical profession and the public health establishment quickly championed the new connection between cardiovascular disease (CVD), high blood pressure, diabetes and obesity.

In June 1951, Dr James Hundley of the US National Institutes of Health (NIH) claimed that 'high blood pressure, heart disease, diabetes and a shortened life span are all associated with obesity'. In 1952, Dr Hundley's boss, Dr W. H. Sebrell, director of the NIH, was quoted in *US News and World Report* as claiming that 'Obesity has replaced vitamin-deficiency diseases as the No. 1 nutrition problem in the United States today.' Dr Lester Breslow, who served as consultant to the President's Commission on the Health Needs of the Nation, even claimed that the weight of average Americans was great enough to lead to excessive mortality. Breslow urged Americans to bring their weights into line with those considered ideal by the MLIC.[11] Indeed, whenever the public health establishment, the government or the medical profession needed substantiation for the message that fat kills, they readily turned to Dublin's MLIC studies. For example, Dr Jean Mayer of the Harvard School of Public Health wrote in a 1955 *Atlantic Monthly* piece that the 'life insurance companies, and in particular Dr Louis Dublin, deserve great credit for having repeatedly called attention to the very serious risks which accompany obesity'.[12]

The limitations of Dublin's supposed correlations, however, were soon evident when other researchers attempted to replicate his findings. For example, from 1952 to 1957 Drake *et al.* studied 3,992 Californian longshoremen, most of whom were overweight by MLIC standards.[13] On average, they were 17 per cent above Dublin's ideals. Drake *et al.* expected to discover that these men would have elevated mortality rates. Instead, they found that the group had significantly lower mortality rates than other Californian males of the same age. However, instead of calling into question Dublin's claim that obesity equates to an increased risk of death, Drake's team were merely 'perplexed' by the data and 'cautious' about drawing conclusions.

Despite Drake's failure to question Dublin's associations, and despite the predictions of massive increases in obesity-related morbidity and mortality, and the frenzied calls for population-wide reductions in weight, the results of the 1950s obesity epidemic were hardly surprising and are, indeed, high-ly instructive as we continue in the second obesity epidemic of the past half century. As the 1960s and 1970s came and went, Americans did not lose significant amounts of weight, though they dieted continuously. They enjoyed better health, while the prevalence of most major diseases declined and longevity increased. In other words, despite the worries of the obesity crusaders of the 1950s, not a single one of their dire predictions about obesity and health came true.

THE OBESITY CRUSADERS AND THE SECOND OBESITY EPIDEMIC

If the first epidemic of obesity was a product, for the most part, of Louis Dublin and his MLIC statistics, and their influence on the medical community and the public health establishment, the second obesity epidemic is also the work of a small number of people from the same circles. They make very much the same sort of claims about the links between overweight/obesity and disease/premature death, and also claim that the obvious answer for better health and longevity is weight loss. Building, perhaps in ignorance, on the legacy of Dublin, these people have completed the process of medicalising obesity so successfully that the debate about obesity, even though it does have significant social, economic, political and even philosophical dimensions, is nevertheless very largely defined as a debate about a medical problem.

Following the lead of one medical sociologist who used the term 'crusader' to describe these architects of obesity, we will call those who have manufactured the second obesity epidemic 'obesity crusaders'. They are the small group of physicians, public health officials and activists who

> work to convince the public and other professionals that obesity is best dealt with as disease rather than deviance. They aggressively make claims to promote the benefits of slimness (focusing on the health justifications more than aesthetic values) and their own ability to treat fatness ... Crusaders work to expand the jurisdiction of

the medical model of obesity by seeking attention for the problem, mobilize resources to support medical claims, publicly and privately press medical claims, and work to counter opposing claims made under other models.[14]

Aside from founding obesity organisations, organising conferences, pushing obesity remedies, writing papers, making pronouncements about the links between obesity and disease and death, and continually warning the press and government about the obesity-caused disasters which lie ahead, the main function of these obesity crusaders is to endlessly repeat the core message of the epidemic: overweight/obesity equals death; weight loss is possible and necessary; the sources of the problem are to be found in corporate misbehaviour, not individual gluttony or sloth; and personal responsibility is insufficient, as significant governmental action is required.

Writing of the success of these crusaders in creating the obesity epidemic, University of Chicago political scientist Eric Oliver notes that

Over the past two decades, a handful of scientists, doctors and health officials have actively campaigned to define our growing weight as an 'obesity epidemic'. They have created a very low and arbitrary definition of what is 'overweight' and 'obese' so that tens of millions of Americans … are now considered to 'weigh too much.' They have also inflated the dangers and distorted the statistics about weight and health, exaggerated the impact of obesity on everything from motor accidents to air pollution. And, most important, they have established body weight as a barometer of wellness, so that being thin is equated with being healthy.[15]

While these obesity crusaders might well be sincere in their belief about the risks of obesity and the efficacy of various treatments, their blatant misrepresentations are neither accidental nor disinterested. Rather, they are driven by enormous amounts of self-interest. This is because the existence of an obesity epidemic offers enormous commercial, financial and power-maximising opportunities ('rent-seeking', in the language of public choice economists) for at least seven groups: the medical profession, academic researchers, the public health community, the government health bureaucracy, the pharmaceutical industry, the fitness industry and the weight-loss industry.

Consider, for example, the benefits that accrue to the public health community and government bureaucracies from an obesity epidemic. Not only does such an epidemic provide an enormous opportunity for them to increase the scope of their power, particularly through interventions to reduce obesity, but it can also provide the justification for substantial increases in their budgets. For the pharmaceutical industry there are enormous opportunities to develop and market new drugs to treat obesity and obesity-related illnesses, while for the medical profession defining obesity as a disease opens up significant new demands for treatment. For the research community, defining obesity as an epidemic offers the prospect of significantly more funding. For the £30 billion a year fitness and weight-loss industries, every newly defined fatty is another potential life-long customer. Indeed, while the economic costs of an obesity epidemic might be substantial, the epidemic is worth tens of billions of pounds to these groups.

The results of such self-interest in manufacturing the obesity crisis can, perhaps, best be seen in the connections between obesity researchers and the weight-loss and pharmaceutical industries, inasmuch as these two industries, along with the government, are the main sources of research funding on obesity. Indeed, it is this intimate connection that is at the root of much of the scientific distortion on which the obesity epidemic is based. As Paul Campos, the American critic of the obesity crisis, notes:

> [G]rant money is scarce, and the process for securing it extremely competitive. One prominent obesity researcher described to me why so many people in the

field seriously exaggerate the known health risks associated with weight. 'This threat to careers may be most important of all. It's more than just being proved wrong', this researcher told me. 'When you apply for a grant ... you have to make a strong case for funding by explaining the significance of the research ... It's in the best interest of many people to portray obesity in the worst way possible. They get their funding: and it goes on and on.[16]

Careers, then, thrive or fail on funding, and the sources of that funding, whether from the pharmaceutical or weight-loss industries, foundations or the government, are powerfully interested not merely in the right areas and questions – ones that have a practical resonance – but in the 'right' results. For example, in her 1997 book, Laura Fraser describes the highly conflicted relationships between many obesity researchers and the weight-loss and pharmaceutical industries:

Diet and pharmaceutical companies influence every step along the way of the scientific process. They pay for the ads that keep obesity journals publishing. They underwrite medical conferences, flying physicians around the country expense-free and paying them large lecture fees to attend. Some obesity researchers have clear conflict of interest, promoting or investing in products or programs based on their research. Others are paid to be consultants to diet companies, and sit on the scientific advisory boards of Weight Watchers, Jenny Craig, or other commercial programs – while they also sit on the boards of the medical journals that determine which studies get printed. What it comes down to is that most obesity researchers would stand to lose a lot of money if they stopped telling Americans they had to lose a lot of weight.[17]

Writing about this 'health-industrial complex', Eric Oliver observes that

Within most of the research institutions and universities where health research is conducted, a significant portion of the salaries of scientists and their staffs is based on grants from foundations and support from private industry or the federal government. The application process for these grants is very political – who gets funded and at what level depends on a number of factors including the importance of the research problem in question and how well it fits within the established health paradigms. Similarly, the funding levels of the CDC, the NIH, and other government agencies depend upon perceptions of the U.S. Congress about the validity of their efforts ... Getting funds to do health research and promotion ... depends largely upon how serious a health problem one is researching.[18]

What we have, then, is a corrupted circular relationship, in which the weight-loss and pharmaceutical industries sponsor researchers whose work will both develop new products and create a market for them. In turn, these sponsored researchers, the new obesity epidemic experts, are recruited by the CDC, the NIH, and the World Health Organization (WHO) to serve as consultants to define, explain and solve the obesity epidemic. The 'scientific' conclusions of the CDC, the NIH and WHO, backed now by the authority of national governments and the expert endorsements of the obesity research experts, not only create but legitimise the market for the obesity-treatment products developed – by, of course, the selfsame researchers who were initially funded by the weight-loss and pharmaceutical industries. The success of these new products provides these industries with the funds for a new round of research, which begins the process anew.

Writing about these sorts of relationships, Case Western Reserve University scientists Paul Ernsberger and Richard Koletsky note that

The National Institutes of Health frequently convene panels of experts to discuss important and controversial issues in medicine and to arrive at compromise or consensus statements ... This process has worked well for many topics, as experts representing a spectrum of opinion are brought together and reach agreement on the current state of knowledge in their field. A major problem with consensus panels, however, is that many of the experts represent special interest groups ... This is clearly a problem with NIH panels on obesity, on which the multi-billion dollar interests of the weight loss industry have been well represented.[19]

Ernsberger and Koletsky outline just how these multi-billion dollar interests are furthered by specific findings of the public health community and the government. For instance, exaggeration of the ill effects of obesity favours the interests of the weight-loss industry through the 'facilitation of third-party payments' and 'increased motivation to seek weight control services' by the public. 'Setting body weight standards as low as possible' helps the industry by expanding its 'client base', while 'overstatement of the long-term benefits of weight loss' results in 'increased utilization and reimbursement for services'. Finally, by minimising 'the ill effects of obesity treatments and weight-cycling', the public health community and the obesity crusaders ensure 'repeat utilization of services'. As the authors conclude,

These economic interests are favored by proclamations from government panels identifying obesity as a major health risk, establishing a very low limit for the definition of obesity and minimizing the hazards of treatment. The economic interest of pharmaceutical firms is illustrated by a major grant program initiated by Knoll Pharmaceuticals, manufacturers of the diet pill sibutramine. In a letter addressed to physicians across the nation, the company offered generous grant support 'to advance the understanding of obesity as a major health problem'.[20]

In effect, there is what Thomas Moore calls an 'interlocking system' of self-perpetuating interests, which might be described in less flattering terms as a vicious circle. As Moore writes, 'The same medical school physicians who serve on NIH consensus and other panels also work as consultants to these drug companies and are paid handsome fees to speak at the medical conferences that these companies finance.'[21] 'The drug industry financially supports many researchers who are on the advisory panels to both the WHO and NIH', notes Oliver.[22] Pharmaceutical companies influence the tenor of scientific research and interpretation, both by funding research and by contracting with various health researchers for them to serve as consultants for the companies' various products.

The results of these relationships are hardly insignificant, as they have the potential to corrupt the entire process of defining obesity, deciding whether there is an obesity epidemic, and, most particularly, determining how to treat it. Consider these three examples:

First, in 1997, the NIH's Task Force on the Prevention and Treatment of Obesity – a key group in terms of defining the nature and extent of the obesity epidemic – had eight of its nine members with ties to the weight-loss or pharmaceutical industry.[23] As Professor Paul Ernsberger noted with regard to this group and a similar group at the WHO,

> The WHO panel consisted entirely of physicians who run weight loss clinics. Many of these clinics are largely dedicated to prescribing weight loss pills. The NIH Obesity Task Force ... consisted almost entirely of people running weight loss clinics ... The NIH and WHO assemble panels of doctors and psychologists who have dedicated their clinical practices to promoting weight loss. Indeed, in their reply to my letter [in the *Journal of the American Medical Association*], the NIH has explained that their very definition of an obesity expert is 'someone who runs a weight loss clinic'. These people are then asked to objectively evaluate the threat posed by obesity and the benefit provided by the clinics they run.[24]

Second, one of the most influential articles in advancing the notion of an obesity epidemic was a 1999 *Journal of the American Medical Association* (*JAMA*) study, which concluded that obesity was responsible for 300,000 US deaths in 1990.[25] The lead researcher for the study, Dr David Allison, has received significant funding from the pharmaceutical makers of weight-loss medicines such as Xenical and Merida, as well as from diet businesses like Jenny Craig, Weight Watchers and Slim Fast Foods. Indeed, an article in *Scientific American* notes that Allison has disclosed payments from 148 pharmaceutical and weight-loss companies. As Jerome Kassirer, the former editor in chief of the *New England Journal of Medicine*, observes,

> On the question of obesity, physicians have been extensively involved with the pharmaceutical industry, especially opinion leaders and in the high ranks of academia. The involvement was in many instances quite deep. It involved consulting, service on speakers' bureaus, and service on advisory boards. And at the same time some of these financially conflicted individuals were producing biased obesity materials, biased obesity lectures, and biased obesity articles in major journals.[26]

Third, the deep connections between leading obesity crusaders, their organisations, their obesity claims and the weight-loss and pharmaceutical industry were particularly evident at the end of 2005 in the UK. One of Britain's leading obesity crusaders, Dr Ian Campbell, suddenly resigned as president of the National Obesity Forum, an organisation that he had founded, because he said the Forum had become too dependent on funding from the pharmaceutical industry. In his resignation letter, Campbell noted that the Forum had suffered a 'loss of direction' because of the influence of its drug company funders. Claiming that the effectiveness of the Forum as a voice on obesity was compromised by its involvement with the pharmaceutical industry, Campbell said that the Forum championed 'ineffective' ways of treating obesity, including the use of weight-loss drugs, and tailored its obesity messages to suit its sponsors' wishes.[27]

There is, thus, much more involved here than merely the need to get funding. There is also the imperative of self-enrichment through manufacturing and biasing the obesity debate in order to advance the strategic interests of the weight-loss and pharmaceutical industries. Nowhere is the work of this vicious circle to create an obesity epidemic more apparent than in the campaign to establish a worldwide standard for what constitutes normal, overweight and obese.

FURTHERING THE CORPORATE AGENDA: MANIPULATION OF THE BODY MASS INDEX (BMI)

If obesity is to be defined as a disease rather than as a moral failing, it is imperative that there be an agreed set of symptoms that provide some plausible scientific definition of what obesity and overweight are. The simple and arbitrary description of someone as 'fat' or 'obese' will not work, as it is both too vague and unquantifiable and too transparently subjective. The important work of making obesity appear to be both a disease and an epidemic is carried out by the Body Mass Index (see Chapter 2 for a fuller discussion of the BMI, particularly its problems).

To judge by the official pronouncements of the NIH, the House of Commons Health Committee, or the WHO, the determination that those individuals with BMIs in excess of 25 but under 30 are overweight, and those with BMIs in excess of 30 are obese, is an 'evidence-based' finding of science. Indeed, it is repeatedly alleged by the crusaders of the obesity epidemic that there is clear and overwhelming evidence that these levels are associated with an increased risk of morbidity.

There is, however, compelling evidence that these levels of overweight and obesity – which substantially contribute to the numbers involved in the obesity epidemic – are instead the product of the International Obesity Task Force (IOTF), headed by Professor Philip James, which receives 75 per cent of its funding from the pharmaceutical companies Hoffman-La Roche and Abbott. The IOTF also receives funding from Servier, the maker of the weight-reduction drug Redux.[28] This funding, by an industry that stands to benefit directly from expanded numbers of overweight and obese people, was recently highlighted in the *British Medical Journal*, which noted that, despite 'being widely seen as an independent think tank and having ties to the World Health Organization', the IOTF 'has relied heavily on funding from the drug industry for a decade'.[29] The same issue of the *BMJ* also reported that an 'expert committee', initiated by Dr William Dietz of the CDC (who was also the original chairman of the IOTF group on childhood obesity), was at work to expand the definitions of childhood obesity, despite concerns from some in the public health community that there may be no connection between childhood overweight and future health problems. Under the proposals, children who are currently classified as 'at risk of overweight' would instead be classified as 'overweight', a move that would dramatically increase the numbers of overweight and obese. According to the *BMJ*, the new classifications would mean 25 per cent of American toddlers, and about 40 per cent of children aged 6–11, being treated as either overweight or obese.[30]

On the surface of it, the decision to set the cut-off point for overweight at BMI 25 and obesity at BMI 30 appears to be based on an international scientific consensus, developed under the auspices of the WHO. For instance, the WHO describes the BMI standards for normal, overweight and obese as the product of an expert technical consultation on obesity, held in Geneva in 1997. However, a careful reading of the documents shows that the real work had little to do with the WHO, and was instead done by the selfsame IOTF, which, as mentioned above, receives the bulk of its money from two pharmaceutical companies with significant financial interests in increasing the numbers of the overweight and obese.

As James notes in his article, conveniently titled 'The Worldwide Obesity Epidemic', 'This short meeting [the WHO 1997 expert technical consultation] was organized after the

International Obesity Task Force developed a comprehensive analysis of the problem with a draft report over 2 years, which was the basis for the WHO Technical Report.'[31] So, despite the veneer of scientific objectivity attached to the WHO technical report, the final document was actually the work of James's industry-backed IOTF. Indeed, as James notes in his article, the IOTF's designations of normal, over-weight and obese were already accepted by the WHO in 1995. At the very least, the worldwide scientific consensus to decide what constitutes being normal, overweight and obese was not only headed by a man with deep financial links to the pharmaceutical and weight-loss industries, but was funded by those industries as well.

MANUFACTURING THE OBESITY EPIDEMIC STEP BY STEP

While it is difficult to say with absolute precision when this process of medicalising obesity culminated in the arrival of the obesity epidemic, it is possible to look at six key moments in the manufacture of the epidemic. The *first* of these involved the capture of the most prestigious American medical research agency, the NIH. As a result of careful work on the part of the obesity crusaders, the NIH devoted one of its consensus development conferences to the issue of obesity. The NIH's consensus conference provided an ideal venue for advancing both the medicalisation of obesity and the obesity epidemic, since it offered a forum for obesity claims, the presentation of expert opinion, an influential official publication and enor-mous publicity for the topic in hand. At the February 1985 conference devoted to obesity, an NIH panel of 15 health pro-fessionals listened to 19 expert obesity presentations, from which the panel concluded that 'obesity has become a public health problem of considerable importance in the United States'. An equivalently 'definitive' conclusion was reached in the UK by the Royal College of Physicians.[32]

The *second* key moment in the manufacture of the obesity epidemic came in 1998, when two scientists at the US Centers for Disease Control and Prevention, William Dietz and Ali Mokdad, changed the format in which the CDC tracked and displayed the changes in the prevalence of obesity in the US. Instead of presenting the data in tabular form, Dietz and Mokdad developed a PowerPoint presentation that showed obesity rates in a series of maps. The maps, beginning in 1985, charted the increasing prevalence of obesity in colours ranging from light blue (lowest obesity rates) to dark red (when obesity prevalence topped 20 per cent). The maps were posted on the CDC website and quickly became a staple in defining the 'obesity epidemic'. In a 1999 issue of the *Journal of the American Medical Association* devoted to obesity, the maps figured prominently, along with an article by Dietz about the obesity epidemic.[33]

The CDC maps also figured in the *third* key event in the manufacturing of the obesity crisis – the 2001 report by then Surgeon General David Satcher, *Call to Action to Prevent and Decrease Overweight and Obesity*, which contained not only the first official use of the word 'epidemic' to describe the state of obesity in the US, but clearly positioned obesity as a *public* health problem, as opposed to a *private* problem. Using the CDC's obesity prevalence map (entitled 'The Surfacing of an Epidemic') as the backdrop for his report, Satcher claimed that 'Overweight and obesity have reached epidemic proportions. Both the prevention and treatment of overweight and obesity and their associated health problems are important public health goals.'

Setting out a line of argument about the scope of the problem that would be repeated countless times, Satcher claimed that 'approximately 300,000 deaths a year in this country are currently associated with overweight and obesity. Left unabated, overweight and obesity may soon cause as much preventable disease and death as cigarette smoking.'[34] A public catastrophe equal to smoking clearly demanded a comprehensive series of public health interventions. While Satcher's plan has undergone subsequent revision, his basic outline is still the basis for the war on fat.

The key assumption behind the *Call to Action* is that the causes of overweight and obesity are largely environmental rather than personal, and as such fall squarely within the province of the public health establishment. As Satcher notes, the key to solving the obesity problem is to 'encourage environmental changes that help prevent overweight and obesity'. Though eating is an individual activity, the role of the public health community must be both to 'assist' Americans toward 'healthful eating' and to identify 'effective and culturally appropriate interventions to prevent and treat overweight and obesity'.

While the obesity crusaders in the US were working to establish the legitimacy of an obesity epidemic, a similar, though perhaps more 'nuanced', process was at work on this side of the Atlantic. While obesity had already been defined as a major public health problem by the Royal College in 1983, the definitive judgement about the legitimacy of both describing it as an epidemic and using the extensive powers of the State to combat it did not come until May 2004 with the publication of a report, simply titled *Obesity*, by the Commons Health Committee – the *fourth* key moment.

The committee's report was obviously influenced by the US experience with obesity, since it describes visiting New York to meet Dr Xavier Pi-Sunyer (described by the committee simply as a 'world expert in diabetes', but not identified as the director of the VanItallie Center for Weight Loss, nor as the paid consultant to several diet and pharmaceutical companies) and Marion Nestle (who, curiously, is not identified as the author of *Food Politics*,[35] a stinging attack on the food industry that portrays Big Food as the new Big Tobacco). It also acknowledges discussions with the CDC and the author of the *Call to Action*, former Surgeon General David Satcher.

The work of the committee was also influenced by five 'specialist advisors', including Professor Gerard Hastings, who had previously authored a highly controversial report on food marketing for the Food Standards Agency, and, perhaps most controversially, Professor Phil James, identified as the chairman of the International Obesity Task Force (IOTF). It should be recalled that, though registered as a charity in the UK, the IOTF receives extensive financial support from the pharmaceutical industry. Moreover, Professor James is a well-known anti-obesity crusader who also has a long-standing relationship with the pharmaceutical industry. He was, for example, the principal researcher in the clinical trials of Sibutramine, a weight-loss drug by Knoll Pharmaceutical, and Orlistat, which is made by Roche.[36]

James's close relationship to the weight-loss and pharmaceutical industries was front-page news in 2005, when the *Mail on Sunday* revealed his industry connections:

> The Government's anti-obesity guru was at the centre of a sleaze row last night after it was revealed he has been paid undisclosed consultancy fees by makers of weight-loss drugs. While issuing warnings that obesity has become an 'epidemic', he has been the leading researcher in trials of weight-loss drugs and has been paid fees by pharmaceutical firms that stand to make billions from slimming pills and potions.[37]

The *Mail on Sunday* went on to note that James, who has participated in American conferences designed to promote obesity lawsuits against the food industry, refused to divulge how much he had been paid by the weight-loss industry. James's role in the obesity campaign is significant. He not only chairs the IOTF, which determined the BMI standards for overweight and obesity, but he was hugely involved in developing the UK's war on obesity, including setting up the Food Standards Agency for the Blair government.

It would be astonishing if Professor James's profound connection to the pharmaceutical industry was unknown to the House of Commons committee, or indeed if the latter was unaware of Professor Hastings' anti-advertising bias for certain products. It is equally astonishing, given Professor James's obvious conflict of interest and Professor Hastings' bias, that the committee would employ them as specialist advisors, or indeed describe their work as 'objective'. Their intimate involvement in the work of the committee at the very least destroys the appearance that its working assumptions, its process or indeed its conclusions can be even remotely characterised as objective.

Like its North American counterpart, the committee's report took particular pains to justify the term epidemic as applied to obesity: 'That word is normally applied to a contagious disease that is rapidly spreading. But the proportion of the population that is obese has grown by almost 400 per cent in the last 25 years.' The committee was also eager, like the surgeon general, to place the obesity epidemic in the context of the more familiar tobacco problem, as it noted that 'On present trends, obesity will soon surpass smoking as the greatest cause of premature loss of life.' If this were not enough to frighten the public and the government, the committee, invoking the surgeon general's language of an unprecedented health catastrophe, warned that obesity might well render the NHS unsustainable: 'It will bring levels of sickness that will put enormous strains on the health service, perhaps even making a publicly funded health service unsustainable.'[38]

In some senses, however, the committee was far more explicit in its recommendations than the general principles that were described in the surgeon general's *Call to Action*. Specifically, it envisaged a range of specific government measures to stem the tide of obesity because 'the main factors contributing to the rapid rises in obesity seen in recent years are societal'. Indeed, the committee was emphatic in its rejection of a personal approach and in its commitment to an environmental account of the sources of the obesity epidemic, noting that 'it is critical that obesity is tackled first and foremost at a societal rather than an individual level'. Included in these recommendations were: the adoption of the precautionary principle where evidence is contradictory, consideration of a ban on advertising of unhealthy foods to children, prohibition of the use of celebrity endorsements of unhealthy foods, the introduction of food warnings for unhealthy foods, and the development of a health-promotion campaign modelled on anti-smoking advertising. While attempting to 'take the food industry at its word' as to its willingness to be part of the solution, the committee nonetheless appeared to be sceptical that the industry would take meaningful action, since it recommended 'that the Government reviews the situation in three years and then decides if more direct regulation is required'.

Perhaps the most memorable, not to say sensationalist, part of the report, however, was its claims about children and obesity; claims that, as we shall see, were destined to become perhaps the central feature of the obesity epidemic rhetoric. For instance, the report claimed that failure to deal with the epidemic of childhood obesity would 'condemn future generations, for the first time in over a century, to shorter life expectancies than their parents' – a shocking claim, but one for which no supporting evidence was adduced. In the report's introduction, for instance, the committee recounted the story of a consultant at the Royal London Hospital, Dr Sheila McKenzie, 'who had witnessed a child of three' who weighed 40 kilos 'dying from heart failure where extreme obesity was a contributory factor', and who described the young children in her unit as 'choking on their own fat'.

The image of children 'choking on their own fat' was, as the committee undoubtedly anticipated, instantly seized on by the press and provided an appropriately sensationalist tag on which to preface any discussion about obesity. A simplistic headline summarised the report as 'Three-year-old dies from obesity.' Unfortunately, the story, as writer Brendan O'Neill soon pointed out, was untrue. Dr McKenzie was horrified both at the way the committee distorted the case – the child referenced in the report was, in fact, suffering from a genetic condition that had nothing to do with either parental neglect or obesity – and the way in which the press reported it. But the issue of veracity aside, the committee's intention to highlight a sensationalist story in order to create a moral panic about obesity, particularly childhood obesity, worked well. For instance, an August 2006 Google search on the 'development of the UK obesity epidemic' turned up 517,000 results!

At the same time as the obesity crusaders in the US and the UK were at work creating national obesity epidemics, they were receiving invaluable assistance from a group of like-minded colleagues at the WHO, who were interested in defining obesity not merely as a national epidemic, but as an international one that demanded an appropriately 'global strategy'. The first steps toward such a strategy were taken by the WHO in 2000 with the publication of its expert technical consultation on obesity, entitled *Obesity: Preventing and Managing the Global Epidemic* and regarded here as the *fifth* key moment in the manufacture of the obesity epidemic. That consultation focused on three areas: the health hazards associated with overweight and obesity, the ways in which weight gain might be prevented, and the ways in which overweight and obesity might be treated.

In late January 2002, the WHO convened an expert consultation on diet, nutrition and the prevention of chronic diseases. Under the leadership of the long-time tsar of the WHO's anti-tobacco campaign, Dr Derek Yach, executive director of the WHO's non-communicable diseases and mental health section, 60 experts assembled the evidence on the consequences of 'unhealthy diets and physical inactivity' and then crafted recommendations on how to combat the now global epidemic. The resulting *Global Strategy on Diet, Physical Activity and Health* was presented to, and approved by, the World Health Assembly in 2004.[39]

Three key differences serve to distinguish the WHO global strategy from the national definitions of, and the responses to, the obesity epidemic in the US and the UK. First, the WHO's global strategy, though obviously designed in response to the obesity epidemic which the WHO had identified in its 2000 expert technical consultation, makes few explicit references to obesity, focusing instead on the ways in which unhealthy diet and physical inactivity contribute to disease. Indeed, the entire strategy is framed as a response to the 'heavy and growing burden of noncommunicable diseases', itself an odd area for WHO involvement, given its original and legitimate focus on communicable diseases.

Second, the WHO's strategy moves beyond the more careful language of the US and UK reports (which, for the most part, spoke of the association between obesity and various diseases), and speaks without hesitation about unhealthy diets and physical inactivity being 'among the leading causes of the major noncommunicable diseases, including cardiovascular disease, type 2 diabetes and certain types of cancer' – a sweeping and, as we shall see, hugely contested claim. (There are only two diseases for which there is an overwhelming linkage to obesity – osteoarthritis of weight-bearing joints and uterine cancer in women.)

Third, the WHO's strategy confidently assumes that the 'vast body of knowledge and public health potential' – notice again the pointed absence of any reference to individual responsibility and action – ensures that the 'behavioural and environmental risk factors' for obesity are amenable to change. Given that the increase in obesity seems, on the WHO's own admission, relentless, and given that there is no compelling evidence that any of the measures proposed by the strategy actually work, this is an astonishingly confident claim.

As might be expected of almost any 'strategy' emanating from the WHO, there is an enormous emphasis on laws, regulations and taxes as mechanisms to reduce obesity, as opposed to individual responsibility and action. This follows, of course, from the strategy's assumption that the sources of unhealthy diet and physical inactivity are to be found in the environment. According to the WHO, the strategy draws together the existing scientific evidence about the connections between diet, physical activity and disease in a way that provides the basis for a variety of actions, including food advertising restrictions, warning labels and taxes on unhealthy foods, and limits on the amount of salt, fat and sugar in foods. While these policy options are presented as national 'interventions', there is already talk from Yach (who has since left the WHO) and others of the need to convert the strategy into a global treaty modelled on the Framework Convention on Tobacco Control, which would make the adoption of such policies mandatory. Yach, for instance, along with other obesity crusaders, is keen to characterise the struggle against the food industry as, in some sense, a replay of the tobacco wars, as he draws explicitly on public policy responses to smoking in outlining a strategy for dealing with the obesity epidemic.[40]

For epidemics to work as moral panics they must produce large numbers of bodies. The younger the bodies, the better.

Indeed, the ideal epidemic is a paediatric one, which points to the cleverness of the anti-smoking lobby's description of youth smoking as the major paediatric disease of our time. In part, the work of the UK Commons Health Committee had gone a substantial way to pushing children to the fore and centre of the obesity epidemic. What was needed, in addition to the sensationalist stories about children choking on their own fat, was hard evidence of substantial numbers of people of all ages dying from being overweight and obese. It was one thing for the Health Committee or the US surgeon general to talk of an obesity epidemic; it was altogether something else actually to say where its victims lived.

The task of totalling up obesity's toll – *the sixth and final moment in manufacturing the obesity epidemic* – was undertaken in 2004 by four scientists at the CDC in Atlanta, including its director, Dr Julie Gerberding, who together published an article in the *Journal of the American Medical Association* (*JAMA*) about, ironically, the 'actual' causes of death in the United States in 2000.[41] Due to the tireless publicity efforts of the CDC, the article received enormous worldwide media coverage, and its figures were quickly adopted by US Health and Human Services Secretary Tommy Thompson. The article claimed that poor diet and physical inactivity were responsible for about 400,000 deaths per year in the US. The researchers claimed that, if this trend continued, obesity would overtake tobacco use as the largest single cause of death.

Despite its impressive pedigree, by May 2004 the CDC study was already the subject of debate, most particularly in a critical article in *Science* magazine. By June, the first letters questioning the research's methodology and its conclusions appeared in *JAMA*. In response to the growing criticism of the research, the CDC established an internal review committee to determine where and how the research had gone wrong. In November 2004, the CDC admitted that the 400,000 figure might have inflated obesity deaths by as many as 80,000; in April 2005, the CDC published a new study that said the net number of obesity-related deaths in the US was not 400,000, but only 25,814.[42] Despite these shocking admissions of error, the CDC initially refused to release to the public the report of its internal review committee. But thanks to a Freedom of Information Act request from the Washington-based Center for Consumer Freedom, it was finally forced to post the results of the internal review on its website.

The saga of the CDC obesity mortality numbers is important in two key respects. First, it is *the* crucial moment in the making of the obesity panic. Second, it is so revealing of why most of the claims about an obesity epidemic are closer to science fiction than hard science. The internal review into the CDC's research that had claimed annual US mortality from obesity to be 400,000 makes for depressing reading, in so far as it reveals the sad way in which one of the world's premier scientific institutions appears to have been co-opted into serving political, rather than scientific, ends. Based on the review's findings, it would seem that at least five significant problems contributed to the CDC obesity fiasco.

First, the authors of the CDC's exaggerated claims about obesity deaths were not experts in obesity but, nevertheless, according to the report, 'weighed in on an area that has been a focus of research careers for some CDC scientists'. With a single exception, all of the authors of the CDC's 400,000 obesity deaths per year claim were attached to the office of the director, Dr Julie Gerberding, whose own defence of the CDC's numbers can only be described as challenged.[43]

In other words, rather than choose experts to author perhaps the most widely anticipated obesity report ever, the CDC director had decided to take on the job herself. The review provides no reasons for this unusual decision, but one wonders whether, given the political and policy sensitivity of the issue (obesity had to be seen to be a – indeed *the* – major health problem), the job was felt to be too important to leave to the CDC's obesity experts. After all, without the requisite 'political sensitivities', they might have got the numbers badly wrong. Indeed, this is precisely what happened in April 2005 with the new obesity numbers produced by the CDC's obesity experts led by Katherine Flegal. Unlike her boss's work, Flegal's figures suggest that the policy concerns for obesity –

indeed, the entire war on obesity – are without scientific foundation.

Second, the obesity numbers research at the CDC was, in part, driven not by concerns about good science but by concerns about good politics – always an ominous sign in a scientific undertaking. As one reviewer noted, 'The authors were under some political pressure to get this paper out.' Indeed, it was noted that, given the 'bold statements' of the paper, it 'might have been better off being presented as a policy exercise rather than a scientific study', suggesting that the research was not really science at all. This view was supported by another reviewer, who noted that 'estimation based on best educated guesses should be acknowledged as such up front'. Of course, educated guesses at this point in the obesity epidemic would not have carried the same weight, nor served the same function, as a CDC-sanctioned 'scientific' study. Obesity policy and educated guesses could be debated; obesity 'science' was less susceptible to critique and to being resisted at a policy level. In something suspiciously close to junk science, not only did policy appear to drive science at the CDC (rather than science shaping policy), but policy was also disguised as science, with estimates parading as carefully evidenced facts.

Third, the CDC's obesity numbers were wrong because the Gerberding research team used outdated data, inappropriate methods and incorrect scientific models, despite being warned about the consequences. Particularly disturbing was the reliance on the work of David Allison, whose extensive connections with the weight-loss and pharmaceutical industries we have already seen. For instance, the authors of the revised 2005 CDC study point out that, merely by using more recent data (which the CDC already possessed), obesity-related mortality was reduced by 63 per cent. As the reviewers noted:

> Methods used to calculate number of deaths due to obesity were incorrect and possibly miscalculated ... The use of the improper formula is a rather serious

mistake to make ... I think we should agree from this point forward to bury this model and its inherent weaknesses for good ... Direct comparisons of deaths attributable to different causes is inappropriate due to the variety of methods used ... Following Allison in using incorrect method was not justified ... Calculations of overweight-attributable deaths were done erroneously in Causes paper [the original paper], and as a results [*sic*], the published numbers do not match the methods described in the paper, are not replicable, and are too high by about 80,000 deaths on average ... The authors of the *JAMA* 2004 Actual Causes of Death paper did not provide adequate support from the literature for three key assumptions that are necessary to conclude that overweight, rather than diet and physical inactivity, is the true cause of excess mortality.

Fourth, the review evidence indicates that the CDC authors knew that their work was deeply flawed, but proceeded to publication despite massive internal dissent within the organisation. This is extremely disturbing, as it suggests that the CDC's work was not due to incompetence but rather to a junk-science misrepresentation of reality. For example, Terry Pechacek, associate director for science in the CDC Office of Smoking and Health, wrote in a 30 April 2004 e-mail, 'I am worried that the scientific credibility of CDC likely could be damaged by the manner in which this paper and valid, credible, and repeated scientific questions about its methodology have been handled ... I would never clear this paper if I had been given the opportunity to provide a formal review.' Pechacek's worries were reflected by one reviewer, who noted substantial concerns by CDC scientists who 'did not push further because, given the prominence and reputation of the authors, they did not feel that it would make any difference'.

The reviewers also found evidence that the authors knew about the obesity numbers problems but pushed ahead anyway. One reviewer, commenting on the study's wildly inaccurate numbers, noted that 'it seems as if this bias from the wrong formula was pointed out to the authors'. Another, speaking of the other problems with the research, indicated that these very problems 'were apparently shared with the authors prior to publication'.

A May 2004 *Science* article also reported on the belief within the CDC that the data were insufficient to justify the conclusions about obesity.[44] Perhaps most significantly, in September 2004, in the *American Journal of Public Health*, a team of CDC researchers led by Katherine Flegal, who would go on to produce the CDC's revised obesity numbers, observed that 'Given the present knowledge about the epidemiology of obesity … it may be difficult to develop accurate and precise estimates. We urge caution in the use of current estimates of the number of deaths attributable to obesity.'[45] Flegal's voice of caution was highly inconvenient to the interests of the epidemic, and was therefore ignored.

Fifth, Gerberding and her colleagues chose to ignore masses of conflicting evidence, in this case 40 years' worth of international data that suggest obesity is not a cause of premature mortality. As a reviewer observed, 'Many studies for multiple different disease outcomes have demonstrated that the effect of both diet and physical activity are independent of the effect of BMI or various measures of body size or fat.'

In looking at the CDC's initial and unwarranted claims about the death toll from obesity, and at the internal review of these claims, one of the key questions to emerge is just how the CDC got the obesity problem so badly wrong. Was it simply a question of competence, where the research team led by the director of one of the world's major scientific institutions inadvertently got its maths wrong and came up with about 375,000 too many deaths? Or is this a case of something much more disturbing, a case of corrupted science[46] where policy considerations (that is, considerations that provided impressive support for the obesity epidemic) took precedence over scientific integrity?

Several things that emerge from the internal review suggest that the CDC obesity numbers were the product of corrupted science. First, there is the fact that the regular CDC obesity and mortality experts were not involved in the project, but instead the task was taken on by the CDC director herself, someone who had no experience in specific issues. Second, there is the evidence, cited by several of the reviewers, of the political pressure to get the paper out and to come up with the right conclusions – a sign that policy was driving science rather than the reverse, and also a sign of junk science at work. Third, there was the abundance of bad data, inappropriate methods and unwarranted assumptions – all of which the research team had been alerted to but chose to ignore in the interests of reaching a predetermined number. Fourth, the fact that the CDC team knew that its work had significant problems but chose to ignore the internal dissent, and also to ignore and not even reference the massive amounts of existing literature that reached different conclusions, again suggests corrupted science rather than incompetence.

HEALTH PROMOTION: ROOT CAUSE OF THE CDC FIASCO AND THE OBESITY EPIDEMIC

Given that there is a strong case to be made for believing that the CDC chose to assist in manufacturing a crucial component of the obesity epidemic, the question arises as to what drove this decision. Indeed, what, beyond the imperatives of self-interest, drives the entire process to create an obesity epidemic?

The answer to this question is to be found in the dominant set of beliefs, generally too inarticulate to be called a philosophy, that drives not just the CDC, but also the public health community in general and the obesity crusaders in particular. One can find it, for instance, in the CDC's full name, the Centers for Disease Control and Prevention, and also on its website, which notes that the Centers' central mission is 'health promotion and prevention of disease, injury and disability'. The CDC and the public health establishment, both in the United States and around the world, is as much about preventing disease through the promotion of health as it is about curing disease. It is this conception of, and mandate for, health promotion that is the driving force behind not merely the obesity numbers scandal, but the war on fat as well.

The idea of health promotion, which dates from the 1970s, is, in a sense, the idea of one man, former Canadian Health Minister Marc Lalonde. Pick up almost any national or international document, particularly one from the WHO, on public health policy or prevention strategies, or a book on health promotion published anywhere in the world, and you will find a reference to the Lalonde Doctrine of health promotion. Indeed, if health promotion has anything resembling a philosophical core, it is the Lalonde Doctrine.[47]

Lalonde was something of a visionary, for, as the minister in charge of a massive publicly funded national health system, he was worried about the potential, in the relatively flush days of the 1970s, for unsustainable increases in the cost of health care. He believed that one answer to the sharply rising health care costs was to divert some resources away from the healing of diseases to their prevention. The key to prevention, according to Lalonde, was changing lifestyles. If people could be convinced to change the way they lived – eating less and differently, drinking little (if at all), stopping smoking, and exercising more – then dramatic and permanent reductions in such chronic and costly multifactorial illnesses as heart disease and cancer were possible.

While this is beyond the scope of this book, it should be noted that, quite apart from its dubious philosophical principles, there is little compelling evidence to support the claims that multifactorial illnesses can be prevented, particularly through lifestyle interventions. For the most part, these are diseases of old age, and the evidence is not convincing that preventing them significantly increases longevity. For example, the populations of southern Europe, with their Mediterranean diet, do not live appreciably longer than their northern neighbours; they simply die of something else. Moreover, as Gori and Richter pointed out almost thirty years ago,[48] preventing disease does not necessarily save money.

However, if the prescription for national and individual good health was straightforward, the means for getting the patient to accept the cure were much more complicated. Even in the 1970s, the evidence about the connection between lifestyles and multifactorial illnesses like cancer and heart disease was debatable. The public was constantly bombarded with conflicting scientific information, whether about cholesterol, fat, coffee, salt, or any number of other alleged lifestyle culprits. Last year's scientific 'truth' about lifestyle-caused diseases was quickly overtaken by this year's often contradictory medical pronouncements.

Lalonde also recognised that there was a strong streak of independence in most people when it came to health and personal choice. Arguing that most people believed that they had the right to 'choose their own poison', he noted that 'It is not easy to get someone not in pain to moderate insidious habits in the interests of future well-being.'

Lalonde realised that, if lifestyle medicine (and with it health promotion) were to succeed, two things had to happen. First, the health establishment and the government had to speak with one clear, authoritative voice about the dangers of certain lifestyles and the necessity of change. Even if the science was contradictory or unsupportive, it must be portrayed as backing the imperative of lifestyle change that the health authorities and the government wished to preach. Second, people had to abandon their belief in their right to live their lives as they pleased – ignoring the social implications of their choices – in favour of an acceptance of their moral obligation to follow society's norm of healthy behaviour and living, even if this meant giving up a good many of life's 'small' pleasures.

What this meant in practice was that lifestyle change had to be vigorously promoted, even if the science supporting such changes was incomplete, ambiguous or divided. Taking his text from St Paul's first letter to the Corinthians, 'If the trumpet give an uncertain sound, who shall prepare himself to battle', Lalonde argued that the careful scientific approach was essentially unfitted to the task of health promotion. As he wrote, 'The spirit of enquiry and scepticism, and particularly the Scientific Method ... are ... a problem in health promotion. The reason for this is that science is full of ifs, buts, and maybes while the messages designed to influence the public must be loud, clear and unequivocal.' No matter how useful the integrity and scepticism of science might be in the laboratory, in the political and health establishment world that wanted to change lifestyles, or, to put it more bluntly, wanted to change the way in which whole nations thought and lived, science often produced an 'uncertain sound' that was decidedly unhelpful. Put at its starkest, telling the truth in health promotion is less important than effectiveness.

Lalonde's beliefs about the lifestyle sources of disease and the importance of health promotion in changing lifestyle quickly attracted international attention. His assumptions, goals and implicit methods were adopted by the WHO in its Alma Ata Declaration in 1977, and again in 1986 in its Charter for Health Promotion. More importantly, his conception of health promotion quickly became the dominant idea in schools of public health and medical schools. The result is that today most people involved in health care, research and in public health, particularly in places like the CDC and the WHO, believe the central tenets of health promotion; namely, that science clearly shows that, if people are to be healthy, they must change their lifestyles, and it is part of the job of the health establishment to see that this change takes place, either voluntarily or, if necessary, through various modes of coercion.

Lest this picture be dismissed as extremist nonsense, consider the musing of the Hastings Center's Daniel Callahan in his book *False Hopes*,[49] which deals with the very issue of sustainability that first led Marc Lalonde to formulate health promotion. According to Callahan, 'a sustainable medicine will require an effective continuum of programs of public health, health promotion, and disease prevention, a continuum ranging from education at one end of the spectrum, economic and other incentives in the middle, and some frankly coercive policies at the other end ... Coercive programs will be necessary.' One could not find a better description of the policy menu suggested by the obesity crusaders.

The implications of these health-promotion beliefs for science, public policy and personal autonomy are enormous. For the moment, let us focus on science in general, and obesity science at the CDC in particular. For many of the believers in health promotion, the scientific method is best described as an impediment to healthy living, since so much that it produces can fail to support the message of lifestyle change as essential to good health. For instance, science can produce results that directly contradict the claims about obesity and mortality – as it did with the finding that only about 26,000, and not 400,000, Americans die from obesity each year. Obviously, such a public and significant reduction in the number of obesity-related deaths strikes at the heart of the claims about the obesity epidemic.

Then, too, science can undermine health promotion simply by its ambiguous findings, which fail to produce an appropriately clear message that health promotion can use to advance its agenda. Science that is full of 'ifs, buts, and maybes', as Lalonde put it (and much good science is), is not what is required to provide the 'loud, clear and unequivocal' message that health promotion requires.

For example, in its consistent health-promotion message that obesity is an epidemic equivalent to the Black Death – a claim made by the CDC's director – the CDC has never bothered the public with any of the ifs, buts and maybes of the scientific sceptics who, like the NIH in its 1992 consensus statement, warn of the dangers not of weight gain but of weight loss: 'Most studies, and the strongest science, shows weight loss, although seemingly to reduce risk factors, is actually strongly associated with increased risks of death – by as much as several hundred percent.'[50]

These misgivings about science show yet again that the health paternalist in general (and the obesity crusader in particular) is not overly concerned about scientific accuracy. Indeed, science can 'work' even if it is inaccurate, even if it is distorted, even if it misrepresents the truth about the way things are. As Kersh and Morone, two of the earlier analysts of the obesity epidemic, note, 'The science does not need to be accurate to have an impact. The findings are sometimes reliable ... they may be partially true ... or the science can be entirely fictitious.'[51] As they go on to suggest, the success of the public health crusade rests not on the truth of its science, but on the way in which the 'policy entrepreneurs' use that science to change policy.

This is, in fact, a concise description of how the obesity entrepreneurs have engineered the triumph of the manufactured obesity epidemic over the last five years. No matter that the idea of obesity as a disease is nonsensical (except perhaps for morbid obesity), or that the evidence of an epidemic of obesity, particularly in children, is unsupported, or that obesity will not destroy the health care system, or kill millions, or even that it is not engineered by the food industry. The truth of any of these statements is immaterial compared to the fact that they are made, that they are made by seemingly knowledgeable and authoritative people, that they are endlessly repeated by the media, that those who disagree with them are dismissed as cranks who serve special interests, and that they are acted upon by government.

Placed within this context of health promotion, it is easier to understand not simply how the CDC acted as it did, but also why. For the previous five years, the obesity promoters had been shamelessly and tirelessly claiming that the industrialised nations, if not the world, were in the midst of an obesity epidemic that would kill millions and put health care systems at risk. While there was a smattering of science backing these claims, when subjected to a close analysis it could not support the extravagant predictions of gloom that were at the heart of the obesity crusaders' story. Certainly, they had none of the definitive status necessary to justify the government's intervention in the stomachs of its citizens. What was needed was to follow the recipe outlined by global warming activist Stephen Schneider: that is, to publicise 'clear and unequivocal' science that would show obesity to be a massive and unrelenting killer, particularly of children; science that would 'capture the public's imagination' through 'scary scenarios ... simplified, dramatic statements' which 'make little mention about any doubts we might have'.[52]

Enter the CDC and its director, Julie Gerberding. What could be more convincing, more compelling for the media, and more likely to end, once and for all, any debate about the nature and scope of the obesity epidemic and the crucial imperative for government action than to have the head of the highly respected CDC tell the world, with impeccable scientific credibility, just how bad the fat problem was. The science may have been slightly problematic, or in some instances decidedly unsupportive, but the media are largely uncritical consumers of whatever the health establishment dishes out, the political establishment was lined up behind the idea of an obesity epidemic, and the doctrine of health promotion's ends could readily justify these small concessions to questionable means.

The consequences of this resort to corrupted science by the CDC and the obesity crusaders were substantial – not simply for the war on obesity, but more generally for science in the service of public policy. For one thing, it threatened the integrity not simply of a set of particular findings of science but of the scientific process itself. That is because the business of making corrupted science is, inevitably, one in which the scientific process of collecting, testing and evaluating evidence and claims is itself distorted. One sees this in the comments of the CDC's internal reviewers, who showed how the researchers' incremental decisions about assumptions, methodology, data and interpretation systematically twisted the scientific conclusions in directions fundamentally at odds with the underlying evidence.

Corrupted science, such as the CDC's obesity data, is a threat to science's main virtue in the public policy process: its objectivity. Indeed, without that objectivity, science loses much of its privileged position in the policy process. While complete objectivity may be impossible, science at least professes a fundamental interest in reason, evidence and bias-free judgement, and at the same time offers a publicly defined and accessible method for measuring these things. This marks it out from much of the political process, and accounts both for science's standing in contemporary society and its usefulness in the policy process.

However, it is precisely this utility that science has for the policy process that is threatened by the use of corrupted science. If science ceases to work *outside* the political and policy processes, and instead allows itself to become enchanted by and co-opted by a particular party *within* the policy process, then it ceases to be a tool available to all sides of an issue. If it becomes politicised and ideologically sensitive, as was suggested by the reviewers of the CDC process, then it ceases to have any value in the policy process, because it becomes nothing more than another special pleading, rather than a uniquely rational way to understand the world. In short, it is the uncorrupted character of science that makes it so essential to democratic policy. When corrupted, it taints the entire process.

In the end, of course, the ruse did not work, though it is an open question whether this setback has made any difference to the campaign to make obesity an epidemic. The methodology was too obviously bad, the data too questionable, the assumptions unsupportable, and the critics too sharp and vocal, even for the CDC and its director. But the important lesson for the obesity crusade is that it was tried. One of the world's major scientific agencies was apparently prepared – deliberately, not accidentally – to allow its commitment to the policy imperatives of health promotion to be used in the service of the obesity epidemic and, most alarmingly, to trump its commitment to genuine science and its responsibility to tell the truth.

THE CULMINATING MOMENT: PAEDIATRIC OBESITY AS AN OFFICIAL DISEASE

The final moment in the obesity crusaders' campaign to create an international obesity epidemic came in March 2005, with the publication of a 'consensus statement' on childhood obesity in the *Journal of Clinical Endocrinology and Metabolism*, which recommended that childhood obesity be classified as a disease for 'treatment and insurance purposes'.[53]

While obesity has been classified as a disease by the WHO since the 1970s, the classification has always been controversial. According to the authors of the consensus statement, this is no longer the case. For example, in a *US News and World Report* cover-story article by Amanda Spake on the issue of whether obesity was a disease, Xavier Pi-Sunyer, described only as 'director of the Obesity Research Center at St. Luke's-Roosevelt Hospital', is quoted as claiming that 'there's enough data now relating to mechanisms of food intake regulation that suggest obesity is a biologically determined process'.[54] Spake fails to mention that, as was detailed above, Pi-Sunyer is a highly controversial US obesity researcher who has served on NIH and WHO obesity panels, while also serving on the advisory boards of, and acting as a paid consultant to, several weight-loss and pharmaceutical companies. According to Eric Oliver, Pi-Sunyer has also been 'named in a lawsuit against the drug company Wyeth-Ayerst because he agreed to have his name attributed to scientific articles about the costs of obesity that were actually written by Excerpta Medica, a medical consulting firm, and paid for by Wyeth-Ayerst'.[55] Nor did Spake mention that Pi-Sunyer is also a member of IOTF.

Pi-Sunyer's conflicts of interest aside, it is still unclear why the fact that obesity might be 'biologically determined' makes it a disease. Any number of physiological functions might, for instance, be biologically determined, but this would hardly be sufficient to classify them as diseases. Although the authors of the consensus statement argue that there is a compelling scientific rationale and evidence to classify obesity as a paediatric disease, it seems far more plausible to assume that their major reason has little to do with science and has much more to do with financial interest. As the 8 March 2005 press release from the Endocrine Society notes, 'By classifying obesity as a legitimate disease, the consensus statement paves the way for public funding and insurers' reimbursement for obesity treatment programs.' The March 2004 meeting in Israel that agreed the consensus statement on obesity as a disease was funded by Aventis, Ferring Pharmaceuticals, Eli Lilly, Pfizer, Roche and Teva Pharmaceuticals.

The reasons for scientific scepticism about the legitimacy of obesity as a disease are several. First, the consensus statement has, as its authors admit, no rigorous scientific foundation, since it is not based on any 'formal evidence-based guidelines'. Second, the supposed diagnostic basis of obesity, the BMI, is, as we have seen, wholly arbitrary in that it has no scientifically valid connection with mortality. Third, obesity makes no sense as a disease, paediatric or otherwise, since its supposed effects are only seen as risk factors for other multifactorial diseases such as cardiovascular disease, cancer and type 2 diabetes, none of which can be conclusively linked with it. Indeed, in contrast to real illnesses like cancer and heart disease, it is odd to speak of someone dying of obesity, as opposed to dying from the risk factors associated with obesity. Finally, there is no scientifically agreed evidence justifying any particular course of treatment for obesity. The only time that speaking of obesity as a disease might make sense is in the case of morbid obesity. Therefore, while we have a disease of convenience that works well for the self-aggrandising public health establishment (and its financial interests) and plays to the interests of bureaucrats and politicians, from a scientific standpoint we have a very odd disease – one that has no scientific diagnostic basis, no independent symptoms, no scientifically established connections with morbidity, and no evidence-based course of treatment.

Nonetheless, the consensus statement on childhood obesity served its purpose. With an official recommendation to define obesity as a disease, the obesity crusaders could appear to speak of the pandemic of obesity with some degree of scientific authority.

WHAT THE OBESITY CRUSADERS BELIEVE

In our description of the manufacture of the obesity epidemic, we have already seen something of what the critics of fat believe. It is now time, however, to set these beliefs out in a more systematic fashion, since they serve to define the shape of the rest of this critique. The purveyors of the obesity panic have at least two sets of beliefs. One set is defined by the *tenets of health promotion*, while the other set is a more specific *application of these principles of health promotion to the problem of obesity.* Let's begin with the tenets of health promotion.

Although there are a number of versions of health promotion, it is not unfair to describe its central beliefs as involving the following claims:

(1) Autonomy is not the central value of democratic societies, since considerations of health and collective welfare must frequently take precedence over it.

(2) In matters relating to health, individuals are often uninformed or irrational in their choices, fail to understand their interests, and do not know best how to realise those interests.

(3) This is due, in large measure, to the fact that individuals are unaware of, or are indifferent to, the growing scientific consensus about what it means to be healthy.

(4) Integral to this conception of 'healthy' is the fact that much disease and premature mortality is caused by unhealthy lifestyles, and much of this can be prevented by appropriate behavioural changes.

(5) Hence, individuals are in need of the health promoter's help to discover and realise their 'genuine' health interests, as well as to avoid irrational courses of action that might result in unhealthy consequences.

(6) The central task of health promotion is to disseminate the truth about the connections between health, disease and lifestyle, through educating, persuading and providing the State with a menu of policy options that will change individual and societal beliefs about health and lifestyle.

(7) Individuals have a moral obligation to live their lives in accordance with this evolving scientific consensus about what constitutes being healthy, particularly with respect to the connection between health and lifestyle.

(8) The State has an obligation to ensure that its citizens, even if they are unwilling or unable, conform to the scientific consensus about what it means to be healthy.

What unites these claims is the central commitment to health paternalism, namely that the State is justified in restricting the rights of competent adults in order to protect them from the allegedly harmful consequences of their own insufficiently considered actions. Indeed, the most potent expression in the vocabulary of health promotion is 'it's for your own good'. According to this philosophy, the health paternalist's, and by extension the State's, conception of health (and indeed the value of health) replaces not only the values of the individual, but also the individual's weighting of risk and reward – a not insubstantial trespass on personal autonomy.

Central, too, to this philosophy of health promotion, though not explicitly enunciated except in the nuanced phrases of Lalonde and the occasionally inadvertently candid remark, is a commitment to corrupted science, effectively to trim the evidence to fit the policy imperatives of what it means to be healthy. This emerges most often in discussions about epidemiology and its implications, since it is epidemiology, rather than the gold-standard evidence from clinical trials, that provides the basis for the assertions of health promotion. (For more on the epidemiological foundations of the obesity crusade, see Chapter 2 and the Appendix.)

For example, it surfaces briefly and obliquely in some of the comments by the CDC internal reviewers, which suggest that, rather than objective science, the obesity mortality study was something much closer to corrupted science. One reviewer, for instance, noted that the research 'might have been better off being presented as a policy exercise rather than a scientific study', thus all but acknowledging that the work was advocacy rather than science. Another reviewer noted that the work was essentially nothing more than a series of poorly substantiated and justified guesses, writing that 'estimation based on best educated guesses should be acknowledged as such up front'. Of course, to do so – to admit that one had nothing more than an estimate, rather than a scientific conclusion about obesity and mortality – would have destroyed the entire point of the exercise.

One also sees this implicit commitment to corrupted science when the health promoters speak of epidemiology and what it can and cannot establish. Professor John Last, for example, in his plenary address to the International Epidemiological Association, decried the fact that scientific rigour often impeded the cause of public health by calling into question the pronouncements of health promotion. As he noted, 'Another kind of credibility is more worrying. This is rigid, insensitive application of scientific rigour that disregards the weight of circumstantial evidence, calling into question the validity of epidemiological findings when it is not in the public interest to do so.'[56] Indeed, the last thing that the obesity crusaders would wish is to have rigorous science discount the circumstantial, indeed largely nonexistent, evidence on which the obesity epidemic is based.

Finally, health promotion's ready resort to corrupted science is starkly apparent in the way in which the obesity crusader is prepared to interpret and use the epidemiological evidence on obesity. Perhaps the most egregious example of this behaviour is to be found in the US Institute of Medicine's (IOM) 2005 report *Preventing Childhood Obesity*, which outlines an allegedly 'prevention-focused action plan to decrease the prevalence of obesity in children and youth'.[57]

Apparently sensitive to the fact that the evidence on the nature and extent of childhood obesity (to say nothing of the possible measures to prevent or ameliorate it) is at best scientifically dubious, the report's authors attempted to deflect attention from this weakness with a series of claims that veer between mindless truisms and patent absurdities. For instance: 'As childhood obesity is a serious public health problem calling for immediate reductions in obesity prevalence ... the committee strongly believed that actions should be based on the best available evidence – as opposed to waiting for the best possible evidence.'[58]

There are two problems with this claim. First, the report offered no compelling evidence in support of childhood obesity as a serious public health problem; and second, there is much evidence to suggest that the claim is not true. Moreover, the logic of acting on the best available evidence would suggest essentially doing either nothing or very little, as opposed to the report's contentious and extravagant options, since the evidence does not support the claim of an extensive problem.

Or consider this claim: 'Absence of experimental evidence does not indicate a lack of causation.'[59] This is true, but quite beside the point, for what it means is that, since science is about causal relationships, there is no basis to make any meaningful claims, and hence there is no genuinely scientific (as opposed to corrupt-science) basis on which to proceed. Or finally, 'Given that obesity is a serious health risk, preventive actions should be taken even if there is as-yet-incomplete scientific evidence on the interventions.'[60] This is a favourite of the corrupted-science crowd, and is often referred to as 'acting ahead of the evidence' – a phrase that neatly captures its absurdly unscientific character, since science-based policy acts in response to the evidence. Indeed, given that science is a set of conclusions founded on the evidence, it would be difficult to conceive of what science ahead of (that is, in the absence of) the evidence might be. Of course, if there is no evidence of serious health risk, then there is no basis for preventive actions. If there is no evidence of an effectiveness fit between problem and solution due to 'incomplete scientific evidence', then preventive actions become not simply a waste but potentially counterproductive.

Nor is this refusal to accept the evidence, this belief that the 'absence of experimental evidence does not indicate a lack of causation', only found in the work of the IOM. While the research failed to support the claim that specific foods or diets reduced health risks, a series of studies published in 2006 was still accompanied by an editorial concluding that the work made no difference either to the claims that diet has an impact on disease or to the sort of advice that the public should be given about eating.[61] The writers noted that, 'Despite null findings from the [Women's Health Initiative] Dietary Modification Trial, dietary changes can have powerful, beneficial effects on CVD risk factors and outcomes.'[62] Not only does this statement contradict the evidence of the studies, but it effectively maintains that, despite what the science says, we continue to have *faith* in our unsupported beliefs that diets cause and can prevent disease and premature death. Whatever the evidence, our belief in the religion of diet cannot be falsified.

This belief in health promotion shapes the obesity story that has been manufactured by the obesity crusaders. For instance, at the heart of the story is the assertion that obesity is the major lifestyle disease of our time, the serious consequences of which, both personally and for society, are unappreciated by most people. Also, there is the almost Messianic belief that a few individuals (that is, the obesity crusaders) understand the connection between fat and good health. Again, there is the assumption that the health-promotion community has the major task of 'solving' the obesity epidemic by providing the government with a recipe of plausible interventions that will re-engineer the eating habits of millions. Finally, there is the belief that education and persuasion, as Daniel Callahan reminds us, will not be enough, and that the coercive powers of the State will be required (for our own good, of course) in order finally to make us thin. Personal responsibility is not the answer. As obesity litigator John Banzhaf, fresh from years of tobacco litigation, put it so eloquently to the National Press Club in Washington on 5 August 2003: 'All of these platitudes about "people should eat less," "responsibility," all this crap!'

Having looked at the ways in which the philosophy of health promotion drives the obesity story, we now turn our attention to the specific components of the obesity story itself. Though the story is told by a variety of individuals and institutions,[63] its central features are, by now, remarkably consistent. First, there is a worldwide epidemic of obesity that affects both the developed and, increasingly, the developing world. Second, this pandemic means that obesity is the major health problem of the twenty-first century – one that threatens the existence of the health care system itself. Third, while there have been significant increases in both adult and childhood overweight and obesity, it is childhood overweight and obesity that is particularly epidemic and worrisome, since childhood overweight and obesity results in greater adult health risks.

Fourth, science convincingly demonstrates that there are causal connections between overweight and obesity, as determined by the BMI, and a range of serious illnesses and premature mortality.

Fifth, science also shows that sustained and significant weight loss is possible and that it results in improved health. Sixth, one of the major sources of this obesity epidemic is, as Yale Professor Kelly Brownell puts it, the 'toxic environment', or, as the US Institute of Medicine describes it, the 'obesogenic' environment. While physical inactivity may have a role in creating this obesogenic environment, the major problem is the environmental prompts both to overeat and to eat inappropriately, both of which are a product of a food industry that is, in many respects, analogous to the tobacco industry, particularly in its marketing and advertising activities. Seventh, personal responsibility and individual action are, for the most part, inadequate to counter the effects of this environment; coordinated actions are required from the public health community and the government. Eighth, there are a variety of public policies that can effectively change this environment of overeating and eating inappropriately, and that thus promote reductions in overweight and obesity. These policies include the classification of foods into healthy and unhealthy categories, warning labels for unhealthy foods, taxes on unhealthy foods, ingredient and production controls on unhealthy foods, controls on access to unhealthy foods, and marketing and advertising restrictions on unhealthy foods.

Perhaps the most overlooked, yet crucially important, aspect of this story is its emphasis on children. While the obesity crusaders also refer to epidemic increases in the numbers of overweight and obese adults, it is the epidemic of childhood obesity that figures most prominently in their story. The reasons for this are a mixture of evidence of harm (overweight and obese children allegedly grow up to be less healthy than their thin contemporaries) and the strategic importance of children, particularly with respect to justifying otherwise unacceptable regulatory policies. Children occupy a uniquely privileged position in most societies, not simply because of their potential, but also because of their limitations, which demand that they be protected from the adult world, and particularly from the marketplace. Threats to children therefore assume an immediate and often uncritical priority. By focusing the obesity crusade on children, and indeed by making obesity a 'paediatric disease' like smoking, the critics of fat are guaranteed far more sympathetic attention not only from the media, but also from parents and policymakers. They are also guaranteed a much greater chance of securing many of the more controversial of their policy objectives, such as banning certain foods and curtailing food advertisements, since these policies are much more easily portrayed as justifiably paternalistic when they refer to children.

The elements of this story, particularly its child-focused aspects and its specific policy menu, can be found most obviously in two works, both American. These are Kelly Brownell's *Food Fight* and Marion Nestle's *Food Politics*. Summarising the obesity story at the end of his book, Brownell notes that the main elements include the claims that 'obesity is occurring in epidemic proportions, obesity is a growing global crisis, and environmental factors are primarily responsible for the rapid increase in prevalence'. Focusing on the crucial importance of the 'need to protect children', Brownell claims that the 'prevalence of obesity in children is growing even faster than that of adults', 'obesity in children ... lead[s] to very serious medical problems in both childhood and adult years', and 'food companies [are] doing their very best to attract even the youngest children as customers'.[64]

Nestle agrees with this picture and, if anything, is even more critical of, and hostile to, the food industry than Brownell. For instance, in summarising the causes of the obesity epidemic, she places the blame almost entirely on the food industry, as it has control over all the major causes – advertising, convenience, larger portions, and foods high in fat, sugar and salt – of what she terms the 'eat more' environment. For instance, in describing food marketing to children, she makes the quite extraordinary and unsupported claim that 'marketers will do whatever they can to encourage even the youngest children to ask for advertised products in hopes of enticing young people to become lifetime consumers'.[65]

Brownell and Nestle are also united in their belief that the food industry is very like the tobacco industry in many ways, and that the crusade against the food industry might well replicate important features of the war on tobacco.[66] For example, in the Center for Science in the Public Interest's *Nutrition Action Health Letter*, Brownell writes: 'I recommend we develop a militant attitude about the toxic food environment, like we have about tobacco.' While admitting that smoking and eating are different, Brownell nevertheless observes that 'It is difficult not to notice that modern food companies may be owned by tobacco companies and that money from the two industries is mingled in organizations that fight for both. We should ask whether the behavior of the food industry differs from that of Big Tobacco.'[67] Indeed, Brownell's signature idea – a tax on unhealthy foods (dubbed the Twinkie Tax by *US News and World Report*) – is modelled on cigarette taxes. Nestle echoes this pairing of the industries. She writes that the actions of food companies are 'thoroughly analogous to the workings of any other major industry – tobacco, for example'. She notes that the parallels between the tobacco and food industries 'are impossible to avoid' and that the 'similarities between the actions of cigarette companies and food companies are no coincidence'.[68]

This comparison between the tobacco and food problems is found elsewhere. For example, Kersh and Morone outline a government policy response that is derived from the policy menu developed for tobacco and alcohol.[69] They suggest four regulatory strategies: 'controlling the conditions of sale through direct restrictions or limits (especially aimed at youth); raising prices through sin taxes; government litigation against producers of unhealthy substances with damage awards earmarked for health care or health alternatives; and regulating marketing and advertising'.

To deal with the obesity disaster, Brownell proposes 61 different actions. Included are:

Recognize that personal resources (responsibility) can be overwhelmed when the environment is toxic.

Move beyond the old no good foods or bad foods stance to a public health perspective in which we identify types of foods the nation should consume less or consume more.

Recognize that overnutrition now rivals hunger as the world's leading nutrition issue.

Encourage legislators to prohibit marketing of products to children.

Mandate equal time for pro-nutrition and activity messages to counter those for unhealthy foods.

Find alternatives to snack food, soft drinks and fast foods in schools with the goal of eliminating unhealthy foods entirely.

Use zoning laws to prohibit establishments with unhealthy foods from operating near schools.

Require food labeling at restaurants.

Consider changing the price structure of food, first by lowering the cost of healthy foods and perhaps by increasing the cost of unhealthy foods.

Think of food taxes not as a means of punishing people for bad choices but rather for raising revenue for programs aimed at improving the nation's diet.[70]

Similar proposals are found in Nestle's *Food Politics*, where, for instance, she is more specific about taxes on 'unhealthy' foods, suggesting that city, state and federal taxes be levied on 'soft drinks and other junk foods to fund eat less, move more campaigns'. She has also called for government pricing policies to set the prices of unhealthy foods and beverages.

While such taxes were not part of the Commons Health Committee's recommendations, they did find favour in a paper in the *British Medical Journal* that proposed extending

VAT to particular foods that might raise serum cholesterol levels, and exempting foods that are currently taxed but that are cholesterol neutral. For example, whole milk would attract VAT, but not skimmed milk.[71] As the author notes, 'Biscuits, buns, cakes and pastries, puddings and ice cream could be taxed if they raised cholesterol concentrations but exempt if the ratio of polyunsaturates to saturates ... were more favourable.'

Where Brownell and Nestle part ways in terms of the obesity story is over the appropriateness of litigation as a tool for reshaping the food environment. Despite agreeing that the food industry is the New Tobacco, Brownell rejects litigation, except for deceptive labelling and marketing, warning that other litigation based on claims about health problems allegedly caused by foods has the possibility of creating a 'backlash that finds the public sympathizing with the food companies'.

Nestle disagrees, sharing the belief of fellow obesity crusader Michael Jacobson, executive director of the Center for Science in the Public Interest (CSPI) (on whose board she served for five years), that the only way to solve the problem of a toxic food environment, as well as to 'save people from themselves', is an extensive and unrelenting campaign of lawsuits against the food industry. Both Nestle and Professor Philip James have participated in American conferences on developing a litigation strategy against the food industry. Nestle, for instance, was the keynote speaker at a June 2003 conference that was intended to encourage and support litigation against the food industry.

Litigation against the food industry began in 2002, when New York City attorney Sam Hirsch, advised by John Banzhaf, who still serves as executive director of Action on Smoking and Health (ASH), brought two actions, one against McDonald's, Wendy's, KFC and Burger King on behalf of a 56-year-old maintenance worker, Caesar Barger, and another against McDonald's on behalf of obese children. Hirsch claimed that the fast-food industry had 'negligently, recklessly, carelessly and/or intentionally' marketed foods to children that were high in fat, salt, sugar and cholesterol, while failing to warn them of the deleterious health consequences of those foods.

Since then, the development of a litigation strategy against the industry has progressed substantially. In a 2005 interview with the *Boston Globe*, anti-tobacco crusader Richard Daynard spoke about the way in which he and others intend to use the similarities between tobacco and certain foods as the basis for suing Big Food. 'You are dealing with an addictive product sold to kids', said Daynard. 'You are dealing with a product that, at least when initially produced, was not understood to be deleterious, yet as the evidence kept coming in, companies kept marketing it and stonewalling.' 'Paternalism', he claimed, 'is a dirty word when applied to adults, but it's not a dirty word when it is applied to children.' Moreover, 'The evidence is crystal clear that this is making a substantial contribution to the obesity epidemic and likelihood of developing chronic illness.'[72]

Indeed, in order to ram home the point about the food industry being the New Tobacco, all Daynard needed to add to his story about the addictiveness of fast food was the claim about marketing, since the two As – addiction and advertising – have provided the basis for the 25-year-long campaign against tobacco. Daynard's claims will form part of the basis of a national campaign, coordinated by Jacobson's CSPI, to bring class actions against the makers of fizzy drinks across America, with the first suit in Massachusetts. The actions will allege that the makers of fizzy drinks know that their products carry significant health risks, yet they market them to consumers, particularly children, without disclosing these risks. The Daynard–Jacobson strategy of making Big Food and certain of its products the New Big Tobacco appears to be working. Writing to the *New York Times* in June 2006 about the policy of hospitals in allowing fizzy drinks to be sold on their premises, Dr Paul Plasky advocates making 'sodas the new tobacco'.[73]

For Jacobson and Daynard, the class actions are part of a larger strategy to force the food industry to change its practices by using litigation to support the regulatory and policy process. Both believe that a successful suit could unleash a tidal wave of public distaste for the food industry similar to that caused in the 1990s by tobacco litigation – a distaste that resulted in the US Master Agreement between the tobacco industry and state governments. Unlike some other obesity crusaders, they see policy initiatives and litigation as complimentary, rather than as competing parts of the same struggle. The recent action by the US Department of Justice against the US tobacco industry under anti-racketeering law suggests not only that it is possible for the government to pursue litigation and regulation simultaneously, but also that litigation need not be left entirely to the policy entrepreneurs of the obesity crusade.

Of course, despite this deep interest in the public good, it is still worth noting that the food litigators like Daynard and Banzhaf act as much from self-interest as any of the other obesity crusaders. Though Daynard refuses to disclose how much money he made from 20 years of tobacco litigation, it is known that he demanded 5 per cent of the fees collected by several of the largest law firms in the key cases. This is an enormous figure, which, if replicated in his suits against Big Food, might well dwarf the fees paid to other obesity crusaders like Professor James.

In any event, Daynard, Jacobson, Brownell, Nestle and the other obesity crusaders clearly expect to win their fight with Big Food, and they expect the result of that win to be a food world quite different from the current one. As Jacobson put it in an expansive, and unnerving, 2003 National Press Club appearance in Washington, DC, this Brave New Food World will be one without junk food, Ronald McDonald will be languishing on death row, and people will be allowed only one fizzy drink a day and *fettuccine Alfredo* as a once-a-year treat. Providing scientific justification for this cheery prospect is a considerable task, and it is to this justification that we now turn our attention.

CHAPTER 2

WEIGHING THE EVIDENCE

What is this but the shameful ignorance of
thinking that we know what we do not know?

Socrates

INTRODUCTION

The international crusade on overweight and obesity is poised
to change drastically those traditional ways of life that, in
most developed countries, have witnessed a near doubling of
life expectancy in little over a century, parallel to a steady
increase in average body weight. Since it is claimed that the
crusade is motivated by scientific findings, it would seem reasonable and prudent to make doubly sure that those claims
are factual and trustworthy.

The lion's share of the claim is attributed to epidemiology,
a discipline that addresses population statistics of prevalence
and time trends of overweight and obesity, and inquires about
what might be possible causes. Common sense would expect
epidemiological studies to be based not on nebulous guesses but
on actual measurements of sufficient and stated precision, on
measurements that have measured what is said to have been
measured and not something else, and on conclusions strong
enough to make a difference and that are repeatedly consistent.
In reality, these requirements are virtually never met in epidemiological studies of overweight and obesity.

Most epidemiological studies do not actually measure
overweight or obesity, but instead rely on what people report
about their own height and weight during telephone interviews or in response to written questions. Even when height

and weight are measured, any excess of body mass over an arbitrary threshold of normality is assumed to be fat, when, in reality, it could be muscle, water or heavy bones. Many studies require information about prior dietary habits, invariably obtained by asking study participants to remember what their diet might have been months, years or decades before. Answers of this kind are manifestly illusory, for it is notoriously impossible to recall with any credibility what was eaten a few days past, let alone months and years. More so when answers might be obtained not directly but through next of kin.

If an overweight person dies of lung cancer, it is not possible to say that overweight was the cause of death without asking if the person was a smoker, exposed to asbestos or radiation, or to scores of other possible hazards for lung cancer. Such multiple and possibly contributory causes are called 'confounders', for they would confound the attribution of death to overweight. While a few studies have superficially explored the potential role of confounders, there has been no rigorous examination of the myriad potential causes of death and disease possibly experienced by the study's participants. Ethnic, behavioural, occupational, environmental and many other differences, including level of physical fitness, could easily skew the results and have rarely been addressed. As might be expected from this range of uncertainties, studies often arrive at divergent conclusions, and the weakness of many of the critical associations reported could easily stem from error in measurement or from uncontrolled confounders and biases.

The public's belief in an obesity epidemic is perversely self-fulfilling, in that it conspires to reinforce whatever media messages and visual clues might be attached. In a culture that prizes slimness, obesity is easily exploitable by callous humour and cartoons. At the same time, the politics of personal liberation has encouraged obviously obese people to be at ease in public places, thus reinforcing visual clues that may sustain the image of an epidemic.

Is it truly an epidemic? One could argue that the word is used improperly in the case of a condition like obesity – a condition conveniently declared to be a disease by the same special interests that also wave the epidemic flag. Still, and even allowing for its use, the word 'epidemic' implies that a majority of individuals in a population experience the condition from which all are at risk, and this is demonstrably not the case. In reality, a large majority of people may have gained a very few pounds – apparently healthy pounds – over the past decades. It is only a small fraction (perhaps around 3–5 per cent) of obesity-prone subjects who have registered excessive weight increases. With the appropriate provisos, the same conclusions hold true for children. This means that most people have been impervious to obesity and self-regulate their weight remarkably well. In fact, there is some indication that the secular trend of a small weight gain for the majority of people may be coming to an end, reflecting observations that the average caloric intake may have been decreasing over the last two decades. At any rate, longevity has continued to increase as the weight of populations has increased. With this in mind, and since it is only the very thin and the very obese who experience excess mortality, the majority of people – those who gained a few pounds but who are not very thin or very obese – must have experienced longevity gains much greater than the overall averages. Thus, all the evidence shows that adding a few pounds of weight has probably been advantageous and healthy for the majority of people who are not too thin or too obese.

The claim of an epidemic rests on statistical equivocations, and most of the problem lies in how overweight and obesity are measured and analysed. The common method is a combination of weight and height measures called the body mass index (BMI), for which an arbitrary normality standard of BMI 25.0 has been set.

Even if normal ranges were known, the task of counselling dangerously thin or obese individuals would still be daunting, given the problematic record of current bariatric medicine and surgery, and the pitiable records of obese and overweight people doing something for themselves about their weight. The literature is replete with reports of the dangers of losing weight even under supervised regimens, and besides, it is still a guessing game about which level of overweight and obesity might be hazardous for any specific individual.

What is an intelligent person to make of this? Is it possible that epidemiology is truly powerless in this case, given the barrage of heavyweight endorsements from all sorts of professed authorities? Even the tentative credibility of epidemiologically derived risks depends on many issues to do with how the study is conducted and its structure, but is largely determined by the strength of a reported risk. For instance, the average risk of lung cancer in cigarette smokers is 10 times the risk for non-smokers, and the prime force of its credibility is that possible confounders and biases are, in all likelihood, too weak to cancel out such a large risk differential. Not so for overweight and obesity, where the small risk differentials could easily be trumped by questionable measurements and many uncontrolled biases and confounders. It is only for very thin and obese people that higher risks are consistently recorded and raise legitimate concern.

Lest anyone doubt these remarks – and others to follow – the analysis in this chapter should bring confirmation to anyone willing to look at the evidence with an open mind and eyes. This analysis will highlight the uncertainties and inconsistencies that affect the studies.

WHAT CAUSES OBESITY?

Humans must eat in order to fuel the energy expenditures that living requires. Some of the energy in the ingested food is utilised immediately as energy; some is conserved, mostly as body fat but also as sugar stores; and some remains unutilised and is expelled as waste.[1] One of the functions of body fat is to secure fuel for long-term energy in times when food might be scarce: a function that probably arose as an evolutionary response to what might have been frequent alternations of feast and famine during lengthy periods of primitive hunting and gathering.

It is intuitive that the rate and amount of fuel stored as body fat hinges on the balance between the rate of ingested food, the rate of ingested food that is consumed to produce energy, the rate of ingested food that is discarded as waste, and the rate of energy generated by consuming already-stored body fat.

It is helpful to think of human bodies as machines that need, use, waste and store energy. At the same time, it is clear that human machines are individually different in terms of their energy requirements, functioning conditions and environmental situations. This accounts for the visible and manifold differences in their physical appearance, and in their responses to internal and external determinants of health and disease. In fact, even simple distinctions of age, sex, race, height, weight, blood type, insulin resistance and a host of other characteristics could not begin to describe the profound differences between two individuals that may be similarly classified on BMI scores.

It is those differences that make it so difficult to arrive at conclusions, prescriptions and recommendations that might be generally valid and applicable, or to construe general characterisations – such as overweight and obesity – often linked to concepts of health and disease that are manifestly discretionary. In truth, individuals show huge differences in the rate of energy they require and burn, in the rate at which they ingest food fuel, in the rate at which the ingested food is wasted, in the rate at which food fuel is stored as body fat, and in the rate of utilisation of body fat as fuel. Individuals also have different inherent predispositions to be healthy or not under a range of different levels of stored body fat, which further complicates the task of attributing risk to overweight and obesity, and of justifying warnings and interventions.

It should be plain that the amount of stored body fat ideally suited for good health is specific to each individual, and even for the same individual it would vary depending on genetic factors, age, environmental changes (such as the seasons or travel climate), behavioural changes, transient diseases and other factors. First, however, how is the extent of body fat measured?

MEASURING BODY FAT

The current interest in body weight is specifically directed at body fat, rather than other components of weight, such as muscle, amount of tissue hydration (or water-logging), bone volume and density, and other elements. The reason is that the public campaigns on body weight seek to manipulate dietary recommendations as a way of exploiting the economics of food and diet, relying on the perception that body fat and diet are related.

The visible clue to overweight and obesity is the extent of swelling of a given body's configurations. Again, though, in any discussion of overweight and obesity, it is important to note that such swelling is not always or exclusively attributable to an accumulation of fat, but is also the result of unrelated effects of muscle and organ swelling, and of the conditions of hydration of both muscle and other organs. So it is, for example, that bodybuilders may have little fat in their oversized bodies, while other individuals may be swollen by excessive water that accumulates on account of disease or excessive water intake. Other than body fat, therefore, different components of body overweight and obesity are generally unrelated to food intake and diet composition, and could be linked to lifestyle or disease.

With this in mind, it is apparent that a direct and precise measurement of the amount of body fat in a given living subject is beyond the pale, unless at autopsy. Many indirect methods have been developed over the years to estimate body fat, ranging from a rough and ready assessment of skinfold thickness measured with calipers, to more sophisticated approaches. The latter include underwater or hydrostatic weighing, air displacement plethysmography, or a combination of different measurements such as total body water estimate by deuterium displacement or by bioelectric impedance, dual energy X-ray absorptiometry, total body potassium, magnetic resonance imaging and positron emission tomography.

None of these methods can justifiably claim to measure body fat, separate from muscle and organ swelling and water-logging. Moreover, the methods require expensive and complex instrumentation that precludes their general applicability, with the exception of the crude method of skinfold measurement.

The method of choice for clinical and epidemiological applications has been the BMI, defined as the measure of the weight of an individual in kilograms, divided by the square of the height in metres (kg/m^2). As such, BMI is a representation of proportional body swelling in relation to weight and height, but it is clearly inadequate as a measure of body fat, because it cannot account for the composition of a body's swelling – fat, muscle, organ and water – and is affected substantially by thin or heavy body frames, by the relative length of legs and torso, etc. Again, bodybuilders may score high BMI values, despite scant fat reserves.[2]

BMI also does not account for body frame, for instance the differences between men and generally shorter women; nor is it a good index for children, being strictly dependent on age and body frame.[3] As an example, slightly built, ethnically Sri Lankan children in Australia have more body fat than white Australian children of similar BMI.[4] BMI also does not take account of whether body fat might be well distributed in the body or located at the waist, the latter condition possibly being more linked to health risks.[5]

Still, because of its easy applicability in epidemiological surveys, BMI has been, and still is, universally used in defining underweight, overweight and obesity, despite its manifest shortcomings and ambiguities as an unqualified index of body fat. It follows that epidemiological studies based on BMI are assuredly wrong in assuming that recorded BMI values are factual representations of body fat, and therefore in claiming that BMI values are solely and proportionately linked to food intake excesses and to dietary composition. All the more so when weight and height are not actually measured, but are simply reported by study participants in response to personal or telephone interviews, or mailed questionnaires.[6] Nevertheless, by virtue of its traditional and general use over many decades, BMI has acquired an epidemiological and popular authority of unwarranted validity, and it is commonly used in the public health definitions and perceptions of body-weight problems, and in the prescription of remedial targets.

In effect, and contrary to available evidence, we are asked to accept BMI assessments at face value in the numerous studies that have attempted to link different segments of the BMI range with health and diseases, and to abide by the official public health linkage of BMI differentials with eating disorders and their fanciful, if still vague, remedies.

Health, disease and mortality studies involve largely epidemiological surveys of adults and the therapeutic interests of the medical profession, especially bariatric medicine and surgery. Consistently successful therapies for obese and overweight adults have been elusive, most relief having been temporary and followed by complications, often life threatening, especially for the morbidly obese.[7] Therapy, however, is not the focus of this book, which is more interested in the official crusades about overweight and obesity that are primarily driven by prevention strategies targeted at children and adolescents.

Still, a rational preventive context first needs to establish what a scientifically defensible range of normal body mass might be, and then what elements of diet, behaviour, psychology, environment, physiology and genetics might offer effective and safely modifiable preventive interventions. What follows is, first, an analysis of the loads of mortality and disease attributed to abnormal BMI in adults, mainly to garner some idea of what a baseline range of normal BMI values might be. The all-important issue of children and BMI will then be addressed.

OBESITY AND DISEASE

Claims of an obesity epidemic imply that most people are at risk of becoming obese, but the evidence does not sustain this. Detailed surveys show that most people have gained small increments of weight over the past decades, whereas the relatively few severely obese are the people who show the excessive gains.[8] This being the case, the classification of people in broad segments, such as those over BMI 30, is bound to give a distorted impression, because it lumps together people with widely different characteristics.

Official public health pronouncements speak of four segments within the range of BMI values in open populations. These correspond to low weight, normal weight, overweight and obese individuals. The official BMI threshold of normal weight has been scaled down in the past decade from 29 to 25, below which the health risks associated with being thin are said to increase progressively, and above which the health risks associated first with overweight (up to a BMI of 30), and then with obesity (upward of BMI 30) are also said to increase progressively. Setting BMI 25 as the threshold of normality is, nevertheless, totally arbitrary, for it cannot be objectively justified.[9]

For BMI values over 25, overweight and obesity are said to be associated mainly with greater risk of mortality from cardiovascular diseases, cancers, diabetes and hypertension. Below BMI 25, progressively thinner people are said to be at greater risk of mortality from cardiovascular diseases, cancers and infectious diseases. Are such official characterisations of normal BMI values justified by the epidemiological evidence?

As a first consideration, it should be clear that declaring a specific cut-off point as the threshold for normal weight is wholly arbitrary, given the uncertain meaning of BMI in relation to obesity, and the manifest variability of individuals in relation to normality. Furthermore, the definition of wide segments of the BMI range – as inclusive of underweight, overweight and obese people – is also arbitrary, because it ignores the natural overlapping between those segments. Thus, defining as overweight those with BMI 25 to 30, and obese those above BMI 30, short-changes the people at the high end of the segments and overloads those at the low end. A more appropriate analysis would consider the continuum of BMI values,[10] but such an approach is rare in studies of body weight.

The epidemiological literature on weight, disease and mortality is vast, goes back several decades, and is remarkably inconsistent, except for reports on subjects at the extremes of body thinness and obesity. An exhaustive review of the entire corpus of literature is beyond the scope of this book, given also that a clear picture emerges from the most recent studies – studies that were carried out in the light of previous work and that are, presumably then, of superior design and conduct, and based on larger numbers.

OBESITY AND PREMATURE DEATH

A central tenet of this book is that the link between obesity and certain diseases is not scientifically or even intuitively established. Most illustrative of the vast uncertainties, and of the arbitrariness of BMI classifications, is a study that made headlines in March 2004.[11] The report came from the Centers for Disease Control and Prevention (CDC), an agency of the US Department of Health and Human Services. For an added measure of impact, the report includes the director of the CDC agency among its authors, and was published by the *Journal of the American Medical Association* (*JAMA*), a most prestigious medical and public health weekly. Largely based on four consecutive National Health and Nutrition Examination Surveys (NHANES) by the same CDC, the report asserts that overweight and obesity in the USA cause upward of 414,000 deaths annually, based on a selective review of past epidemiological studies. Predictably, this CDC report enjoyed extensive and alarming media coverage, even though it put the annual death toll at 134,000 more than a previous report that had also been published in *JAMA* in 1999.[12]

Astonishingly, the 2004 report was contradicted a few months later by a second report, also from the CDC agency and also published in *JAMA*.[13] This second official study from the same government agency severely criticised the previous one because it:

[U]sed adjusted relative risks in an attributable fraction formula appropriate only for unadjusted relative risks, and thus only partially adjusted for confounding factors, did not account for variations by age in the relation of body weight to mortality, and did not include measures of uncertainty in the form of [standard errors] or confidence intervals (CIs). [It] used data from a variety of studies to estimate relative risk, but the studies had some limitations. Four of the 6 included only older data (2 studies ended follow-up in the 1970s and 2 in the 1980s), 3 had only self-reported weight and height, and 1 study included only women. Only 1 data set, the National Health and Nutrition Examination Survey (NHANES) was nationally representative.[14]

Using what was billed as a more credible approach, the study concluded that in the US, relative to a normal weight category of BMI between 18.5 and 25.0, obesity over 30 BMI was associated with 111,909 excess deaths, while underweight was associated with 33,746 excess deaths. Surprisingly, it also found that, for the category of BMI between 25.0 and 30.0, overweight reduced mortality by 86,094 units annually. Such a report of reduced mortality unequivocally shows that the 'normal' reference range of BMI 18.5 to 25.0 selected in this study was too low, and that the actual normal range should have been extended to values much higher than BMI 25.0. Actually, a table in the report (reproduced on next page), which included data for non-smokers, lists one mortality hazard ratio (0.77) that indicates a reduction in mortality for values above BMI 30.0, meaning that the BMI range of normality may well extend above BMI 30.0. Indeed, if the apparent mortality protection of body fat extends into the BMI 30.0–35.0 category, it means that the estimated lives saved by body fat could be more numerous than the study reported for the BMI 25.0–30.0 category alone.

Notice, in any event, that the mortality risks reported are extremely weak and are mostly without statistical significance. Data are also much weaker for non-smokers than for smokers and non-smokers together, which raises the question of how much weaker the data might be if the innumerable causes known to affect mortality had been accounted for in the same way as the study accounted for smoking. Even for the confounders that were accounted for, the authors note

TABLE 2.1

Relative Risks by Age Group and BMI Level from the Combined
NHANES I, II and III Data Set

| BMI Level | Relative Risk (95% Confidence Interval) by Age Category | | |
	25–59y	60–69y	≥70y
	Overall		
<18.5	1.38 (0.82–2.32)	2.30 (1.70–3.13)	1.69 (1.38–2.07)
18.5 to <25	1.00	1.00	1.00
25 to <30	0.83 (0.65–1.06)	0.95 (0.80–1.13)	0.91 (0.83–1.01)
30 to <35	1.20 (0.84–1.72)	1.13 (0.89–1.42)	1.03 (0.91–1.17)
≥35	1.83 (1.27–2.62)	1.63 (1.16–2.30)	1.17 (0.94–1.47)
	Never-Smokers Only		
<18.5	1.25 (0.29–5.49)	2.97 (1.17–7.54)	1.50 (1.11–2.02)
18.5 to <25	1.00	1.00	1.00
25 to <30	0.66 (0.38–1.16)	0.81 (0.56–1.16)	0.90 (0.79–1.04)
30 to <35	0.77 (0.46–1.28)	1.21 (0.83–1.77)	1.13 (0.96–1.31)
≥35	1.25 (0.76–2.06)	2.30 (1.47–3.59)	1.12 (0.87–1.45)

Abbreviations: BMI, body mass index (measured as weight in kilograms
divided by the square of height in metres); NHANES, National Health
and Nutrition Examination Survey.   Source: Flegal et al., 2005.

that '[b]ecause of errors in confounder measurement, our estimates of relative risk for BMI categories may be subject to
residual confounding'.[15] Which brings the authors to note
also that 'estimates give numbers of excess deaths associated
with different levels of body weight, but the associations are
not necessarily causal'. Moreover, the authors and other
studies also warn of the extreme sensitivity of excess deaths
calculations to very slight changes in the estimates of relative
risks.[16] Also, the overall conclusions of the study are based on
three consecutive NHANES surveys (1971–75; 1976–80;
1988–94), and the study shows that mortality decreased from
the first to the last survey, a trend that implies much lower
mortality rates in more recent years and today. Within statistical error, the study reports virtually no increase in mortality
for the elderly over 60 years of age, even for obesity levels of
over BMI 35. Figure 2.1 clearly shows that, for the last two
surveys and for all surveys combined, there is no statistical
excess of mortality for the category of BMI 30–35.

FIGURE 2.1

Semiparametric mortality estimates for 1995, by gender and body mass index (BMI), derived from self-reported height and weight: US adults aged 18–64 years in 1987 or 1989

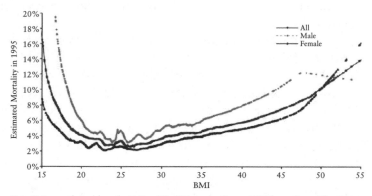

Note: Data were derived from the National Health Interview Survey 1987 Cancer Control Supplement File, 1989 Diabetes Supplement File and 1995 Multiple Cause of Death File. Plots represent predictions for an average individual at a given BMI according to semiparametric regression results (bandwidth = 0.15). All covariates other than BMI were treated parametrically. Analyses were limited to respondents aged between 18 and 64 years with available mortality, BMI and smoking information. All mortality estimates were adjusted, via stratification, for race, age, limited smoking history, education level, income level and marital status.

Source: Gronniger, 2006.

Indeed, a 1999 epidemiological study dealing with the different subjects of the large Cancer Prevention Study (CPS-II) of the American Cancer Society essentially agrees with this second CDC report, as does a study of life expectancy and other studies.[17] What are we to make of the contrasting CDC reports? A commentary published in the same issue of *JAMA* as the second CDC report expressed shock, noting that 'The magnitude of the differences cries out for an explanation of the reasons behind these differences. Some might wonder: If well-intentioned efforts to calculate this number can result in such widely varied estimates, is it worth trying to do at all?'[18]

Further clarification came from a 2006 study of US data from a nationally representative survey, where BMI and mortality were treated not in segments, but as continuous variables. This preferred non-parametric approach allowed the study to conclude that 'Normal weight individuals of both genders did not appear to be relatively more long-lived than mildly obese individuals (BMIs of 30–35) whereas overweight people (BMIs of 25–30) appeared healthiest of all.' Within statistical error, the study concluded that there are negligible differences in mortality risk in the range of BMI 20–35.[19] Similar conclusions were reported in earlier analyses of NHANES data.[20]

A reasonable conclusion is that the excess mortality attributed by Flegal *et al.* (2005) to the category over BMI 30 would be reduced considerably for the more current and meaningful state of affairs of the year 2000, if the category of BMI 30–35 were analysed separately for the more recent NHANES III survey. This is because a higher BMI reference category would be selected in view of the reduction in mortality reported for the BMI 25–30 category, because of other results listed in the study and the volatile uncertainties inherent to the data and their analysis, and because of the extreme sensitivity of the analysis to risk estimates. Under these conditions, the category of BMI 30–35 would not show significant excess mortality for the NHANES III survey, as was suggested in Flegal *et al.* (2005), and an excess of mortality might be attributable only to the category over BMI 35. In fact there are reports that the risk of obesity may be noticeable only above BMI 40.†

The studies by Gronniger and others also raise intriguing implications with regard to longevity, which continued to increase as the weight of populations increased. It would seem obvious that, if the very thin and very obese were excluded, the majority of people, who gained only a few pounds, must have experienced longevity gains much greater than overall averages. Clearly, adding a few pounds has been advantageous and healthy for the majority of people who are neither too thin nor too obese. Some epidemic, indeed.

In any event, it is sobering to recall that all reports rely on the precarious meaning of BMI, and none could account for the effects of changing lifestyles, medical improvements and

---

† K. McTigue *et al.*, 'Mortality and cardiac and vascular outcomes in extremely obese women', *JAMA* 2006 (296): 79–86.

other causes of mortality during the periods of observation. Still, in general, the majority of studies conflict with claims of significant excess mortality for body mass levels of BMI 20–35.

An earlier meta-analysis[21] summary of US survey data (also by CDC investigators) concluded that the mortality risk increased below BMI 23 and above BMI 28 for men, but it found no association between BMI and mortality for women, even among non-smokers.[22] A study of 115,000 US nurses found that, among non-smokers, the group below BMI 19.0 had the lowest mortality, while mortality increased progressively with BMI, up to a relative risk[23] of 2.2 for BMI in excess of 32.0.[24] By contrast, a large-scale Canadian study among women found an increased risk of mortality for subjects of BMI below 18.5, and a progressive increase in the risk for BMI values above 22.0, up to a relative risk of 1.4 for subjects with BMI 35.0 and over.[25] A study of over 19,000 alumni of Harvard University found no increased mortality risk for lean men, but an increase in risk for subjects above BMI 22.5.[26]

A Polish study of 5,200 men and 5,600 women controlled for age, place of residence, blood cholesterol, hypertension and smoking over a mean period of 10 years. For men at BMI of below 20.0, the risk of death was 2.2, compared to the low-risk group of BMI 20.0–32.0, while the risk was 1.4 for the group at BMI 32.0–35.0, and 1.7 for those with BMI of over 35.0. Women, by contrast, had an increased risk of mortality of 1.66 below BMI 20.0, but no increase in risk for higher BMI values.[27] Similarly, a study of 7,900 European men found that the relative risk of mortality among people with BMI of below 18.5 was 2.1, compared to the group of BMI 25.0–30.0, and a relative risk of 1.8 for people with BMI of over 30.[28] A study of 16,000 Japanese men and women concluded that 'Taking only never-smokers, the highest risk for all-cause mortality was observed in the lowest BMI category for men and women.'[29]

In a study of 2,100 Finnish men and women, 'BMI did not prove to be an independent factor for mortality', but physical fitness did. The study controlled for age, marital and employment status, and smoking and alcohol consumption.[30] Somewhat different relationships were reported for a group of 5,500 men and 5,800 women from Japan. For subjects with BMI of below 18.5, the study reported an increased mortality risk of 2.66 for men and 3.14 for women. For the highest group over BMI 28.0, only women showed an increased risk of 3.25.[31]

An Italian study of 32,700 men and 30,300 women controlled for age, smoking and systolic blood pressure, but failed to demonstrate in all cases a relationship between BMI and mortality, except for some differences between young (higher) and mature (lower) women. The study concluded that 'uncommon high values of BMI carrying the minimum risk of death seems to be in contrast with weight guidelines'.[32] A study of Aboriginal Australians found that 'BMI and mortality are inversely associated in Aboriginal adults in a remote community. Individuals with relatively higher BMI have a lower risk of death.'[33]

High BMI values seem of less concern for elderly subjects. A recent study found that nursing-home residents with BMI of over 28.0 had a lower relative risk of mortality (RR=0.89) compared to controls. It concluded that this suggested '*a higher BMI may be protective among long-stay residents*' (emphasis added), in line with the findings of an earlier study by the authors.[34] Also, a study of 6,400 elderly Norwegian men and women found that 'BMI was not associated with all-cause mortality' – mortality being highly correlated with hypertension.[35] Similarly, a study of 3,700 elderly Japanese-Americans from Honolulu, Hawaii, found '*a consistent inverse association*' (emphasis added) of BMI and mortality risk – increasing BMI values related to decreasing mortality risk.[36]

What can epidemiological studies of BMI and mortality tell us? The uncertainties and ambiguities should not be of surprise in the context of population surveys that cannot certify what they purport to have measured, and cannot control for the very numerous competing hazards that affect mortality. Indeed, prominent authors have been keen to warn of the pitfalls in analysing and interpreting studies of over-weight and mortality.[37]

In light of previous considerations on the limitations of epidemiology, it is also necessary to recall that many primary surveys have not actually measured height, weight and other characteristics of the individual approached. Rather, they have collected such information from the subjects themselves or their next of kin, who were responding to a written or tele-phone questionnaire, or to a verbal interview. Such data do not qualify as measurements, cannot lead to the calculation of justifiable error rates, and therefore do not deserve the term 'scientific', let alone 'objective'.

Moreover, as has already been discussed, BMI is an ambiguous measure of body fat, being corrupted by several conditions of age, sex, body structure, relative organ and muscle mass, tissue hydration, and more. Such conditions could relate to mortality rather than body fat itself, or body fat might be a contributor of unknown and variable potency to a constellation of conditions that affect the overall mortality experience, from which the quantitative or qualita-tive contribution of BMI could not possibly be extracted. Most of these conditions are likely to be unrelated to over-eating and to excessive intake of caloric food, meaning that focusing on diet as a measure by which to reduce weight and retard mortality could be misguided, ineffective or even dangerous.[38]

In general, studies of BMI and mortality associations have divided the BMI range into segments, for example as BMI below 18.5, between 18.9 and 28, and 29 and above, with dif-ferent studies adopting segmentations of different length. Essentially, those studies calculate and compare mean values of the data for each segment, and are therefore unable to offer useful information about the likely overlapping of different segments. The notable exception is the recent study by Gronniger,[39] which takes into account the continuum of the BMI range, resulting in what appears to be a more explana-tory account of the relationship between BMI and mortality.

As has been noted, such an analysis of data from a broad survey of the US population indicates that mortality rates are lowest in the range of BMI 18–35 – the study attributing to data noise whatever little random variation might show up within that range. It is only below and above that range that mortality rates begin sharply and consistently to increase.

All studies report observational associations and do not amount to a verifiable causal link between BMI and mortality. Indeed, the apparent association is questioned by several studies that show that mortality may be exacerbated by a deliberate attempt to reduce BMI through dietary restrictions, and studies consistently indicate that mortality is definitely enhanced following involuntary weight loss and weight cycling, especially in the elderly.[40] In fact, there are reports that even being morbidly obese confers survival advantages in certain disease situations.[41]

Whatever meaning the studies of BMI and mortality may have in relation to body fat and diet, they are silent about what diseases may be responsible for the excess mortalities claimed at the lowest and highest BMI categories. According to the World Health Organization (WHO), overweight and obesity are mostly associated with cardiovascular disease (CVD) and cancer risks, the risk of hypertension, and of non-insulin dependent diabetes mellitus (NID diabetes).[42] Still, there are dozens of known cancer hazards, hundreds of hazards for cardiovascular diseases, and many more conditions besides body weight that influence hypertension and diabetes. None of the epidemiological studies offer a comprehensive analysis of these hazards, meaning that their claims remain just as perplexing as in the case of the association between BMI and mortality.

OBESITY AND CARDIOVASCULAR DISEASE

Although they did not measure CVD incidence itself in 2005, investigators from the US Centers for Disease Control and Prevention reported on US trends in the prevalence of major CVD risk factors, using data from five nationally representative surveys conducted between 1960 and 2000. The authors of the report concluded that '[e]xcept for diabetes, CVD risk factors declined considerably over the past 40 years in all BMI groups. Although obese persons still have higher risk factors than lean persons, the levels of these risk factors are much lower than in previous decades.' They went on: 'Total diabetes prevalence was stable within BMI groups over time, as non-significant 1–2 percentage-point increases occurred between 1976–1980 and 1999–2000.'[43] The study categorised BMI as less than 25, 25 to 30, and over 30 – a segmentation that likely missed important and potentially revealing overlaps, as is suggested by the aforementioned Gronniger report.[44]

According to the Gregg *et al.* study, the prevalence of high cholesterol, high blood pressure, and cigarette smoking has declined by 21, 18 and 12 percentage points, respectively, since 1960–62 for obese persons with BMI of over 30. Those risks were lower for obese persons in 1999–2000 than for lean people in 1960–62. At the same time, the study reported that overall BMI values, and the prevalence of overweight and obesity, had increased by more than 10 per cent from 1960–62 to 1999–2000; it also noted that several official reports had documented a much greater decline in CVD over the same period.[45]

Mindful of the limitations of epidemiological surveys that explore possible BMI roles, these contrasting trends strongly suggest that the claimed association between CVD and BMI is at least questionable, and may be a mirage caused by contingent hazards that are only incidentally related to overweight and obesity, and therefore unrelated to diet. In fact, at least two studies indicate that CVD mortality in obese subjects that are physically fit is comparable to that of normal-weight individuals: a finding that would seem to exonerate obesity itself as a cause of CVD mortality.[46]

While there are earlier reports associating CVD and BMI, more recent and arguably better studies tend to indicate no association, or even a protective effect of BMI on CVD. A US study of 15,000 patients suffering from coronary heart disease found that 'Overweight and obese BMI classifications were associated with better intermediate-term survival after acute coronary syndromes than normal weight and very obese, but deaths after myocardial infarction were similar.'[47]

A large French study of 140,000 men and 104,000 women concluded that, with regard to mortality, '[i]n both genders, the association of overweight with diabetes alone or hypercholesterolemia alone did not increase the risk. By contrast, in the presence of hypertension, cardiovascular mortality dramatically increased in overweight subjects with hypercholesterolemia ... or diabetes', again indicating a major role of hazard factors other than high BMI.[48]

A US study of 7,700 patients that had experienced heart failure (HF), but were in a stable condition, found that

> Crude all-cause mortality rates decreased in a near linear fashion across successively higher BMI groups, from 45.0 percent in the underweight group to 28.4 percent in the obese group (P for trend <.001). After multivariable adjustment, overweight and obese patients were at lower risk of death (hazard ratio [HR], 0.88; 95 percent confidence interval [CI], 0.80–0.96, and HR, 0.81; 95 percent CI, 0.72–0.92, respectively), compared with patients at a healthy weight (referent). In contrast, underweight patients with stable HF were at increased risk of death (HR 1.21; 95 percent CI, 0.95-1.53).

The study concluded:

> In a cohort of outpatients with established HF, higher BMIs were associated with lower mortality risks; overweight and obese patients had lower risk of death compared with those at a healthy weight. Understanding the mechanisms and impact of the 'obesity paradox' in patients with HF is necessary before recommendations are made concerning weight and weight control in this population.[49]

This study was corroborated by independent and similar evidence.[50]

A Swedish study of elderly subjects found that high BMI values were a hazard for strokes in men, but not in women.[51] A meta-analysis study of 13 international surveys of elderly subjects concluded that '[m]ost studies showed a negative or no association between BMI and all-cause mortality'.[52] Also, a study of over 900 patients with coronary disease found that the electrocardiograms 'of overweight and obese coronary patients showed no significant differences when compared with electrocardiograms of normal-weight patients'.[53]

The massive MONICA study conducted by the WHO in 38 different communities found no association in women between BMI and coronary heart disease – the major subset of CVD – and a declining risk for men as BMI increases.[54] A study of 5,000 male physicians concluded that the 'findings indicate that elevated BMI may not be strongly associated with total cardiovascular mortality among men with pre-viously manifested coronary disease'. In fact, none of the weak associations was statistically significant in this study.[55]

Taking 2,600 subjects in a US Health Maintenance Organization who had experienced myocardial infarction, during a follow-up examination three to four years later it was found that people in the highest quartile of BMI values had the highest rate of re-infarction, but the lowest rate of mortality.[56] A similar study of 2,000 Welshmen who had suf-fered myocardial infarction found the highest mortality rate in the leaner group (BMI 15–24) and a lower mortality risk for all subjects with higher BMI values.[57]

A study of 6,100 obese German subjects concluded that 'morbid obesity (BMI of > or = 40) was a strong predictor of premature death due to CVD. Excess mortality risks associat-ed with gross obesity (BMI from 32 to <40 kg/m^2) were con-siderably lower than hitherto assumed; moderate degrees of obesity (BMI from 25 to <32 kg/m^2) were not significantly associated with excess mortality'.[58] Such results are remark-ably in line with the studies of Flegal and Gronniger already cited.[59]

It has also been noted that numerous overweight and obese people – and more likely the unfit ones – have long been self-medicating for weight loss with phenylpropanolamine (PPA) and food supplements, especially those containing ephedrine, many of which were recently banned on account of having been linked to heart problems and stroke.[60] Although these findings have been contested in the case of PPA,[61] none of the studies on overweight and obesity have controlled for the use of weight-control dietary supplements, despite their obvious interest.

Thus, and while some earlier and arguably less experienced studies may have hinted at a correlation between BMI and CVD, more recent and probably better-run studies tend to play down the correlation, and many actually suggest that obesity may exert a protective influence in CVD, especially in the elderly. Obese people who are physically fit may not experience an increased risk of CVD. Thus, it is likely that independent CVD hazards, such as hypertension, hypercholesterolaemia or cigarette smoking, were more prevalent in the obese in decades past, when they caused diseases and mortality that was erroneously imputed to overweight and obesity. Indeed, more recent studies find a marked decrease in those hazards that previously accompanied high BMI, a substantial reduction in CVD mortality, and also a noticeably increased BMI average – a convergence of circumstances that tends to exonerate BMI as a significant risk factor for CVD, with the possible exception of unfit, obese individuals.

OBESITY AND CANCER

As was noted above, most studies of BMI, disease and mortality divide the BMI range into two or three segments, the average values of which are then compared to assess the relative risk of each segment. Clearly, such an exceedingly broad segmentation ends up erroneously attributing risk to overlapping BMI values. The Gronniger study and other studies avoided segmentation by considering the continuum of BMI values, and for the population surveyed – representative of the US population – the study noted overall mortality rates that were essentially the same in the range of BMI values of 18–35, with mortality risk surging at both ends of that range.[62] If, instead, the study had selected a segment of, say, all subjects with BMI of over 27, such a segment would have included subjects at no risk, as well as morbidly obese subjects at the extreme of risk, which would have resulted in a composite risk assessment that could not do justice to the true risks at the lower and the higher ends of that range. Such a problem is common in the majority of studies that seek a possible correlation between BMI and cancer, and therefore eclipses their meaning and interpretation.

In a recent example, a Swedish study of 25,000 women and 33,000 men found no association between BMI and over-all cancer in men, but it did find an increase in cancer in women with BMI of above 27.1 – much too broad a segment of the BMI range. This leaves open the all-important question of whether the risk progresses linearly from BMI 27.1 onward, or at what point over BMI 27.1 the risk may begin to increase.[63]

A worldwide WHO study that included seven World Bank-defined regions found an increased incidence of cancers of the colon and uterus, and of post-menopausal breast can-cer, in relation to body mass scores in excess of BMI 21 – also an excessively broad category that provided no credible or useful guidance as to the specific shape of the relationship or possible public health action.[64] A study of 18,000 middle-aged London men, who were tracked for an average of 35 years, found an increase in the incidence of cancers of the rectum, bladder, colon, liver and lymphoma for obese and overweight people with BMI of over 25 – results that clearly cannot be properly interpreted to provide sensible guidance for possible weight control.[65]

By contrast, a large Japanese study of 42,000 men and 46,000 women with a 10-year follow-up found a U-shaped association between BMI and cancer incidence in men, with the lowest risk for the BMI interval at 23–24.9. The risk was most significant for underweight males with BMI of 14.0–18.9. Remarkably, the study found no association between BMI and cancer risk in women.[66]

With a median follow-up of 14 years, investigators at the US Centers for Disease Control and Prevention studied breast cancer mortality trends in a group of nearly 4,000 women who had been diagnosed with breast cancer. The study found a slightly increased risk of mortality in women with BMI of above 22.9, but concluded that '[f]urther study is needed to determine how these findings might affect recommendations to reduce breast cancer mortality' – a highly appropriate conclusion, given the unjustifiable range of the segment of BMI values considered.[67]

A study of women with breast cancer in Hong Kong found that 'present BMI and BMI 5 years before diagnosis were poorly associated with breast cancer risk among pre- and post-menopausal women'.[68] A French study followed nearly 70,000 women aged 45–70 years. It found a non-significant reduction in breast cancer at higher BMI values among pre-menopausal women, and an equally non-significant increase in breast cancer at increasing BMI values in post-menopausal women.[69]

A study by the American Cancer Society followed 900,000 male and female adults who were free of cancer when first interviewed in 1982. The study found that, in relation to normal-weight people, there was a 52 per cent increase in the incidence of cancer among men with BMI of over 40 in 1982, and a corresponding 62 per cent increase among women. The specific cancers were of the stomach and prostate for men, and of the breast, uterus, cervix and ovary for women. The study found no increased cancer incidence for underweight people. Being a study of mortality, rather than of incidence of cancer, the reported risks could be inflated by other independent mortality risks, including obesity – which prompted the authors to warn that '[i]t is also likely that the stronger associations seen in our study reflect a greater effect of body mass index on mortality than on incidence of cancer at some sites'.[70] Indeed, a multi-country study by the International Agency for Research on Cancer, a part of the WHO, found that 'increasing body weight may confer a protection against ovarian cancer'.[71]

Another study followed 8,000 Japanese men for 15 years and found an increased risk of colon cancer in relation to increasing BMI among subjects who were 55 years of age or older at the initial examination. The study found that '[n]o other cancer had a significant positive association with either BMI at the time of examination or with weight gain since age 25'.[72]

Hence, the picture of a possible association between BMI and cancer is anything but clear and consistent. In the available epidemiological studies, the pervasive methodology of dividing the BMI range into segments that are too broad is bound to distort the interpretation of a possible association. Given the observation that baseline mortality rates are essentially stationary in the BMI range of 18–35,[73] one might think that an eventual association between body mass and cancer could show a heightened risk at BMI levels below and above that baseline range. Such an assumption may not hold if there is a tradeoff between – for instance – reduced mortality for CVD and increased mortality for cancer, but all the information currently available is unable to shed light on that issue. In any event, and with a possible exception of the morbidly obese, the epidemiological record is ambiguous about a possible association between BMI and cancer.

OBESITY, HYPERTENSION AND DIABETES

Many metabolic and physiological functions act in a concerted fashion, influence each other, and, in the process, may influence hypertension and diabetes. These functions include appetite, hunger, food intake, food utilisation as energy, storage of energy as body fat or glycogen, release of stored energy, body water retention, kidney function efficiency, insulin and glucagon release in response to blood levels of sugars and other signals, dilation or constriction of blood vessels and airways, kidney diuresis and sodium retention, and heart integrity and pumping rates. The expression of any particular function at a given time is mediated and regulated by a complex sum of signals derived from the assembly of body functions located in different organs, and under the constraints dictated by the underlying genetic makeup.

Blood pressure, for instance, is controlled directly by the degree of constriction of arteries, capillaries and veins, by the volume and osmolarity of the blood, and by the heart's pumping power. In turn, such conditions continuously send and receive modifying signals of a hormonal, chemical and electrical nature to and from virtually all other body functions, but especially to and from the kidneys, the adrenal gland, muscle activity, brain emotional signals, diet and salt intake, and many other conditions.

The end result is a concerted effort by various body functions to maintain a blood pressure that is compatible with the requirements of the moment, in ways that will also vary in relation to genetic traits. Thus it is that people of African descent are more prone to develop high blood pressure or hypertension after migrating and living in temperate climates, probably on account of earlier genetic adaptations to retain sodium – the result of evolution under conditions of reduced access to salt and in hot and arid climates that favour a high rate of perspiration.[74]

Obesity and overweight are often linked to what is defined as the metabolic syndrome: a cluster of metabolic and vascular deficiencies. The syndrome lacks a set of generally accepted diagnostic criteria, but is usually attended by hyperglycaemia, elevated blood triglycerides, low HDL-cholesterol, hypertension, impaired insulin sensitivity and abdominal obesity. The syndrome may affect especially the older segments of populations of affluent countries, and carries an increased risk of diabetes and CVD, as a result of which it may also affect mortality. It is clear, though, that the syndrome results from many more conditions than the few just mentioned, each of the latter being itself determined by a network of more or less manifest disorders and countervailing repair mechanisms.

Within such a muddled web of causative and protective interactions, it would still be impossible to define even approximately what may be the causes and what the effects.

All things considered, hypertension and diabetes mellitus may be more prevalent in obese people, but it is still an unresolved question whether they may depend on obesity, whether obesity itself may depend on them, or whether each of those conditions may derive from even more remote determinants.

CHILDHOOD OBESITY

For adults, the prevalence of overweight and obesity – defined by what are inconsistent segmentations of BMI ranges – has increased in many countries.[75] In many countries, too, a similar increasing trend has been observed in children and adolescents.[76]

These gains should be seen as a continuation of a trend in body-weight increases that was apparent over many decades of the last century, parallel to a steady increase in life expectancy.[77] Moreover, recent increases in body mass have occurred over the entire spectrum of BMI values in adult populations, while gains are mostly confined to the over-weight and obese segments of child populations. Children of normal weight have not experienced significant gains in body mass.[78]

It is intuitive that an increase in stored body fat results when the rate of ingestion of food calories is not counter-balanced by a commensurate consumption of energy, or by a heightened amount of ingested food energy discarded as waste. Still, despite the reported BMI increases, most (but not all) American reports show that the amount of calories ingested by children and adolescents has declined over the time span in which average body mass has increased. Reports from other countries tend to show that energy intakes have remained virtually unchanged as body mass has increased.[79]

We remind the reader that dietary surveys are among the weakest of epidemiological exercises, dependent as they are on the vague individual recall of dietary intakes in previous months and years. As a result, dietary intakes are not mea-sured, but are simply guessed at, and no statistical deftness could remedy the intrinsic uncertainty. That said, studies leave the general impression that dietary calorie intakes may not have changed much over the last four decades in many countries, and might have decreased in the US.

Public health crusades and media attention have tended to focus concern on foods that are simply caloric (for example, fizzy drinks, dietary fats, dairy products), on the issue of regular meals versus frequent nibbling and snacking from vending machines, and on the reduced expenditure of energy due to lack of exercise, television, computer games and so on. Such public information, however, is not sustained by epidemiological reports that are inconsistent and often contradictory. A review of the most recent studies illustrates the rather confusing record.

An American study of beverage consumption from school vending machines found 'no impact on BMI by removing [regular carbonated soft drinks] consumption in schools'.[80] A US study followed, for a year, nearly 11,000 2–3-year-old children who were consuming sweet drinks. For children of normal weight at the start, the consumption of sweet drinks made no significant difference to weight gain, but for children who were classified as overweight at the outset, the consumption of two to three drinks a day increased significantly the risk of overweight. The results suggest the role of susceptibility factors that are independent of the consumption of sweet drinks.[81]

A longitudinal Norwegian study between 1981 and 1999 followed subjects aged 15–33 in relation to their consumption of carbonated fizzy drinks, and found 'no differences in body mass index, overweight or obesity in 1999 between long term high and low consumers'.[82] A counterintuitive Nebraska study followed 164 children for two years, and found that more 'diet' fizzy drinks were consumed by subjects who were overweight at the start and by those who gained weight after two years. The study left it unclear how 'diet' fizzy drinks, which are without caloric content, could account for an increased BMI score.[83]

A Tennessee study concluded that fruit juice intake in children aged 2–5 years 'was not associated with either stature or overweight'.[84] The Bogalusa Heart Study followed the sweetened-beverage consumption of 1,500 children from 1973 to 1994, and concluded that 'there was no linear relationship between sweetened-beverage consumption and BMI and total energy intake'.[85]

A Harvard study tracked over two years the consumption of sugar-added beverages and weight gain among 10,000 boys and girls aged between nine and 14 years in 1996. No significant differences were observed after adjustments were made for total energy intakes.[86] A North Dakota study of 1,300 low-income pre-school children aged two to five years found that weight change was not related to intakes of fruit juices, milk or sugared fizzy drinks. The same study found no significant associations between BMI and energy-adjusted dietary fat or fibre.[87]

In a German study of 4,300 children aged five to six years, '[a] protective effect of increased daily meal frequency on obesity in children was observed and appeared independent of other risk factors for childhood obesity', even though the study also noted 'a higher energy intake in nibblers compared to gorgers'. The authors attributed the difference to a possible increased mobilisation of insulin.[88] At the same time, a US study came to different conclusions and recommended limiting food intake to 'no more than six times per day'.[89]

A study at the Children's Hospital in Boston, Massachusetts, asked why some adolescents who frequently ate fast food did not become overweight. In the study, all subjects 'over-consumed fast food regardless of body weight, although the phenomenon was more pronounced in overweight participants'. The implication is that characteristics of susceptibility are likely to play a role in overweight beyond diet itself.[90] A Harvard study of some 13,000 adolescents found that children who drank the most milk gained more weight, but that dairy fat was not responsible for weight increases.[91] By contrast, a contemporary Italian study found 'a significant inverse association between frequency of milk consumption and body mass in children'.[92]

Again in Boston, a three-year study followed some 14,000 children aged nine to 14 years at the outset, on the basis of self-reported questionnaire data. The study found virtually no differences in the consumption of fried food away from home (FFA). Subjects who consumed one or no FFA per week had an average BMI of 19.1; for FFA consumption of 1–3 times a week the average BMI was 19.2; and for consumption of four to seven FFA per week the average BMI was 19.3.[93] In a different study, the same authors followed the same cohort of children to investigate the relationship between the frequency with which they had dinner with the family and BMI. The study found that the frequency of eating a family dinner was slightly (RR=0.85) inversely associated with overweight prevalence at the start of the study, but that such an association no longer held true at the end of the three-year observation period.[94]

A study of 137,000 children aged 10–16 years from 34 countries (mostly European) concluded that overweight 'was not associated with the intake of fruits, vegetables, and soft drinks or time spent on the computer'.[95] Another 10-year study followed 196 non-obese girls aged eight to 12 years at the outset, to investigate the relationship between BMI and the intake of energy-dense snacks (EDS) such as baked goods, ice cream, crisps, sugar-sweetened fizzy drinks and sweets. At entry, the girls consumed an average of 2.3 +/– 1.7 servings of EDS per day, amounting to 15.7 +/– 8.1 per cent of total energy intake. After 10 years of observation, no relationship was detected between body fat (BMI) and consumption of EDS foods. The study also found a significant association between EDS intake and time spent watching television: a finding that seems to exonerate television viewing as a cause of BMI gain, given that the study found no association between EDS consumption and BMI.[96]

Another large-scale American study spent three years tracking almost 15,000 boys and girls aged 9–14 years at the start, to investigate the relationship between BMI and the consumption of fruit and vegetables. As with other work, this study relied on questionnaire data self-reported by the children themselves. After controlling for developmental variables, no correlation was found between intake of fruit and vegetables and BMI scores. The study concluded that 'the recommendation for consumption of fruit and vegetables may be well founded, but should not be based on a beneficial effect on weight regulation'.[97]

Under the aegis of the European Commission, a British study among young adults found that different individuals displayed different susceptibility to obesity, depending on several characteristics, including: weak satiety response to fatty meals, preference for high-fat over low-energy food, a hedonic attraction to palatable foods and eating, low basal metabolic rate, a binge preference, different profiles of allelic variations in a variable number of genes, differences in hormonal responses to food and to fat accumulation, and so on. The consequences of susceptibility traits would be enhanced in a permissive environment, but subjects who were not susceptible would maintain normal weight even in a permissive environment.[98] Although the study examined young adults, there is no reason to doubt that susceptibility characteristics would also be common in children.

In fact, a study of 3,000 children who were tracked from age 1–8 years suggested further conditions of susceptibility in children, and concluded that 'prenatal characteristics, particularly race, ethnicity, maternal smoking during pregnancy, and maternal pregnancy obesity, exert influence on the child's weight states through an early tendency toward overweight, which then is perpetuated as the child ages'.[99] Another study followed a separate cohort of 3,000 children between the ages of four and 24 months. It reached the somewhat divergent conclusion that infants that eat small portions eat more frequently, and vice versa. The study warned about 'the potential adverse effects of coercive feeding behaviors ... on children's innate ability to regulate energy intake. This includes not only admonitions to "clean your plate", but overrestrictions of intake that may be motivated by concerns that children are overeating.'[100]

The studies reviewed here leave a rather ambiguous impression about the possible role of excess food intake and the observed variations of BMI scores in children. They seem to hint at underlying conditions of susceptibility to overweight, especially in permissible environments – conditions that are possibly linked to genetic, environmental and behavioural characteristics of individual children. Such a conclusion would also be compatible with the observation that BMI enhancements have been mostly apparent in children who were already decidedly overweight or obese, but not in children who were in the normal BMI range.[101]

If, in fact, BMI scores have increased at the same time as caloric intakes have remained flat or have actually decreased, the reasonable conclusions would be: first, that most children have an innate capacity to self-regulate food intake, despite the easy and abundant variety at hand; and second, that the observed BMI enhancements may be more specifically related to a decline in physical activity and energy expenditures.

Most, but not all, studies find a correlation of overweight and obesity with low physical activity and time spent with the television and computer. A 2004 meta-analysis of previous studies – for what a meta-analysis is worth! – found that 'a statistically significant relationship exists between TV viewing and body fatness among children and youth, although it is likely to be too small to be of substantial clinical relevance'. The study concluded that 'Relationships between sedentary behavior and health are unlikely to be explained using single markers of inactivity, such as TV viewing or video/computer game use.'[102]

More recently, a British study found that physical activity among young people can both decrease and increase BMI at different stages of development, but offers little guidance about possible causes and remedies.[103] Other studies have found a modest reduction in BMI values associated with self-reported increases in physical activity.[104]

A group of over 8,000 Japanese children were tracked from age 3–6 in a study of their BMI and body build and lifestyle data, as obtained by questionnaires filled in by parents and carers. 'Significant factors associated with overweight children were diet (eating rice, green tea, eggs, meat, but less breads and juice), rapid eating, short sleep duration, early bedtime, long periods of television viewing, avoidance of physical activity, and frequent bowel movement.'[105] A Swiss study found that in 'this sample of children living in Switzerland, the use of electronic games was significantly associated with obesity, independently of confounding factors. The association of obesity with television use and lack of physical activity confirms results from other populations and points to potential strategies for obesity prevention.'[106]

By contrast, a US study found that 'In a national sample of preschool children, mothers' perception of neighborhood safety was related to their children's TV viewing time but not to their outdoor play time or risk for obesity.'[107] A British cohort was followed up at five, 10 and 30 years of age from 1970, and the subsequent report concluded that 'Weekend TV viewing in early childhood continues to influence BMI in adulthood. Interventions to influence obesity by reducing sedentary behaviors must begin in early childhood.'[108] A national representative sample of 6,500 Finnish children aged 14, 16 and 18 found that overweight was associated with television and computer use (RR=2.0 for over four hours daily), but not with the playing of video games.[109]

A study of UK children found that watching television for more than eight hours per week at age three was one of eight factors associated with the risk of overweight/obesity at age seven (RR=1.55).[110] A US study of children aged 3–7 found that:

> Physical activity and TV viewing were the only significant predictors (other than baseline BMI) of BMI among a tri-ethnic cohort of 3–4-y-old children followed for 3 y, with both physical activity (negatively associated) and TV viewing (positively associated) becoming stronger predictors as the children aged. It appears that 6 or 7 y is a critical age when TV viewing and physical activity may affect BMI. Therefore, focusing on reducing time spent watching television and increasing time spent in physical activity may be successful means of preventing obesity among this age group.[111]

A study of 137,000 young people aged 10–16 years from 34 mainly European countries – based on self-reported data from questionnaires – found that overweight was associated with television viewing, but not with time spent on a computer.[112] A group of over 1,000 New Zealand children was followed from birth and every two years from age three to age 15. The study concluded that 'Time spent watching television is a significant predictor of BMI and overweight in childhood. Although the effect size appears small, it is larger than the effect sizes commonly reported for nutritional intake and physical activity. Television viewing should be regarded as an important contributing factor to childhood obesity.'[113]

All in all, it makes sense that reduced physical activity would contribute to reduced energy expenditure, and thus to an accumulation of body mass, even though available studies are incapable of producing reliable quantitative estimates of the relationship. Direct measures of physical activity by accelerometry techniques might offer better quantitative insights,[114] but their meaning would relate to immediate local conditions, and may still be unable to provide crucial longitudinal evidence over periods of time.

Other studies also highlight the likely role of psychosocial, socioeconomic and environmental factors that are independent of dietary intake, and are likely to interfere significantly with an understanding of the relationship between physical activity, overweight and obesity.[115] Such interferences are most likely to be of material significance, given that physical activity, psychosocial, socioeconomic and environmental determinants seem all to have comparable effects and a similar small force on BMI scores. Could food and excess body weight be the product of self-therapy attempts in the face of complex psychosocial stressors?[116]

Generally overlooked has been the likely contribution to population weight gain of the progressive decline in cigarette smoking over the past two decades. Smokers are notoriously lighter than non-smokers, and a review of the literature has concluded that smokers weigh from 1.18 to 9.79 kilograms less than non-smokers.[117] Such differentials amount to average deficits considerably in excess of population weight gains registered over the last two decades. In addition, there is much evidence that smoking cessation can result in weight gains that average several kilograms.[118] The evidence suggests that the decline in smoking has probably made a significant contribution to the population weight gain of the past two decades, both in adults and adolescents. It is worth noting that the weight gain attributable to the decline in smoking could not be unhealthy, for it lifts former smokers up to the weight of presumably healthier non-smokers.

In any event, and with regard to adolescents and children, it appears that the spike in overweight has been mostly confined to children who were consistently overweight over time, and was not apparent in those in the normal weight range.[119] The observation again suggests the likely influence of susceptibility traits of genetic, physiological or pathological origin, which are apt to conspire with dietary habits to cause a fraction of children to become overweight. Recent reports that viral infections might play a part in the onset and maintenance of obesity add another intriguing dimension to the problem.[120] The potential of such a constellation of susceptibilities is reinforced by the observation that children with excessive BMI are prone to be overweight when they reach adulthood.[121]

Therefore, the picture emerging from the available studies on children and BMI is anything but clear. The comparatively smaller fraction of heavy and susceptible children seems to have become heavier within the span of some two decades, but normal-weight children may only have gained a few normal pounds. This observation seems congruous with the observation that overall caloric intake was probably either constant or slightly reduced during the period. Remedies for the children at risk are not clear. The feared roles of dietary components such as fizzy drinks, fast-food items, milk, fats and high-calorie snacks were not confirmed in several studies, with a possible exception for the heaviest children. At the same time, the presence of conditions of susceptibility independent of diet – such as physical activity, viral infections, psychosocial and other stressors – seems to be confirmed.

The basis for a rational and decisive course of action is not immediately apparent, and a plethora of uncertain signals demands caution. Conceivably, remedial action should focus on the heavier children, for whom a reduction in caloric intake would seem the easy answer. Still, the long clinical and anecdotal experience of voluntary weight loss is less than reassuring and is fraught with alarming safety issues; it requires extreme caution and personalised attention, rather than sweeping generic guidelines. It is to be hoped that safe, new interventions will emerge from genetic studies, and from the understanding of the intricate physiological and psychological conditions that influence appetite, energy utilisation and waste, and storage and release of energy as body fat.

THE FAT GENE

While the human genome has been successfully dissected and illustrated, the steps by which it is transcribed into live and functioning individual people are virtually unknown. We know how genes code for different proteins and how, in some cases, genes and their proteins have been linked to specific physiological functions or to specific disorders and disabilities. However, the big picture, as it coalesces into a complete organism, is still very elusive.

What is becoming increasingly apparent is a proclivity of genes to influence each other's expressions, and to act in concert like an orchestra, rather than as independent soloists. Just as clusters of kindred instruments produce different resonations in an orchestra, so gene clusters resonate to express different functions, even as they are influenced by, and contribute to, the resonation of other clusters. With so many genes and possible functions, the complexity of interactions is mind-boggling.

The physiology and underlying genetics of appetite control, energy intake, energy utilisation and energy storage are being studied quite intensively, and certain elements of the puzzle have been identified. How those elements may work together to result (or not) in overweight and obesity is still much less clear, and still far from being useful in counselling real people or in setting public health policies.

A recent review presents a summary of many known functions that work either for or against appetite reduction and energy storage as body fat:

> The signaling network underlying hunger, satiety and metabolic status includes the hormonal signals leptin and insulin from energy stores, and cholecystokinin, glucagon-like peptide-1, ghrelin and peptide YY3-36 from the gastrointestinal tract, as well as neuronal influences via the vagus nerve from the digestive tract. This information is routed to specific nuclei of the hypothalamus and brain stem, such as the arcuate nucleus and the solitary tract nucleus respectively, which in turn activate distinct neuronal networks. Of the numerous neuropeptides in the brain, neuropeptide Y, agouti gene-related peptide and orexin stimulate appetite, while melanocortins and alpha-melanocortin-stimulating hormone are involved in satiety. Of the many gastrointestinal peptides, ghrelin is the only appetite-stimulating hormone, whereas cholecystokinin, glucagons-like peptide-l and peptide YY3-36 promote satiety. Adipose tissue provides signals about energy storage levels to the brain through leptin, adiponectin and resistin. Binge-eating has been related to a dysfunction in the ghrelin signaling system.[122]

A class of cell nucleus receptors, the peroxisome proliferators-activated receptor gamma (PPARgamma), is involved in the regulation of bone metabolism, turnover of atherosclerosis lesions, and other functions, including the differentiation of fat-containing cells (adipocytes). PPARgamma are also connected with the metabolic syndrome affecting most obese individuals and characterised by insulin resistance, abdominal obesity, irregularities in blood lipids (dyslipidaemia) and hypertension.[123] Adipocytes secrete leptin, a hormone that signals the brain's hypothalamus, calling for appetite control and maintenance of a stable body weight. Genetic and pathological imbalances that reduce the efficiency of leptin can have a role in promoting obesity, and in fact most obese people are leptin-resistant.[124]

The literature also reports that infectious agents are among the significant mediators of obesity.[125] The hepatitis B and C viruses have been implicated in weight gain and lipidaemic profiles.[126] Many adenoviruses express an enzyme that leads to increased food intake and obesity, even with increased levels of leptin and insulin. The effect has been well described in animals and is associated with obesity in humans.[127] This raises the possibility that hereditary susceptibility to obesity may have originated from the encoding of hazardous viral genes into a progenitor's genome. This field is new and fascinating, but so far has been poorly researched.

The complex network of appetite and weight-gain controls includes mediators that can also influence the development of diabetes mellitus, a frequent disorder in morbidly obese subjects, and also the metabolism of fatty acids or lipids. Lipids, in turn, can have various influences on the expression of many genes that can affect obesity itself.[128] The complexity of functions that can lead to obesity is further enhanced by genetic studies in twins that have identified a number of genes acting in concert (polymorphism) in the determination of obesity, and which seem to display an effect superior to, and independent of, behavioural, environmental, and now probably infectious influences.[129]

Still, it would be out of place here to engage in a detailed analysis of the genetic and physiological complexities that impinge on the maintenance of normal weight and ultimately on the development of obesity. Such an analysis would require an intimate understanding of physiological and genetic issues that are still at an evolutionary stage of research, and a command of the highly specific vocabulary used in researching those issues.

Even in the absence of such specialisation, however, it is possible to reach the overall conclusion that the regulation of appetite, energy intake and energy storage as body fat –

complex as it may be – is remarkably efficient and successful for a majority of what appear to be normal individuals in a population, while its aberrations only become apparent in the small fraction of people who may become morbidly obese. Given this, admonitions to 'take yourself in hand' and to take personal responsibility may be hopeless for the morbidly obese, for whom only specialised medical attention might be appropriate, if and when bariatric medicine becomes more competent than it has been thus far.

CONCLUSION

An obesity crusade that focuses primarily on dietary changes and restrictions would seem counterfactual to a secular historical trend that, in little more than a century, has seen unprecedented advances in food quality, safety and availability, and that has come about in parallel with a near doubling of life expectancy and rapidly declining mortality rates. This occurred in the wake of unprecedented economic development, rising standards of living, and a steadily expanding average height and weight of the population. In fact, advances in food production, quality and distribution hold the promise of liberating mankind for higher pursuits by virtually eliminating the toil of food gathering, and, as such, they must count among the most significant milestones of civilisation since hominids emerged from Africa.

With obvious exceptions for the minorities who are very thin or morbidly obese, tampering with the current dietary habits of the overwhelming majority of people would be foolhardy, unless it was based on a more than secure scientific footing. The studies reviewed in this chapter prove that such a footing is not presently available. What is known is that the web of interacting functions and signals that determine body weight is extremely complex. It encompasses: genetics, body structure, body energy requirements and expenditure, micronutrient requirements, digestive dynamics, physiological determinants of storage and release of energy to and from stores that include body fat, physiological and neurological controls of appetite, psychological and cultural determinants of personal aesthetics and appetite, and probably viral infections and the effects of sleep deprivation. Given those complexities, at the present rate of discovery it will take a long time before it may be possible to say safely, and with objective confidence, what might be healthy dietary and body-weight changes and restrictions (if any), and what might be their long-term consequences for the vast majority of people who are not too thin nor too obese.

If losing weight were indeed desirable, what seems surprisingly overlooked in the entire obesity literature is the opportunity for sustaining and increasing the excretion of unwanted calories by decreasing the bowel transit time, namely the time during which digested food remains in the absorbing section of the digestive tract. Considerable research, going back decades, has shown that over 20 per cent of ingested calories could be eliminated by the addition of suitable fibre supplements to the diet.[130] To function properly, our digestive systems need to be properly filled, but recommending a greater intake of dietary non-caloric roughage would raise a new series of unresolved nutritional questions.

What is quite apparent is that generic dietary and body-weight guidelines are dangerously arrogant, and are based on the foolish assumption that populations are made up of uniform individuals. Nothing short of individual attention is acceptable, yet public health authorities keep insisting on standard dietary guidelines and a general threshold of BMI 25.0 for normal weight, reflecting statistical readings that have nothing to do with real lives.

There are indications that there is a range of normal body mass, rather than a point threshold. In fact, the indications are that there are different normal ranges for different ages, sexes, ethnicities and other markers, including different conditions of lifestyle and stress, and different historical times. Normality ranges will be moving targets, for they are bound to change as culture, technology and affluence change. Therefore, it is high time studies determined what the current ranges of normality are, for without such information public health and clinical efforts are powerless, if not presumptuous and dangerous. To do so, epidemiological studies of the kind performed until now should be halted, for they have nothing more to offer besides the same equivocal results. More of the same studies would be an irresponsible waste of public funds. Epidemiology will have to get smarter and become subservient to the testing of more specific clinical and laboratory work, much as it did in the advancements against infectious diseases.

Advice about dietary and nutritional requirements is of little use unless it can be specifically tailored to each individual. The current inability to do so is one of the principal reasons why bariatric medicine and surgery have a patchy record in reducing and controlling the weight of obese people. Education and individually tailored and reliable information ought to be more successful in the long run, especially in following individual children through their early development and into the stability of adulthood.

Children would undoubtedly be the best subjects for study because of the relative plasticity of their conditions and development. Such plasticity, however, remains individual and is determined by genetic traits and environmental and cultural pressures, which in turn are apt to determine what is desirable body mass and diet. Today, no one in good faith and with testable data ready to hand could claim to know what the preferred body mass and dietary goals of a child ought to be. The standard growth charts currently in use remain simplistic approximations based on outdated records of development that will have to be revisited in view of the historically sudden and profound changes in behaviour, stress and affluence that child populations have experienced in developed and developing countries. Those changes are here to stay and will cause even more change, simply because they portend what is perceived as an inevitable and fatally attractive new way of life.

In this context, it is fair to ask whether much success can be expected from hopeful exhortations to greater physical activity. Much could be gained if, in fact, such activity increased meaningfully, but much may militate against that goal – information technology, the innumerable labour-saving gadgets, increasingly cheap energy, amusements and work patterns that mimic and take the place of physical activity, food there for the asking. In contemporary British society, there also exists an ease of life that makes less evident the need for learning and work; relaxed and casual learning methods; increased opportunities to enter make-believe professions; less emphasis on focused personal goals; transient and superficial social connections; broken families; poverty; and unsafe neighbourhoods. All this, and more, is linked to health and disease and to ideal body mass and diet, although our knowledge of these complexities is sketchy indeed.

Even if sweeping government impositions were conceivable in a free society, no one can be said to possess the firm and transparent knowledge that would be needed to justify changing diets and lifestyles that have allowed over two billion people to reach levels of health and longevity unprecedented in human history. Perhaps weight change might be desirable for the majority who are neither too thin nor too obese, but scientific – or even practical – knowledge is woefully inadequate. The available knowledge is sufficient merely to label as reckless any crusade by self-appointed and self-serving public health authorities that profess to know what they plainly do not.

CHAPTER 3

AND NOW A WORD FROM OUR SPONSORS: HOW THE FOOD ENVIRONMENT MAKES US FAT

> Marketers will do whatever they can to encourage even the youngest children to ask for advertised products.
>
> Marion Nestle, *Food Politics*

INTRODUCTION

At the core of the obesity crusaders' story is an account of why there is suddenly so much obesity everywhere in the world. The answer to this question is that obesity is largely, though not completely, the result of a contrived food environment, an environment of unhealthy, inexpensive and heavily promoted foods served in enormous portions; an environment engineered by the food industry. The problem is not one of caloric expenditure, which might just as well explain obesity, but one of consumption. People are consuming more calories than they are expending. Of course, this account is not the only environmental explanation that might be offered for obesity. For instance, it could plausibly be argued that, while it is true that the environment does play a role in the 'obesity epidemic', it is not so much the *food* environment as the generally *sedentary* environment of most of modern life, including such things as the work environment, the school environment, the recreational environment, the technological environment, or even the built environment of cities and towns. For instance, Philipson and Posner argue that techno-logical change provides a 'natural' explanation of what they see as a long-term growth in obesity stretching back to the last century – a growth that they see as having taken place with 'little or no increase in long-run calorie consumption'.[1] As Prentice and Jebb note, 'Evidence suggests that modern inactive lifestyles are at least as important as diet in the aetiology of obesity and possibly represents the dominant factor.'[2] Environmental explanations for obesity, in other words, need not focus either primarily or exclusively on the food environment. Environmentally induced sloth, not gluttony, might be the culprit.

Nor, of course, are environmental explanations themselves the only way to explain obesity. As we have noted, before its medicalisation, obesity was routinely explained as a product of individual choice: individuals chose to become fat, or at least allowed themselves to get fat. The major cause of obesity was to be found in individual moral agency, not the environment. There was, for instance, an abundance of food on many Victorian and Edwardian tables, particularly on formal occasions, but no late nineteenth- or early twentieth-century person of substance would have attributed his expanding stomach to being a 'victim' of a toxic food environment.

For the obesity crusader, however, neither the alternative environmental account nor the explanation of obesity as an outcome of individual choice would secure the public policies he wishes. The alternative environmental account, with its emphasis on the ways in which our various environments conspire to make us sedentary, suggests, for the most part, things that are too diffuse, too difficult and too large to be easily brought within the regulatory ambit. It is difficult, for instance, to think how one might practically and economically re-engineer the way in which cities are built and run so as to make those who live and work in them less sedentary. Again, it is difficult to envision how regulatory policy might reshape a culture built around such sedentary, and supposedly fat-inducing, devices as computers and televisions.

Then, too, the alternative environmental explanation for obesity fails to work as a lever for policy because it is difficult to find within it a single, powerful and threatening entity – preferably a business that can become an enemy that is easily identified and readily vilified as the plausible source of the obesity problem. While, for example, the computer industry or the automobile industry might each contribute to, and thus share some environmental responsibility for, obesity, neither Microsoft nor General Motors could be convincingly portrayed as the causal mastermind behind the 'obesity epidemic'. The same, of course, is not true of Big Food.

Nor does the explanation of obesity as a product of individual choice work as a foundation for the policy aspirations of the obesity crusader. This is because, if obesity is a problem brought about by something that individuals choose to do, rather than by something that is done to them by their environment, then it is much more difficult to justify involving the government in solving the problem. There are ways, however, of diminishing the difficulties posed by regarding obesity as a personal decision. Individual liberty is not an absolute right: it is generally qualified by provisions that require its exercise to do no harm to others. And this, as in the case of public smoking, opens up the possibilities of significant government restrictions. For instance, it might be argued that, while being fat is a personal choice, it is a choice that imposes significant costs (harms) on others, and as such should be subject to some degree of government control. Some obesity crusaders with a particularly strong commitment to health promotion would go further, arguing either that no rational person who fully understood the implications of obesity for health would choose it, and hence the decision to become fat was not really 'my' decision at all (this would certainly be the case for children), or that one's moral responsibility to live a healthy life allowed for the State to intervene to overturn even a freely made decision to become fat.

However, the preferred course of action for those behind the obesity crusade is to root the primary cause of obesity neither in the general environment, nor in the misguided choices of individuals, but instead in the corrupted food environment engineered by the multinational food industry. As Kersh and Morone write in a recent article about obesity and the new politics of public health:

Some critics take the next step and identify corporate villains. Food merchants cynically manipulate children. They put soda machines in schools and fast-food outlets in the lunchrooms. Nothing moves the political system like tales of greed and profit – especially when they menace kids. As the most ardent critics put it, a cynical industry targets children, reshapes their eating habits, and causally sponsors an obesity epidemic.[3]

Big Food, as it is increasingly described, presents a wonderfully easy target. It is highly visible, universally recognised, supposedly powerful, rich, media sensitive and the master of an array of dubious fat-making practices, particularly in the ways in which it advertises its products to children and young people. While the claims of someone like Marion Nestle that 'marketers will do *whatever* [emphasis added] they can to encourage even the youngest children to ask for advertised products' might appear rather extreme, it is nonetheless a fair representation of how the obesity crusaders wish to portray the industry. Even the supposedly more restrained commentary from groups like the US Institute of Medicine (IOM) tends to present food advertising, particularly food advertising to children, in a highly unfavourable light. As the IOM notes in its recent report *Food Marketing to Children and Youth: Threat or Opportunity?* 'the prevailing pattern of food and beverage marketing to children in America represents, at best, a missed opportunity, and, at worst, a direct threat to the health of the next generation'.[4]

HOW BIG FOOD CREATES THE TOXIC FOOD ENVIRONMENT

The case against the food industry for its supposed creation of a food environment that causes overweight and obesity, particularly in children, is composed of at least four claims. (There appear to be fewer advocates of restrictions on advertising intended for adults; the major policy tool for changing adults' food preferences appears to be warning labels on food: see Chapter 4.) First, adults and children are too fat. Second, their (particularly children's) obesity is caused both by eating too much (excessive caloric intake) and by eating the wrong foods – 'unhealthy foods'. (There is some confusion in this argument about whether unhealthy foods are unhealthy because they lead to obesity, and through obesity to other diseases, or because they directly cause other diseases.) Third, their consumption of the wrong foods is, to a significant extent, a function of the advertising of the food industry. Fourth, overweight and obesity can be reduced by placing restrictions or bans on food advertising.

The causal connection between obesity and overweight in adults and children and the food industry is thus allegedly fourfold: it is a product of the sorts of food produced by the industry; of the ways in which those foods cause obesity and disease; of the food advertising by the industry; and of the relationship between advertising restrictions or bans and a decline in overweight and obesity. For the story to work, all of these causal connections must, in fact, hold. The foods produced and marketed by the food industry must be shown to cause obesity and disease, and the consumption of these foods must be shown to be caused by the food industry's advertising. As we shall see, there is an enormous amount of sloppy reasoning in this story about the food environment, in that causal connections are often assumed rather than argued for, let alone established. In many instances, arguments are advanced in which the causal thread is entirely absent.

We wish to argue that this story about the supposed causal connections between (particularly) children's diets, weight and food advertising, told over and over again by the obesity crusaders, the media and a number of 'academic' reviews, is at the least unproven and at the most false in each of its claims. We shall examine the first three claims of this story here and the fourth claim in Chapter 4.

As we have seen, the claim that adults and children are too fat is plagued by at least two substantial problems. The first, as we saw in Chapter 2, is that the idea of 'too fat' is derived from the body mass index or BMI, which lacks a substantial scientific basis. The second is that, even allowing for the legitimacy of the BMI in determining the meaning of 'too fat', the evidence fails to support the claim of an epidemic of obesity in Canada, the US or the UK.

For instance, according to an analysis from the US National Center for Health Statistics, the weight of the majority of Americans has increased by only six to seven pounds over the last decade, apart from in the case of the already obese.[5] Most Americans have weights that vary within a 10-pound range in any given year. According to Hedley, the prevalence of overweight and obesity in US children showed no statistically significant increase from 1999 to 2002, and there was no statistically significant increase in adult weights during the same period.[6] As Campos *et al.* noted recently in the *International Journal of Epidemiology*:

> [W]hat we have seen, in the US, is a relatively modest rightward skewing of average weight on the distribution curve, with people of lower weights gaining little or no weight, and the majority of people weighing ~3–5kg more than they did a generation ago ... While there has been significant weight gain among the heaviest individuals, the vast majority of people in the 'overweight' and 'obese' categories are now at weight levels that are only slightly higher than those they or their predecessor were maintaining a generation ago. In other words, we are seeing subtle shifts rather than an alarming epidemic.[7]

As the authors note, the 'obesity epidemic' in the United States translates into about 10 extra calories a day.

A similar lack of compelling evidence about too much fat is found in the UK. The Health Survey for England, published in December 2004, found that the average weight of boys (aged 3–15) in 2003 was 31.9 kg, compared with 32 kg in 1995. The average weight of girls was 32.4 kg in 2003, as against 32 kg in 1995. Comparing BMI results between 1995 and 2003, the increase in average BMIs for boys was 0.5 and for girls 0.6 points, a statistically insignificant increase.[8]

So we are left with a truly puzzling claim: during the time in which food advertising is supposed to have made people fat, the numbers of fat adults and children has not increased significantly.

Nor is there a stronger evidentiary basis for the claim that the reason for all this fat is that too much is being eaten. For example, in a 2004 study of weight gain and consumption in the US, the National Bureau of Economic Research noted that, while there was an increase in weight, there were 'only modest gains in calorie consumption'.[9] Indeed, as Harnack *et al.* observed in a 2000 analysis, 'Energy intakes per person were 7 percent lower in 1994 than in 1977–78.'[10] Again, as Salbe and Ravussin observed in 2000, 'there is considerable evidence showing that fat intake has actually been decreasing as the prevalence of obesity has been rising'.[11] Moreover, the alleged connection between excessive eating and obesity is further undermined by studies which show that the caloric intake among the obese is not more, and indeed may be less, than among the non-obese:

In fact, several investigators report that the caloric intake of obese persons ... is not greater and may be less than the intake of non-obese persons. Body weight, body fat, and lean body mass were also not associated with caloric intake in our study of obese men ... [W]e conclude that the nonsignificant correlations between obesity measure and total caloric intake suggest that variations in the level of obesity among these sedentary overweight men cannot be directly related to caloric consumption.[12]

And the evidence is equally clear about paediatric obesity and overeating. Writing in the *Journal of Clinical Endocrinology and Metabolism*, Slyper observed that 'It is often assumed that the increase in pediatric obesity has occurred because of an increase in caloric intake. However, the data do not substantiate this.'[13] Kimm *et al.*, in an article in the *Lancet*, noted that 'The composite findings from [the

National Growth and Health Study] so far indicate that the drastic decline in habitual activity during adolescence might be a major factor in the doubling of the rate of obesity development in the USA in the past two decades, since no concomitant increase in energy intake was apparent.'[14] The same finding – no increase in calories – is found in a study, published by Troiano *et al.* in the *American Journal of Clinical Nutrition*, of the energy and fat intakes of children, which noted the 'lack of evidence of a general increase in energy intake among youths despite an increase in the prevalence of overweight'.[15] Lest this lack of connection between supposedly too much fat and overeating be thought to be confined only to the United States, Jebb, writing in the *British Medical Bulletin*, observed that 'there has been no relationship between either total energy intake or fat consumption in the prevalence of clinical obesity over the last 60 years'.[16]

So, here is another curious claim: during the time in which food advertising was making people fat, the amount of food being consumed did not significantly increase.

What, then, of the claim that the problem rests not in too much eating, but in the wrong kind of eating, namely the consumption of 'unhealthy' or bad foods? The authors of *The Consensus Statement on Childhood Obesity* argue that there is a causal connection between childhood obesity and the consumption of such unhealthy foods as fizzy drinks and fast foods:

> In terms of dietary content, there is an inverse
> relationship between calcium intake and adiposity.
> The consumption of high carbohydrate soft drinks is a
> major contributing factor to high calorie counts ...
> Additionally, fast food consumption now accounts for
> 10 percent of food intake in children in US schools,
> compared to 2 percent in the 1970s. Children who
> frequently eat fast food consume more total energy,
> more energy per gram of food, more total fat, more total
> carbohydrate, more added sugars, less fiber, less milk ...
> and fewer fruits and vegetables than children who eat
> fast food infrequently. Those who are overweight are

particularly vulnerable to adverse health effects of consuming fast foods.[17]

The implicit assumption, of course, is that these sorts of unhealthy foods are causally connected with certain diseases, either directly or by producing obesity. But, despite these confident, sweeping and, it should be noted, thinly evidenced assertions, when one begins to examine the scientific basis for the claim that certain foods are unhealthy, in that they cause either obesity or disease, it becomes apparent that the notion of unhealthy or bad foods as a scientific claim is one that is open to question. Contrary to what the obesity crusaders say, science does not speak with one voice about what constitutes healthy and unhealthy, good or bad foods.

First, the claims supporting the characterisation of foods as unhealthy are, for the most part, based on nutritional epidemiological studies, which, as was argued in Chapter 2, are highly unreliable for a variety of reasons. This is acknowledged even by nutritional epidemiologists themselves. For instance, Tim Byers, writing in an issue of the *American Journal of Clinical Nutrition* devoted to nutritional epidemiology, noted that, because animal nutritional studies have limited usefulness as the basis for determining unhealthy foods (because animals are fed foods in such large quantities that they have little relevance to human eating patterns), and because there are very few controlled human studies of specific foods and specific diseases, 'most of our inferences about the roles of foods and nutrients in the prevention of chronic diseases must be based on observational epidemiology'.[18] Note that Byers characterises the link between foods and disease as an 'inference', unlike the obesity crusaders, who describe it as an established scientific fact. In other words, since animal studies are not helpful in establishing a reliable causal link between specific foods and diseases in humans, and since there are few controlled studies in humans – for example, there are no such studies that link dietary fat to cancer – one is left to the 'inferences' drawn by observational epidemiology.

Second, even with the already problematic field of epidemiology, nutritional observational epidemiology suffers its own additional problems. Byers notes that 'The classic criteria for causation are often not met by nutritional epidemiologic studies, in large part because many dietary factors are weak and do not show linear dose-response relations with disease risk within the range of exposures common in the population.'[19] Thus, even the epidemiology studies that purportedly link certain unhealthy foods with certain diseases fail to establish a causal connection between the supposedly unhealthy food and the disease.

Third, the specific claims about unhealthy foods and disease are highly contradictory. In the 1930s and 1940s, for instance, the medical profession recommended a diet high in fat, though by the 1950s dairy fats and meats were implicated as causes of heart disease. Despite this, in 1966 the US National Research Council and the US National Academy of Science still reported that there was not enough evidence from reduced fat consumption to justify advising the public to cut down on fat. The move to classify foods as good and bad depending on their supposed links with disease received official standing in 1970, when the anti-cholesterol crusader Jeremiah Stamler provided detailed diet instructions for every American to avoid butter, egg yolk, bacon and lard – instructions that were officially adopted by the American Medical Association and incorporated into successive dietary guidelines issued by the government. In 1976, the British Royal College of Physicians and the British Cardiac Society produced similar guidelines, including a recommendation to reduce fat consumption to a total of 35 per cent of one's diet. Both sets, however, failed to provide scientific evidence that avoiding these supposedly unhealthy foods would reduce mortality, which was supposedly their original justification.[20] As Jon Robison observes of this constantly changing, conflicting and ill-supported advice:

[O]ur interpretation of what the research suggests to us about how foods or specific components of foods relate to our health, is constantly changing. Remember just a few years ago when all fats were considered to be *bad*? Then it was only saturated fats that were *bad*; then only some saturated fats. Most recently the villain *de-jour* is trans fats. Carbohydrates on the other hand – what we were supposed to be eating instead of the *bad* fats – were considered *good*. But now, only a few years later, they are *bad*. But not all carbohydrates are *bad*. Some carbohydrates are *good* and some are *bad*. Sugars are particularly *bad*. But some sugars are better than others; sucrose is not as *bad* as fructose, and so on and so on. Quite maddeningly, these confusing flip-flops have become a common occurrence with all different types of foods.[21]

By the early 1990s, the 'worldwide consensus' on healthy and unhealthy foods was that fat should make up no more than 30 per cent of a diet, with an equal ratio of saturated, monounsaturated and polyunsaturated fats (though this is now subject to controversy); cholesterol intake should be less than 300 milligrams a day; and sodium consumption no more than 3 grams per day. Again, these recommendations about healthy foods were not widely supported by evidence of population-wide health benefits. To take but one example, the claim that polyunsaturated fats should make up 30 per cent of one's daily fat intake was contradicted by the Seven Countries Study – the main evidence supposedly supporting such dietary advice – which showed that the lowest rates of heart disease were in populations that received less than 30 per cent of their calories from such fats. Again, Crete, with one of the lowest rates of heart disease in the Seven Countries Study, had a dietary fat intake of 40 per cent.

Fourth, many of the claims advanced by the obesity crusaders about the nature of so-called 'unhealthy' foods are false. For instance, despite what is often claimed, all foods have nutritional value – even fats and sugars, which are constantly demonised as bad foods. Sugar is a carbohydrate and, as such, is a nutrient. Or, for example, consider Coke, perhaps the most demonised of 'unhealthy' foods. Coke contains the same amount of sugar per litre as unsweetened orange juice and roughly the same amount of calories (39 calories per 100 ml for Coke, compared to 36 for orange juice). What exactly makes one healthy and the other unhealthy? Again, there is frequently the implication, if not the direct suggestion, that some foods are so inherently bad that they should never be consumed, or consumed in greatly reduced quantities. But there is no compelling scientific evidence to support this link between any one food and a specific disease.[22]

Take the argument about dietary salt, which is always linked with sugar and fat as an 'unhealthy' food component. Some organisations, like the US-based Center for Science in the Public Interest, have asked the Food and Drug Administration (FDA) to classify salt as a food additive, in order to limit its use in foods, on the basis that a reduction in dietary salt in the US would save 150,000 lives a year. Susan Jebb, head of nutrition and health research for the UK's Medical Research Council, has also called for substantial reductions in salt use, arguing that salt reductions could reduce blood pressure and dramatically improve Britain's health.

The science about salt as 'unhealthy' is significantly different from the claims made by the critics of 'bad' foods. To begin with, there is no study showing population-wide net health benefits from low-sodium diets. Since 1995, at least ten studies have looked at whether reduced-salt diets provide a public health benefit. All these studies have found that, in the general population, there is no health benefit to be derived from a reduction in salt intake, even though some sub-groups may benefit from reduced salt intake. Indeed, on a population-wide basis, there is little evidence that a reduction in 'unhealthy' salt intake results in fewer strokes or heart attacks, or in reduced risk of premature mortality. In fact, for some groups such reductions actually *increase* certain risks. For example, analysis of the MRFIT (Multiple Risk Factor Intervention Trial), which followed the lives and deaths of

12,866 American males for an average of 12 years, found there were no health benefits from low-sodium diets.[23]

Nor is the MRFIT analysis an anomaly. A meta-analysis of randomised controlled trials of dietary salt reduction, published in the *British Medical Journal* in 2002, found that significant salt reduction led to only very small reductions in blood pressure; the degree of salt reduction and change in blood pressure were not related; and there were no health benefits. The researchers did find certain risks associated with reduced salt intake, including effects on vascular endothelium and serum total and low-density lipoprotein cholesterol. As they noted, 'lower salt intake in people with hypertension has been associated with *higher* [emphasis added] levels of cardiovascular disease and in general populations with greater all cause mortality'.[24]

This absence of benefit is also found in the 1997 Dietary Approaches to Stop Hypertension (DASH) study.[25] In the original DASH study, subjects consumed a diet high in fruit, vegetables and low-fat dairy products, in which the salt content remained the same. After three weeks, the DASH diet reduced blood pressure by 5.5/3.0 mmHg in mild hypertensives and 11.4/5.5 mmHg in those with extreme hypertension. Since the salt content was constant, the reductions had nothing to do with the blood pressure changes.

In the second DASH study (DASH-Sodium, 2000), researchers examined the effects of the DASH diet at three levels – 8, 6 and 4 grams a day – of salt intake. For the hypertensives in this study, the DASH diet, combined with a sodium restriction of 4 grams, reduced systolic blood pressure by 11.5 millimetres; given that the original DASH study, which used normal sodium levels, reduced systolic blood pressure for this group by 11.4 millimetres, this is a non-significant difference. For those with normal blood pressure, eating the DASH diet with a low salt intake produced little difference in blood pressure.

A comprehensive analysis of 114 study populations found that the effect size of sodium reduction on blood pressure 'does not justify a general recommendation for reduced sodium intake'. The researchers also found that the benefits of sodium reduction for hypertensives were significantly less than could be achieved by using anti-hypertensive drug therapy.[26] In an article published in 2005 in the *American Journal of Hypertension*, which looked at data from the US National Health and Nutrition Examination Survey (NHANES), researchers found that top-number hypertensives (those with systolic blood pressure of more than 140 mmHg) already have the lowest intakes of salt, calcium, potassium and magnesium.[27] What this group needs is a diet that increases these minerals, not that reduces them. Telling them to reduce salt is obviously unwarranted, and shows the danger of the indiscriminate population-wide health advice on so-called good and bad foods that is offered by the obesity crusaders. As the authors note, 'the emphasis of national nutrition policy on sodium restriction for hypertension is not consistent with these findings'.

Fifth, the appropriateness of a particular food is more often the result of the context in which it is eaten, rather than any inherent aspect of the food. Jon Robison notes that many people might consider broccoli to be intrinsically healthy and pizza to be inherently unhealthy:

> On a given day, however, if an individual has eaten no protein, but consumed plenty of fruits and vegetables, eating only broccoli might contribute less to health because the body in this context needs protein, not more fiber and antioxidants. If that same individual happened to be in prison for 6 months with the same two food choices: healthy broccoli or unhealthy pizza, which choice would best promote health? The answer is clearly the unhealthy pizza. In fact, choosing the healthy broccoli might just be fatal.[28]

Sixth, the claimed links between specific foods and obesity in children and adolescents is highly questionable. There is, for example, no clear and consistent connection between fat intake and obesity in children. As Professor David

Ashton notes, 'Epidemiological studies do not show a consistent association between dietary fat and adiposity in children and young adults.'[29] Though there is much speculation about the link between dietary fat (which is the most energy-dense nutrient) and obesity, the relationship between the two is, in fact, not scientifically established. As Ludwig and Ebbeling admit, the 'Findings of epidemiological studies do not consistently show an association between dietary fat and adiposity in children and young adults.'[30]

Of course, the culprit linking specific foods and obesity in children might not be fat but rather carbohydrates. Some observers have noted that the decline in fat intake has been compensated for by an increase in carbohydrate consumption among children and young people, especially through things like breakfast cereals, breads, pastries and fizzy drinks. But the evidence for this is not at all decisive. It is not at all clear how the consumption of carbohydrates like breakfast cereals contributes to paediatric obesity. One theory is that high glycaemic-index foods like cereals and fizzy drinks lead to hormonal changes, which in turn cause hunger and lead to overeating. There are, however, no clinical trials that have substantiated this theory.

Equally important, there are a number of studies that count against the claim that such heavily advertised carbohydrates as fast foods and fizzy drinks lead to fatter children. For example, a 2005 study from researchers at the Health Behaviour in School-Aged Children Obesity Working Group looked at the supposed connections between overweight and obesity and diet and physical activity in 137,000 schoolchildren in 34 countries. The researchers found that there was a 'negative relationship between the intake of sweets (candy, chocolate) and BMI classification in 31 out of the 34 countries ... such that higher sweets intake was associated with a lower odds of overweight'. In other words, the children who ate larger amounts of so-called unhealthy and heavily advertised foods, like fizzy drinks, actually had less chance of being overweight. Again, 'overweight status was not associated with the intake of fruits, vegetables, and soft drinks'.[31]

This research confirms the findings of several other studies that have also found that fizzy drinks and 'junk food' do not cause childhood obesity. For instance, Field *et al.* from Harvard looked at the eating and physical activity habits of 14,000 American children aged 9–14 over a three-year period, and found that eating so-called junk food did not lead to obesity among children.[32] However these foods were defined, with or without fizzy drinks, the researchers were unable to find a link between these heavily advertised 'bad' foods and obesity. As the authors noted, the 'inclusion of sugar-sweetened beverages in the snack food category did not meaningfully change the results. Regardless of the definition of snack foods, there was not a strong association between intake of snack foods and weight gain.'[33] Indeed, as Field *et al.* note, their findings provide no support for the theory that high glycaemic-index foods promote weight gain.

Nor do the results of a Canadian study that examined the eating and physical activity habits of 4,298 schoolchildren in an effort to determine which risk factors were important for overweight and obese children. The researchers included questions about whether the children ate breakfast, whether their lunch was brought from home or purchased at school, how often they ate in fast-food restaurants, whether there were regular family dinners, and whether dinner was eaten in front of the television.[34]

They found that eating in a fast-food restaurant, supposedly a major source of childhood obesity, was not statistically significant as a risk factor in obesity, even in children who ate in such restaurants more than three times a week. There was also no statistically significant association between the availability of fizzy drinks at school and the risk of children being overweight or obese, or between schools having food vending machines and the same risk.

Similar evidence was found by researchers at the Centers for Disease Control and Prevention (CDC) and published in the *International Journal of Obesity* in 2005.[35] They noted that 'Evidence for the association between sugar-sweetened drink consumption and obesity is inconclusive ... [N]ational data showed no association between sugar-sweetened beverage consumption and BMI.' This finding was replicated in an earlier study by Forshee *et al.*, which looked at the association between BMI and milk, fizzy drinks and juices, where the authors reported that 'BMI was not associated with consumption of milk, regular carbonated beverages, regular or diet drinks/ades, or non-citrus juices.'[36] In a more recent study, Forshee, using data from NHANES, found 'no statistically significant association [between fizzy drink consumption and BMI], and, in fact regular carbonated soft drinks accounted for less than 1 percent of the variance in BMI'.[37]

Here is another curious fact. The evidence linking specific foods, or even whole diets, to specific diseases and obesity is highly tenuous, yet it is claimed that advertising of these products makes us both fat and sick. We have emphasised this lack of compelling scientific evidence about causation, since reports such as those by Hastings and the IOM, and the obesity crusaders, routinely claim that there is a self-evident connection between so-called 'advertised diets', high in salt, sugar and fat, and childhood obesity and disease. But if it is not obviously the case that these foods are linked to childhood obesity and disease, then the case against advertising of such foods cannot proceed, any more than the case against advertising tobacco products could proceed in the absence of evidence that smoking causes disease.

However, let us suppose for the moment that at least one aspect of the toxic food environment story is true: namely, we are getting fatter. Might there be an arguable explanation for this, other than the obesity crusaders' claim that it is due to the eating of too many unhealthy foods produced and promoted by Big Food? In other words, might we concede the claim that adults, adolescents and children are gaining weight without having to accept that this weight gain is caused by a toxic food environment? The answer is yes, as there is a significant amount of evidence that a plausible alternative cause of increased weight is the decline in physical activity in industrialised countries over the past century.

The evidence of such a decline in energy expenditure is considerable. As Lee and Paffenbarger observed back in 1996, 'Almost 60 percent of all U.S. adults today engage in no physical activity or only irregular physical activity.'[38] The same problem is to be found in the UK, as the House of Commons Health Committee observed in its 2004 *Obesity* report that 'only around 37% of men and 25% of women currently achieve' the Department of Health's activity targets. 'Levels of activity in the UK', commented the report, 'are below the European average, which is part of the explanation for higher obesity rates.'[39] Moreover, in both countries, this pattern of minimal and irregular physical activity is also found in children. According to the US Department of Health and Human Services, 'Only about one half of US young people (ages 12–21 years) regularly participate in vigorous physical activity.' The Department also found that 'More than a third of young people in grades 9–12 do not regularly engage in vigorous physical activity. Daily participation in high school physical education classes dropped from 42 per-cent in 1991 to 29 percent in 1999.'[40]

The sources of such a decline are various, ranging from changes in the types of work people do and the physical demands of their work, to the increased use of cars, to the ways in which people spend their leisure time. For instance, according to the US National Bureau of Economic Research (NBER), there has been a significant decline in physical activity from 'technological changes in home and market pro-duction'.[41] Similarly, the US Urban Institute, in a report on the changing requirements of work, observed that 'Using Labor Department data, we estimate that the percentage of workers in physically demanding jobs has dropped substan-tially – from about 20 percent in 1950 to almost 8 percent in 1996 ... Our estimate probably understates the decline because it does not take into account the possibility that even jobs classified as physically demanding today are less strenuous than jobs in the past.'[42] Or, as Jebb notes in the *British Medical Bulletin*, 'there has been no relationship between either total energy intake or fat consumption and the prevalence of clinical obesity over the last 60 years, whilst proxy measures of physical inactivity (TV viewing and car ownership) are closely related'.[43]

There is also evidence that links this decline in physical activity to weight gain. The Harvard Institute of Economic Research, in a comparison of physically active and more sedentary jobs, found that 'After 14 years of working, those in the least sedentary occupations have about 3.5 units of BMI less than those in the most sedentary ones.'[44] The NBER attributes 60 per cent of America's weight gain to declining physical activity.[45] Again, as Troiano et al. concluded on the basis of the NHANE Survey, 'The lack of evidence of a general increase in energy intake among youths despite an increase in the prevalence of overweight suggests that physical inactivity is a major public health challenge in this group.'[46]

The same link between physical inactivity and weight gain was observed by Kimm et al., writing in the Lancet in 2005: 'These results suggest that habitual activity plays an important role in weight gain, with no parallel evidence that energy intake had a similar role ... The composite findings from [the National Growth and Health Study] so far indicate that the drastic decline in habitual activity during adolescence might be a major factor in the doubling of the rate of obesity development in the USA in the past two decades.'[47] And this was also observed in a recent study by Patrick et al., which examined the connection between overweight, obesity and seven dietary and physical activity factors.[48] The authors note that 'Of the 7 dietary and physical activity variables examined in this cross-sectional study, insufficient vigorous physical activity was the only risk factor for higher body mass index for adolescent boys and girls.' The same link between physical inactivity and overweight and obesity is found in a consensus statement about physical activity and unhealthy weights published in 2003, which concluded that 'A decline in daily physical activity levels (PALs) is clearly a major factor contributing to the current obesity epidemic.'[49]

FOOD ADVERTISING, FOOD CHOICE, DIETS AND OBESITY

Thus far, the evidence of causal connections, which constitute the claim that the toxic food environment engineered by Big Food is responsible for the 'epidemic of obesity' (and particularly the epidemic of paediatric obesity), is decidedly weak. As we have seen, it is not at all clear that most people have got significantly fatter; or if they have, that this is because they have eaten more, or even because they have eaten 'unhealthy' foods. It now remains for us to examine the central argument about obesity and the food environment: that food advertising is why people, particularly children and adolescents, eat unhealthy foods and get fat.

The case against food advertising consists of two arguments: first, that food advertising to children and adolescents causes them to eat a diet that makes them overweight, obese and unhealthy, and second, that, regardless of its effects, in the case of children such advertising is deceptive. These two arguments are advanced in different ways by two different groups of obesity crusaders – one that might be called the 'unsophisticated', 'rhetorical' advocates, who offer the arguments without any substantial analysis of the evidence supporting them, and who, indeed, at times appear to believe the arguments are self-evident; and a second group, made up of official bodies such as the US Institute of Medicine and the UK's Food Standards Agency, both of which have commissioned substantial academic reviews of the scholarly research on the purported effects of advertising, and who consequently claim that their arguments about advertising and obesity are consistent with the standards of 'evidence-based medicine'.

Food Advertising Causes a Diet that Produces Overweight and Obese Children

Typical of the first group are anti-food advertising claims advanced by Marion Nestle in her book *Food Politics*,[50] Susan Linn in her book *Consuming Kids*,[51] and Kelly Brownell and Katherine Horgen in their *Food Fight*.[52] Despite the unsophisticated and rhetorical nature of their anti-advertising advocacy, Brownell, Linn and Nestle are academics (Brownell is at Yale University, Linn at Harvard, and Nestle at New York University) who presumably understand the ways in which scholarly arguments are made.

Nestle bases her policy proposal to 'restrict television advertising of foods of minimal nutritional value' on the claim that 'televised commercials influence the food choices, preferences and demands of children – particularly young children', something she says 'has been well understood since the early 1970s'. Moreover, she implies that much of the food advertising directed at children is unfair, since 'prior to the age of 9 or 10, children do not readily understand the difference between commercials and programs'. Indeed, according to Nestle, 'Even high school students have difficulty distinguishing between commercials and programming.'

In support of these sweeping and highly controversial claims, Nestle provides six pieces of evidence, the most recent of which is 15 years old, with one study coming from 1964 and another from 1974. For example, her support for the claim that children cannot distinguish TV advertisements from programmes until they are nine or 10 years old, and that even high-school students cannot distinguish between commercials and programming, is based on a single, non-peer-reviewed study from 1964. Moreover, it is contradicted by a substantial number of recent studies, which show that children as young as three or four can distinguish an ad from a TV programme. As Dale Kunkel, lead author for the American Psychological Association's Task Force on Advertising and Children, has observed, 'by age 3 or 4 most children are able to differentiate an ad from a program'.[53]

Nor is Nestle's evidence about the ways in which televised food advertising affects the food choices and preferences of children any more compelling. For instance, in support of this claim, she references a two decade-old study by Dietz and Gortmaker on the connection between obesity and TV viewing.[54] Unfortunately, the study was not about the causal connection between viewing TV food advertisements and obesity, but about the connection between TV viewing and obesity. Indeed, since Nestle's main example of an advertising effect relates to brand preference advertising (the effects of which are not in dispute), she seems unaware of the distinction between this and claiming that food advertising affects children's food choices.

Linn's arguments are equally unsophisticated and unsupported, despite the fact that her book *Consuming Kids* is supposed to present a critique of the effects of advertising on children. For instance, she argues that 'When it comes to food, children are targets for everything from edible checkers to battery-operated lollipops. No wonder 25 percent of American children are overweight, obese or at risk for obesity.' Linn obviously believes that the causal connection is intuitive, since she offers no evidence that moves one from the claim that children are the targets of food advertising to the conclusion that this is what makes them overweight or obese. Indeed, the only support she provides for this connection is a reference to the UK Food Standards Agency's Hastings Review, which we consider below, and a review by Horgen, Choate and Brownell.

Despite Linn's reliance on them, Brownell's arguments for the causal connection between food advertising, children's diets and overweight and obesity are decidedly curious: the author advocates a ban on food advertising to children, even as he admits that 'there is only circumstantial evidence that the ads cause poor eating'. Having reviewed a small portion of the extant evidence, Brownell, despite finding this selected evidence 'circumstantial', nonetheless argues that 'We can conclude that more TV means more food ads, and with more ads comes deteriorating diet.' How such incomplete and circumstantial evidence establishes a causal connection between food advertising, children's diets and obesity, let alone supports a ban on food advertising, remains unexplained.

Even more curious is Brownell's support for the claim that food advertising is 'deceptive' and 'exploitative'. Despite the complexity of this issue, and despite the extensive research literature, Brownell's sole argument is from authority. As he writes,

> When the country's main pediatrics association, a broad coalition of organizations concerned with child welfare, an organization for media and children, a leading nutrition watchdog group, and a top medical journal conclude that advertising practices are deceptive, exploitative, and harmful to the health and well-being of our children, there is reason for the nation to take notice.

Thus far, the claim that food advertising aimed at children leads to a diet that results in overweight and obesity is much closer to rhetoric than to evidence-based science. What, then, of the major academic reviews of the supposed causal connection – the Hastings Review of the UK's Food Standards Agency[55] and the Institute of Medicine's *Food Marketing to Children and Youth*?[56]

Both the Hastings Review and the report by the IOM make much of the fact that they follow the principles of evidence-based medicine in order to ensure that their judgements are both rigorous and objective. However, before we turn to the two reports, it is important to note that, given the nature of obesity, they share a central and definitive flaw in their understanding of what counts as demonstrating causality.

If defining obesity as a disease is to make any sense (and we have argued that it does not), then it can only be as a multifactorial disease, similar to cardiovascular disease or cancer. (By multifactorial we mean a disease with multiple risk factors.) This recognition of the multifactorial nature of obesity is evident in most reports that attempt to explain it, even those that assign greater weight to one risk factor. Though there is no comprehensive list of the risk factors for obesity, the literature, including the pronouncements of the obesity crusaders, typically includes the following:

- birth weight
- parental adiposity
- gender
- race

- working in a job requiring little physical activity
- living in a city
- living in a suburb
- owning a car
- earning less than $30,000 per year
- not having access to a park or playground
- having less than 12 years of education
- living in a single-parent family
- having a mother who works outside the home
- eating in front of the TV
- taking a bus to school
- attending a school without a physical education programme
- eating a school lunch
- using a school vending machine
- eating breakfast
- living in a home with regular family dinners
- buying food in a corner shop or convenience store
- having type 2 diabetes
- having cardiovascular disease
- eating food away from home
- engaging in little exercise
- consuming fizzy drinks
- seeing TV advertisements for food
- eating a diet high in fat
- eating a diet high in carbohydrates
- eating a diet high in sugar
- eating fast foods
- having access to inexpensive food
- shopping for food while hungry
- having little access to healthy food

- eating food other than at mealtimes
- owning/watching a TV
- owning/using a computer
- attending a school without a nutrition education programme
- playing video games

This means that, in order to identify a causal connection between a particular risk factor and obesity, one must design a study that controls for all the other risk factors that might lead to obesity. Unless this is done, one's causal hypothesis is improperly specified and it is impossible to say which factor is the causal one. The implication of this for the claims of a causal connection between food advertising, children's diets and obesity are significant, in that most of the studies that purport to establish such connections have not controlled for even a handful of these factors.[57] This means that, whatever claims may be made by the authors either of these reports or of the Hastings Review and the IOM report, no scientifically valid evidence can be provided of a causal connection between food advertising, children's diets and obesity.

The Hastings Review

The Hastings Review (after Professor Gerard Hastings of the Centre for Social Marketing at the University of Strathclyde) is the product of an extensive literature search that initially yielded almost 30,000 papers on food advertising, children's diets and obesity. These were then reduced to a shortlist of 120 papers considered appropriately scientific. Of these 120 papers, 46 were used to answer the question of whether there was a causal link between food advertising and the diet of children. On the basis of this evidence, the Review concludes that:

(1) There is a lot of food advertising to children.
(2) The advertised diet is less healthy than the recommended one.

(3) Children enjoy and engage with food promotion.
(4) Food promotion is having an effect, particularly on children's preferences, purchase behaviour and consumption.
(5) This effect is independent of other factors and operates at both the brand and category level.

Following the submission of the Review, the FSA convened an academic panel to assess what it had established. The panel concluded that the Hastings Review 'had provided sufficient evidence to indicate a causal link between promotional activity and children's food knowledge, preferences and behaviours'. This conclusion is, of course, somewhat different from that of the Hastings Review, since it is accepted by almost everyone in the debate that advertising affects knowledge, preferences and behaviour. The relevant question is whether this occurs at the level of the brand or, as Hastings asserts, the diet (category).

In addition to the general problem about causality in this debate, there are seven problems with Hastings' findings: problems which vitiate any claim that the Review provides compelling evidence of a causal connection between food advertising to children, children's diets and obesity. *First*, the claim that there is a 'lot of food advertising to children' is a curious one. In the UK, for instance, ad-spend on food and drink has been falling in real terms since 1999, and is now at roughly 1982 levels. In 1982 food and drink ads constituted 34 per cent of the total TV advertising in the UK, whereas in 2002 they made up 18 per cent.[58]

In the US, one finds a similar trend. According to the Federal Trade Commission, advertising during children's TV programming has declined by 34 per cent in recent years.[59] Data from Nielsen surveys show that food advertising on television has declined by 13 per cent since 1993. Additionally, TV viewing has itself not increased during the period of the 'obesity epidemic', and some observers suggest that it has not changed for children and adolescents for the last 40 years.[60] There is some evidence that the time children spend watching TV has actually declined in recent years.[61]

Nor can it be assumed that TV viewing is a legitimate proxy for advertising exposure, since the two are not equivalent. Though this is recognised by some reviewers, few studies of children's exposure to advertising actually measure advertising exposure, as opposed to TV viewing.

Thus, the mere assertion that there is a 'lot of food advertising to children' is difficult to credit against the actual data, and the data on falling amounts of food advertising to children on TV are difficult to reconcile with a causal thesis in which such advertising has supposedly led to the recent rise in childhood obesity.

Second, the Review appears to ignore the evidence, which suggests that children see a far more balanced presentation of foods and diet than is maintained by the critics of food advertising. For instance, a unique British study looked at the food references and messages in regular programming, as opposed to those contained in food advertising.[62] The study found that there were as many references to food within regular programming as during the commercial breaks. It also found that the food references in regular programming watched by children were far more centred on so-called healthy foods. For example, fruit and vegetables were the most frequently portrayed foods in regular programming.

Third, it is difficult to understand what is meant by the claim that the advertised diet is 'less healthy' than the recommended one. Most obviously, there is no such thing as an 'advertised diet'. Food advertising is advertising about brands, not diets. Moreover, the Review provides no evidence to support its distinction between a healthy diet and an advertised diet that is less healthy. As we have seen, there is no compelling scientific evidence to link a diet or an individual food to a particular disease. Ultimately, the claim that most food advertising is for an 'unhealthy' diet is not substantiated in the Review. Some of the largest advertisers in both the UK and the US are supermarkets, which extensively advertise fresh foods – presumably 'healthy', according to the Review.

Fourth, the Review completely ignores, as does the IOM report, some important research that undermines its implicit view that children are passive and uncritical consumers of advertising. The Review's belief that advertising has almost magical powers to affect what children eat is especially challenged by a two-year project on the Development of Television Literacy in Middle Childhood and Adolescence, funded by the UK Economic and Social Research Council and carried out by Professor David Buckingham.

Buckingham's findings, reported in his book *Children Talking Television*,[63] focus on the ways in which children aged seven to 12 actually talk about television. His findings are based on a variety of activities undertaken over 15 months by small groups of between two and five children. The sample included 90 children, with equal numbers of boys and girls recruited from four British schools and chosen to provide a balance of race and class. Two schools were in the London inner city, and had a majority of children from working-class backgrounds and a high proportion from single-parent homes. The two suburban schools were in a comparatively affluent outer-London borough, with a majority of children from middle-class, two-parent families.

In the session devoted specifically to TV advertising, the children were first of all shown four advertisements taken from a commercial break in a children's programme. The interviewer then asked the children questions about what they would normally do at home during a commercial break, what they liked and disliked about the ads, why they thought there were ads on TV, what the ads were for, and whether they had purchased things that had been advertised. Specific questions about the four ads focused on who the children thought the ad was aimed at and why the advertisers chose the people they had chosen to be in the ads. In summarising the children's discussion of the advertising, Buckingham notes:

> The children demonstrated a clear awareness of the functions of advertising, and in many cases a profound degree of scepticism. Their 'defences' were very diverse and often extremely forceful. What emerges here is an image of children, not as vulnerable and innocent, but

on the contrary as 'streetwise' and highly cynical about advertising – and indeed as more than capable of protecting themselves from its alleged effects.

For instance, when the children were asked about the purpose of advertising, replies included this from Ben (aged 8): 'they're trying to persuade people to buy things or do things'; and from Nancy (8): 'Buy all the things, that's why they advertise it, cause they can't get anyone to buy it, so they just try and get it, make it look really good.' Note the implicit assumption in Nancy's comment that she realises there is some element of deception – or at least embellishment – in advertising, in that advertisers attempt to make things look better.

In some cases, Buckingham notes, there was a generalised rejection of advertising. Ivor (8), for instance, said 'I think they just want our money', while others described advertising as a 'con' or 'rip-off'. Children clearly understood that there was a discrepancy between the real world and the world shown in advertising. In a washing powder ad, the children suggested that the results were 'faked', and with toy advertisements many said that the claims made were false.

The children were also sceptical about food advertising. Justine (8) claimed that, although there were different brands, all crisps were 'just the same'. Several children were sceptical about the implication from a Diet Coke ad that drinking Coke would make you beautiful:

Charlotte (8): 'Diet Coke makes you fat. If you sort of like have ten bottles of Diet Coke, cause you think it's absolutely brilliant, you'll walk around like this [imitates fat person].'

Diana: 'It makes your teeth go bad.'

Nancy: 'Beautiful people, they only get [film] them from a distance, because they've got no teeth!'

Anne (10) suggested that Diet Coke was 'bad for your brain' because it contained artificial sweeteners, while Sonia

(8) argued that sweet drinks were 'not good for you, they haven't got no vitamins in, they make you hyperactive'. Justine described how she studied the ingredients listed on the packets of cereals, yoghurts and fruit drinks, looking for information about sugar and additives. As Buckingham notes, the most cynical comment on food advertising came from Anne:

> 'Kellogg's Oat Bran isn't good for your heart. Even though it's in a heart-shaped bowl, and it's supposed to be a sensible breakfast, it's got just as much crap in it as Coco Pops.'[64]

The children's food advertising literacy was particularly apparent with respect to the use of celebrities to endorse products – something increasingly under attack by the obesity crusaders. Consider the comments of two 10-year-olds speaking about Diet Coke and Lucozade advertisements using celebrity footballer John Barnes:

> Adele (10): 'I think they choose those people, cause they get actors or very talented people, but they have to be slim and beautiful cause it's an advert for Diet Coke, and they think, [mocking voice] you can drink this without doing exercises and you'll get to look like her.'

> Tracey (10): 'I know why they've got him [John Barnes] to do that advert because he's a famous footballer and they thought, they think that if they drink that drink and play football, they will score something and it will give them more strength.'

> Interviewer: 'And, do you believe that?'

> Tracey: 'No!'[65]

Fifth, there is little evidence adduced to support the key conclusion that advertising affects children's diets. For example, the Review, in examining the evidence about

whether food promotion influences children's food consumption behaviour, refers to 11 studies supporting the conclusion that it does. Yet, of the 11 studies, nine provide no
evidence in support of the claim. Again, in support of the
claim about dietary impacts, the Review relies extensively on
a study by Bolton (modelling the impact of television food
advertising on children's diets), a 20-year-old study that
involved a sample of 262 Ohio children and found that exposure to food advertising reduced the quality of their nutritional intake, but had no effect on their caloric intake.[66] In
other words, there was no connection in the study between
the supposed effect of food advertising and childhood obesity. Even on the issue of advertising's effect on nutritional
intake, the study found that advertising accounted for only
2 per cent of the differences found in the children. More
importantly, the influence of parents on children's food
choices was found to be 15 times more important than advertising. All of which makes it difficult to conclude that this
study constitutes evidence of a causal connection between
food advertising, children's diets and childhood obesity.

Sixth, the Review's evidence suggesting a causal connection between food advertising and children's diets fails completely to establish such a link. The primary reason for this is
that, although the Review claims that the effect of advertising
on diet is 'independent of other factors', this is not established. As we noted previously, to determine that advertising's
effect is independent, one would have to control for the other
factors that influence children's diets. Yet none of the studies
presented as evidence by the Review does this. Indeed, the
Review concedes that 'no studies addressed this question
directly'. Nevertheless, it adduces 13 studies as evidence of
this crucial connection. Five of these studies fail to touch on a
connection at all. The remaining eight do not deal with diet;
they look at advertising in terms of such categories as salt content, sugar content or fat content (none of which constitutes a
dietary category), rather than at advertising of all snack
foods, for instance, which would at least come closer to
approximating one aspect of a diet. Furthermore, all that the

studies show is that children preferred one product to another, rather than one diet to another.

Seventh, the Review completely ignores a number of econometric analyses of the case for a causal connection between food advertising, food consumption and diet. For example, Peter Kyle of the University of Lancaster examined the impact of food advertising on food consumption in the UK and found no evidence to support the 'popular myth that advertising will increase market size'.[67] There is also the work of Martyn Duffy of the University of Manchester, who looked at the supposed impact of advertising on 11 food categories from 1969 to 1999, precisely the question at issue in the Review. Duffy found that not only did advertising have no effect on food demand, but also that it had virtually no effect on the demand for any individual food. As he notes, 'This study joins the accumulating number of studies that have found little or no evidence to support the view that advertising can affect the product composition of total food demand.'[68] In 2003, in a second attempt to inform the growing debate on whether restrictions or bans on food advertising were justified, Duffy again looked at the issue of food advertising. Again, he found that 'there is very little evidence here to support the view that advertising is a potent force in the determination of consumer preferences'.[69]

Duffy's conclusions are hardly exceptional. For example, Henry carried out two studies into the effect of advertising of such items as breakfast cereals and biscuits, both frequently cited as culprits in the childhood obesity epidemic. One study looked at advertising of such products from 1975 to 1983, and the second at marketing of the same products 10 years later. Henry's conclusion in both studies was that advertising did 'not over the years affect market size in any general way or to any material extent'.[70]

Similar conclusions about the effects of food advertising are also found in Yasim, who looked at the effect of advertising on 31 frequently purchased foods, including many that are supposed to be connected with childhood obesity, such as breakfast cereals, biscuits, desserts, chocolate, fizzy drinks, crisps, ice cream and prepared snacks.[71] He found that there was no relationship between advertising and market growth, and no relationship between advertising and market size.

It might be argued, of course, that these studies are large-scale analyses that involve multiple foods, and as such they might well miss the impact of advertising for a single 'unhealthy' food that might be part of a dietary pattern. Consider, then, a study that looked at the influence of advertising on just one such food – chocolate confectionery. Eagle and Ambler looked at the impact of advertising on chocolate consumption in five European countries, in order specifically to test the claim by European public health authorities that a reduction in advertising would reduce 'inappropriate' food consumption.[72] They found no statistically significant association between the amount of advertising and the size of the chocolate market. As the authors observe, 'It seems likely that those calling for curtailing advertising are seeking a convenient scapegoat rather than attempting to understand either how advertising works or when it increases category demand.'

Thus, despite the claims of the Food Standards Agency that the Hastings Review provides compelling evidence that food advertising to children affects their diet, the evidence put forward by the Review fails to provide any sound reasons for believing that there is a causal connection between food advertising, children's diets and childhood obesity.

What, then, of the more recent IOM report?

The Institute of Medicine report
Like the Hastings Review, the IOM report bills itself as a comprehensive and rigorous examination of the evidence concerning the effects of food advertising on children and adolescents. This is important for the IOM, inasmuch as it labels itself the science 'advisor to the nation'. Like the Hastings Review, the report makes a number of claims about the supposed effects of food advertising on the diets of children and young people, and also on their weight. And, as with the conclusions of the Hastings Review, the conclusions of the IOM

report are often misrepresented for ideological purposes by the obesity crusaders.

For instance, one of the report's more appropriately cautious scientific conclusions (that the 'current evidence is not sufficient to arrive at any finding about a causal relationship from television advertising to adiposity among children and youth') is quickly lost in the comments of the committee chairman, Michael McGinnis, who told the press conference at the launch of the report that 'There is strong evidence that television advertising influences the diets of children.' A careful reading of the report reveals, of course, that McGinnis's claim is not true – even on the report's own terms, which are themselves suspect. Of course, the question of dietary influence by itself is still not the really important question. The principle question is whether food advertising makes children fat. And the answer to that in turn requires a causal link between advertised foods and weight gain – something, as we have seen, for which there is no conclusive evidence.

Of course, McGinnis's comments reveal much about the real purpose of 'scientific' reviews like those by Hastings and the IOM. They are not intended to enhance our scientific understanding of a highly complex issue, but rather to impart to a collection of highly contentious claims a scientific veneer tough enough to provide a policy basis for significant restrictions on food advertising. The problem with veneers, of course, is that they are liable to crack. McGinnis's ideological take on the IOM report is not unique. Fellow committee member Aimee Dorr of the University of California, Los Angeles, opined that the report was the 'nail in the coffin' of food advertising. If so, both the nail and the coffin are very strange indeed.

The faux science at work at the IOM is seen most obviously in the fact that several of the report's authors had already come to their conclusions about both obesity and food advertising before they examined the evidence and produced their report – something that suggests a substantial bias at work in determining the direction of the IOM report. For instance, two decades before, Aimee Dorr had already concluded, when writing about the importance of mandatory regulation of advertising, that 'research information ... can help shape voluntary and involuntary regulations of programs and commercial advertising to children', a view, with its assumption that advertising should be regulated, as unsupported by Dorr in 1986 as it is in 2006.[73] Another author, Dale Kunkel, argued in 1989 that the 'most sound policy for our nation's children would be to ban advertising from children's programs altogether'.[74] The disturbing thing is that, rather than a scientific report produced by means of a process that at least strives to be objective, we seem here to have a report whose work is shaped by authors whose prior advocacy of a particular policy position is not revealed.

We are not told that the report committee's chair, Michael McGinnis, had, prior to the start of the committee's work, reached conclusions about the weight of Americans, its causes and its consequences. Nor are we told how completely wrong he was. Through his co-authored 1993 study, 'Actual Causes of Death in the United States', for example, McGinnis was one of the key figures in the creation of the obesity crusade. The study claimed that 'diet and activity patterns' were the second leading cause of death in the US, being responsible for 300,000 deaths a year, second only to tobacco.[75] This figure, of course, provided the platform for the ill-fated 2004 Mokdad *et al.* study, which claimed that diet and lack of physical activity were responsible for 400,000 deaths annually, a figure that exceeded tobacco deaths.[76] Unsurprisingly, McGinnis and Foege, in an editorial accompanying the Mokdad study, lauded the latter's figures on overweight and obesity as providing a 'stronger measure of confidence' in the effects of overweight and obesity.[77] They argued, without any evidence, that a 'substantial proportion of early deaths among the US population is preventable through lifestyle change', and claimed that the decisions about 'what kinds of food to consume' were the 'results of strong cultural and commercial signals'.

This confidence in the Mokdad obesity-death numbers was, of course, entirely misplaced: a year after publication of the study, the Centers for Disease Control and Prevention retracted the 400,000 annual deaths from diet and activity patterns, and admitted that the figure for net obesity and overweight-related deaths in the US was not 400,000, nor McGinnis and Foege's 300,000, but rather 25,814.[78]

McGinnis assumed his role as chairman of the IOM report committee already committed to several key components of the story about food advertising, children and obesity, namely that: Americans, including children, are too fat, and this fat is not only making them sick, but is killing them; their obesity is, to a large extent, a product of the food they eat; and the food they eat is a result of those 'commercial signals'. This is not to suggest that McGinnis, Kunkel or Dorr are not entitled to their views about food advertising, obesity and children; it is simply to say that they did not approach their work without substantial bias, and that the reader was not informed of this bias.

Turning to the report itself, the essential problem with it is twofold: its evidence fails to support its claims, and this in turn creates a mismatch between its claims and the policy recommendations that stem from those claims. In some sense, the report's authors appear to understand this, since, instead of talking about the critical question of whether food advertising makes children fat, they talk about the influence of advertising on children's food preferences. But this is to miss the point. No one in this debate denies that advertising affects children's food preferences; what is at issue is whether it affects their diets and whether it causes obesity – two quite different questions. To have a child's diet (and hence his weight) affected, his food preferences have to be realised. And since most children do not purchase the bulk of their food, this realisation depends on the parents. So, if there is a causal connection linking food preference to diet to weight, it necessarily involves parental decision-making.

Indeed, the authors seem to realise that they have failed to provide a scientific, rather than an ideological, basis for proposing restrictions on food advertising. This is because, when all is said and done, science is about demonstrating causal connections; connections that are, as we have argued, measurable, reproducible, and that specify their margin of error. And, by its own admission, the evidence assembled by the report fails to reach this standard. As it notes, 'the current evidence is not sufficient to arrive at any finding about a causal relationship from television advertising to adiposity'. In other words, however much the authors try to distract us by answering non-relevant questions, the answer to the central question is contained there, and it indicates that there is no justification for the policy menu advanced by the report.

In reality, the report says more about the IOM's pretensions to science and objectivity than it does about the role of advertising in childhood obesity. Rather than reading like a scientific report, the IOM's work appears more as an ideological document written by a group of people who have strong and, for the most part, unsupported views about advertising, definite biases about what constitutes good/healthy and bad/unhealthy foods, and a serious misunderstanding of how the scientific method moves from hypothesis to conclusion. Instead of carefully moving from data to conclusion, the report's evidence fails to support its conclusions. To arrive at the report's public policy recommendations on restricting food advertising, readers must make a purely speculative leap from what the evidence shows to what the report demands. As even Aimee Dorr admits about her nail in the coffin, 'It is not the perfect golden spike, but it is sufficient to take action.'

These causal failings are evident throughout the report, but most particularly in two instances. First, though the report discusses the foods that children aged 2–18 eat, it fails to provide any causal evidence that these foods are linked to children being fat or diseased. For instance, one of the report's tables lists the top 10 food sources of energy among American children and adolescents aged 2–18 in 1991: milk, yeast bread, cakes/cookies/quick breads/donuts, beef, ready-to-eat cereal, carbonated soft drinks, cheese, potato crisps/ corn chips/popcorn, sugars/syrups/jams and poultry. Yet the report provides not a shred of evidence that causally links any of these foods with cardiovascular disease, cancer, diabetes or premature mortality.

Second, the lack of causality is apparent when the crucial question is addressed of whether food advertising causes children's diet. In evaluating the evidence on this, the report looks at 24 studies, *none* of which is statistically significant with high causal validity. Furthermore, the report looks at studies into whether TV food advertising causes children's diets by age group: for younger children aged 2–5, older children aged 6–11, and teens aged 12–18 years. *None* of the studies is statistically significant with high causal validity. The report concludes from this evidence that 'There is moderate evidence that television advertising influences the usual dietary intake of younger children ages 2 to 5 and weak evidence that it influences the usual dietary intake of older children ages 6 to 11. There is also weak evidence that it does not influence the usual dietary intake of teens aged 12 to 18 years.' It is, of course, strange that the report speaks of weak evidence that advertising does not influence the dietary intake of teens, rather than reporting that there is weak evidence that it does. So, even on the report's own terms, there is no compelling causal evidence that food advertising causes the diets of young children, older children or teens.

This leaves us with one group – children under two – for which the report produced no evidence. However, in a 1996 review of the effects of food advertising on children's food choice produced for the UK Ministry of Agriculture, Fisheries and Food, Brian Young of Exeter University observed that children's food acceptance patterns and some eating preferences develop in infancy and so pre-date the influence of parents, peers and advertising. He writes:

> The infant brings to the eating situation a preference for
> the sweet taste and an innate ability to learn the
> relationship between consuming specific foods and their
> energy value, both of which appear to be highly
> adaptive. These mechanisms contribute to food
> acceptance patterns early in the child's development and

can explain, in part, the tendency for children to like foods which are sweet, high calorie and high in fat. Clearly these influences occur early in the child's development before any input from outside influences including parents, peers, and the wider social context such as the media.[79]

The IOM report appears to accept Young's conclusions, since it cites the same sources he uses and acknowledges a 'biological predisposition to prefer sweet, high fat, and salty foods'. Thus, whatever the claims about advertising influencing children's food preferences and behaviours, it is impossible for advertising to create children's basic preferences for sweet, high-fat and salty foods. If children do prefer foods that are sweet, high in fat and salty, it is not because those preferences have been created by advertising.

Gathering together the evidence about whether food advertising causes children's diets and their obesity, we find the following:

● For children aged under two, there is no evidence that advertising causes their diet. Indeed, children's food preferences for sweet, high-calorie and high-fat foods appear to be innate, and certainly pre-date their exposure to advertising. The report is silent about the implications of these pre-advertising preferences for the claim that advertising creates children's diets and obesity.

● For children aged 2–5, there is no evidence to show that advertising causes their diets.

● For children aged 6–11, there is no evidence to show that advertising causes their diets.

● For adolescents aged 12–18, there is no evidence to show that advertising causes their diets.

● There is no evidence for children and adolescents aged 2–18 to show that advertising causes adiposity.

The Hastings Review and the IOM report share two quite fatal flaws in establishing a causal link between advertising and children being overweight, obese and diseased. First, neither shows that the main foods that children now eat are the cause of obesity or of diseases such as cardiovascular disease, cancer or diabetes. Second, neither provides studies about the supposed connection between advertising and children's diets and obesity that have properly controlled for the multiple risk factors for obesity. Thus, neither can properly draw a causal conclusion about the relationship between advertising, children's diets and obesity.

The Ofcom report

In addition to the Hastings Review and the IOM report, there is a third major study of the influence of food advertising on children's food choices. It stems from a research project carried out by Ofcom (the UK government's Office of Communications) in response to the secretary for culture, media and sport's request for the agency to consider 'targeted and proportionate proposals for strengthening the existing code on TV advertising in respect of food and drink to children'. However, unlike the Hastings Review and IOM report, the July 2004 Ofcom report, *Childhood Obesity: Food Advertising in Context*, attempts to assess the influence of food advertising within the context of the other influences on children's food preferences.[80]

For instance, the report notes that 'there is a general consensus of opinion that food preference, consumption and behaviour are multi-determined'. The primary factors that help to determine children's food preferences, according to the report, are:

- psychosocial factors (e.g. food preferences, meanings of food, food knowledge)

- biological factors (e.g. heredity, hunger and gender)

- behavioural factors (e.g. time and convenience, meal patterns, dieting)

- family (e.g. income, working status of mother, family eating patterns, parental weight, diet and knowledge)

- friends (e.g. conformity, norms and peer networks)

- schools (e.g. school meals, sponsorships, vending machines)

- commercial sites (e.g. fast-food restaurants, stores)

- consumerism (youth market and pester power)

- media (food promotion, including television advertising)

While this list is not complete, it does signal a sharp break with the approach taken by the Hastings Review and IOM report, in that it begins by accepting that there are multifactorial influences on children's food preferences, and that advertising is, at best, simply one influence, and not the dominant, or even primary, influence.

One can see how this approach produces a much more balanced picture of the influences on children's diets in the report's discussion of how the 'food culture' of British children develops. According to the report, the current food culture is a product of at least nine distinct trends:

(1) a steady rise in incomes
(2) longer working hours
(3) an increase in the number of working mothers
(4) an increase in the number of time-poor/cash-rich parents
(5) an increase in the consumption of pre-prepared convenience foods
(6) an increase in out-of-home eating
(7) a trend toward a 'snacking/grazing culture' amongst children
(8) an increase in children-only meals
(9) the increasing influence of children over their food choices

In addition, there are four trends in children's activity levels:

(1) an increase in media ownership in the home and in children's rooms
(2) an increase in parents' fears for the safety of children outdoors
(3) an increase in sedentary indoor pastimes (watching TV, playing computer games)
(4) a decrease in physical activity amongst children

When the former nine trends are added to the latter four, one begins to see how these various factors affect children's diets.

But the report also devotes considerable attention to the role of parents' beliefs about themselves and their health and diets as critical factors in shaping what children eat. For example, using data from quantitative surveys (1,000 interviews with parents and their children) commissioned by Ofcom, the report looks at parents' beliefs about their own health, using the common social psychological measure known as 'locus of control'. Locus of control, which is widely used in health research, measures the degree to which an individual believes in chance/fate against the value the individual places on health and the degree to which they assume responsibility for their own health. A composite score is produced that distinguishes those whose locus of control is internal from those whose locus is external. Individuals with an internal locus of control believe that they are responsible for their own health, while those with an external locus of control see their health as the outcome of powerful others and/or fate.

These results were then correlated with data about parents' eating habits, attitudes to health, and media consumption to produce three groups: light consumers, healthy consumers and heavy consumers. Parents who were termed 'light consumers' have an internal locus of control, take responsibility for their health, and tend to eat and serve their families more vegetables and fruit than other groups. However, they also tend to eat high levels of foods with fat, salt and sugar.

Parents judged 'healthy consumers' have a slightly lower internal locus of control and attach a strong importance to healthy eating. Their children are less likely to eat snack foods, other than fizzy drinks, and they are also more active than children in other groups with lower BMIs.

Parents termed 'heavy consumers' have an external locus of control and believe that factors outside their control determine their health. They attach less importance to healthy eating, 'show unhealthy eating patterns in that they are higher than the other groups in their mention of confectionery food and fast foods', and report that their children are less active than those in the other two groups and have higher BMI scores.[81]

While the limited sample size makes it impossible to draw any definitive conclusions, it is interesting that Ofcom's research found that a majority of parents (mothers were seen to be the parent more responsible for food) tended toward an external locus of control, in which health and healthy eating were seen not as their responsibility, but as the result of outside forces. Most parents had little interest or confidence in influencing their children's food choices. At a population level, this has clear implications for what children eat, since it suggests that many parents have effectively abdicated the parental role in shaping children's diets.

Despite this, the Ofcom research clearly shows that parents see parents, and not the government, the media or broadcasters, as having the primary responsibility for improving children's diets. As the report notes, 'People see parents as primarily responsible for improving children's diet. School and food manufacturers are also seen to play an important role. The role of government, the media, supermarkets and broadcasters is not perceived to be as important as these three.'[82]

What about advertising as an influence? Only having carefully examined the influences of the food culture of families and the other trends that have substantially reduced children's physical activity levels does the report turn its attention to the influence that advertising might have on children's food choices. Unlike the hyped conclusions of the Hastings Review and IOM report (which bear little resemblance to what the evidence actually suggested), the Ofcom report restricts itself to conclusions that follow from the evidence. These conclusions are that 'TV advertising has a modest direct effect on children's food choices'. While it might have indirect effects that are larger, it is difficult to determine what these are and what their size might be. This modest effect, moreover, needs to be placed in the context of the other factors that influence children's eating decisions. As the report notes, 'For example, to parent and child alike, the child's own taste preferences are paramount and price and familiarity are also important. Peer pressure ... is also a notable influence on food choice for children. Parents are influenced by the healthiness of the products, although when actually serving food or drink, convenience is a more powerful motivator.'[83] Furthermore, the modest effect is found, according to Ofcom's own quantitative survey, in obese children, who noted that, 'Food promotion generally, and television advertising in particular ... play a very small role in their decisions.'[84]

When attempting to quantify the extent of this modest effect, the report cites research that suggests food advertising 'in the broad array of factors that influence eating habits, independently contributes up to 2 per cent of the variance explained' – hardly a significant contribution by any measure. Moreover, it is unclear from the literature precisely what weight should even be attached to this effect, as 'many studies are designed to identify correlations, not causes' and are thus useless at answering the key question about the effect of advertising. As the report notes, many of the studies have 'small samples, simple measures, paucity of longitudinal designs and few replications'.[85] Most crucial, however, is the fact that the research is unable to offer any evidence to demonstrate that advertising has a dietary impact in terms of food categories, as opposed to brand impact.

Therefore, what is most striking about the Ofcom report, when it is compared to the Hastings Review and IOM report (or the report by the American Psychological Association

(APA) discussed below), is its objective and non-ideological character. Looking at much the same evidence as the other reports, it appears to be guided by what the evidence actually reports, rather than taking an *a priori* position on advertising. It thus finds that advertising's influences on children's food choices is much more modest than those reports whose findings are based more on their authors' prejudices than on the evidentiary record.

Food Advertising to Children Is Inherently Deceptive

The second part of the case against food advertising aimed at children is that such advertising is inherently deceptive: children do not understand the persuasive intent of advertising and are thus uniquely susceptible to its influence.

For instance, the IOM report appears to support Nestle's claim that even older children do not really understand advertising in a manner that allows them to fully 'defend' themselves against it. As the report notes:

> [T]he ability to recognize persuasive intent in television advertising begins to appear in its most basic form at approximately ages 7–8, but it is not consolidated and consistently applied until later years. Indeed, several studies have demonstrated that even when older children and adolescents possess mature knowledge about advertising's persuasive intent, such understanding is not consistently applied to effectively defend against commercial claims, appeals and persuasive outcomes.[86]

Unfortunately, such arrogantly paternalistic conclusions are typical of much of what passes for scientific research on the issue of children and persuasive intent. In much of this research, what counts as a failure to understand persuasive intent is nothing more than a persuasive outcome – i.e. a purchase decision that the researcher disagrees with. Indeed, were we to use the definition of 'understanding persuasive intent' that is employed by many of the critics of advertisers, we would find most adults to be advertising illiterate!

The usual story about children and advertising: the
American Psychological Association's report
The most extensive and influential recent discussion of children's limited understanding of persuasive intent, and of the
case for banning the advertising of food to children, is to be
found in the American Psychological Association's report on
advertising and children.[87]

In one sense, there is nothing particularly original about
the APA's attack on advertising to children, for one can turn
to a variety of previous work that makes the same case. For
instance, in a 1984 report, Smith and Sweeney note that
advertising prohibitionists find advertising to children objec-
tionable because young children are unable to understand
persuasive intention and are thus vulnerable; advertising leads
children to unreasonable expectations and creates family
tensions; advertising creates a demand for junk food; and the
advertising industry is unable to manage itself through meaningful self-regulation.[88]

The advocates of banning children's advertising present a
picture of children that is reassuringly old-fashioned and sen-
timental in character, in which children, despite the now
decades-long contraction of innocence and acceleration
toward adolescence, if not quite adulthood, are portrayed as
essentially naive and malleable by advertisers. Thus, the APA
tells us that children aged eight and younger 'lack the cognitive skills and abilities of older children and adults, they do
not comprehend commercial messages in the same way as
do more mature audiences, and … are uniquely susceptible to
advertising influence'.[89] It is worth noting that the first of
these claims is a truism, the second is true but is not necessarily decisive for this debate, and the third does not follow from
the first two. Nevertheless, it is the third claim that carries the
argumentative weight embodied in the word 'susceptible',
with its implication of manipulation. The claim is a rehash of
the Federal Trade Commission (FTC) staff research review of
1978, which argued that advertising directed at children
below a certain age is unfair, that is to say deceptive, because
these children cannot distinguish it from television program-

ming or understand what it is designed to do.[90]

The usual story is thus a combination of a certain picture of children and how they develop, a series of assumptions about how children understand and react to advertising, and finally, a view, often not enunciated and almost always undefended, about advertising itself, particularly its capacities to persuade and shape behaviour. All of these are necessary for this second part of the case against advertising to children to be sustained. If the model, the assumptions or the view of advertising are open to question, then the case weakens, if not collapses. Put in its most direct form, the case against advertising to children on the grounds of its inherently deceptive character resolves itself into the claims that:

(1) TV commercials encounter children who, because of their limited cognitive development, cannot understand the manipulative nature of the advertisement.
(2) As a result of this encounter, children form wants for the things advertised.
(3) This leads them to demand that their parents purchase these things.
(4) This can, in turn, result in parent–child conflict.
(A similar model is developed by both Goldstein[91] and Furnham.[92])

The crucial claim of the argument – that children's limited cognitive abilities necessarily mean that advertisements manipulate them – is generally broken down into two separate claims: first, that certain children are unable to distinguish between commercials and television programming, and, second, that children do not understand the intention of commercials. As the report notes, 'Children must acquire two key information-processing skills in order to achieve mature comprehension of advertising messages. First, they must be able to discriminate at a perceptual level commercial from noncommercial content; and second, they must be able to attribute persuasive intent to advertising and to apply a degree of skepticism to their interpretation of advertising messages consistent with that knowledge.'[93]

Since this claim is central to the report's case, it is particularly odd that it is neither referenced nor properly argued. Though it is true, by definition, that children do not possess a 'mature comprehension of advertising messages' it does not follow from this that their comprehension leaves them open to manipulation. Indeed, to demand that young children must have a mature understanding of advertising before they can be exposed to it is to beg the question. Children might possess something less than mature comprehension and yet still understand enough of what advertising is about so as not to be open to manipulation. For instance, it is uncontroversial to say that young children fail to understand some aspects of advertising, such as humour, product symbolism and ambiguity. It does not, however, follow that this failure leaves children open to manipulation. If mature comprehension is a necessary condition for dealing with advertising, then we need to know why this is the case.

One suspects that the reason for such sloppy logic is that the authors of the APA report, particularly the lead author Dale Kunkel, have made the case so often. For instance, here are Huston, Watkins and Kunkel in a 1989 policy piece: 'A convincing body of research accumulated during the 1970s demonstrated that preschool children typically fail to distinguish program material from advertising. Children below about age 8 do not understand the persuasive intent of advertising and are, therefore, particularly vulnerable to its appeals.'[94] The same claims are repeated by Kunkel and Roberts in a 1991 article in which the notion of persuasive intent is firmly linked to the idea of intrinsic unfairness.[95]

The degree to which children are able to recognise persuasive intent has been a dominant focus of research on children and advertising. Its importance derives from the legal argument that, if young children are unaware of persuasive intent, then all commercials aimed at them are, by definition, unfair and/or misleading. Of course, if they are unfair or misleading, then such commercials might legitimately be banned, as Huston, Watkins and Kunkel concluded in 1989:

'The most sound policy for our nation's children would be to ban advertising from children's programs altogether.'[96]

Underlying this picture of children and these assumptions about how children react to advertising is, of course, a view about advertising itself. The view argues that advertising effects changes in an individual's attitudes and these attitudes are translated into purchasing behaviour, not just with individual brands but with entire product categories. The process of precisely how advertising changes attitudes is generally left unspecified though, if push comes to shove, it often parrots a version of the now 80-year-old 'hierarchy of effect' model.

According to this model – which comes in multiple versions – advertising succeeds in persuading and shaping behaviour because it is able to move a consumer from reading or seeing or listening to an ad to believing it, to remembering it, finally to acting on it. However, the model, in whichever version it appears, is always more assertion than explanation, in that it never explains precisely how an advertisement moves one through the supposedly successive effects, and never provides actual examples of how an advertisement supposedly changes attitudes and how these changed attitudes are reflected in purchasing behaviours. Indeed, the model is often described as 'self-evident' and based on common sense. For instance, it is assumed, as part of the model, that causality is always one way – that changes in attitude about a product lead to its purchase rather than follow from its purchase (despite considerable evidence to the contrary); or that attention to advertisements leads to interest in a product, rather than vice versa.

But the most significant problems with this conception of advertising as the determinant of attitude and behaviour are to be found in the sturdy empirical facts about how advertising is actually used and how often it 'works'. For instance, of the 9,000–10,000 brands being advertised in a given year, the average consumer will buy only about 400.[97] Moreover, the data on individual marketing campaigns suggest advertising campaigns for established brands are successful only 20–30 per cent of the time.[98] Campaigns for new brands are successful even less often, and one author has noted that four out of five new brands fail in the marketplace.[99] As Murray notes in discussing the failures of this view of advertising's supposed power,

> And yet the shortcomings of the hierarchy of effect model of how advertising works were always apparent. It did not account for the uncomfortable fact that a very high proportion of new brands ... fail in the market-place. And that they fail despite the fact that they are most frequently launched by major companies, who have researched both product and market: who often have experience in the market, through the marketing of complementary products; who have the marketing muscle to achieve the desired levels of distribution; who have sales force and merchandising power; and who have the financial resources to mount, and sustain, heavy advertising and promotional campaigns.
>
> Nor did it explain the survival of small firms, with low advertising budget, in the face of the very heavy competition of the market leaders. Nor did it explain the relative stability of most markets, where market shares, and shares of total advertising, do not differ significantly from year to year. It gave no explanation of the fact that product group advertising is rarely effective; nor did it explain why social issue advertising has such little effect on the population's attitudes and behaviour. There is almost a total absence in the literature of case histories of how advertising changed attitudes, and how those changed attitudes affected sales.[100]

Indeed, what the case-history literature demonstrates is something quite different. For instance, for the last 20 years the UK's Institute of Practitioners in Advertising has published case histories of advertising campaigns as part of the Institute's Advertising Effectiveness Award programme, which is designed to showcase both how advertising campaigns are created and the effectiveness of such campaigns. The case histories, published in the series *Advertising Works,*[101] now include over 200 examples, and there are several hundred more examples as yet unpublished. Commenting on these case histories, Mike Waterson has observed that

> Careful examination of these case histories makes it absolutely clear that the overwhelming majority of the advertising campaigns submitted for this competition are firmly brand-orientated and that most of the non-brand campaigns are not for products at all, but government information, charity, recruitment and other such-like campaigns ... The overwhelming majority of evidence suggests that campaigns are not directed to changing overall market sizes and do not accidentally result in overall market changes, except in some very specialist and small product areas.[102]

The empirical evidence, then, suggests that the critic's view of branded advertising as an irrationally persuasive force with the capacity to change attitudes and behaviour, whether in adults or children, is mistaken. 'The main role of advertising', observes Murray, 'is defensive. It follows, therefore, that criticisms of advertising on the grounds that it is irrationally persuasive ... are unsound.'[103]

The usual story: the evidence about children's understanding of advertising

Even allowing for the APA report's inadequately argued definition of mature comprehension and its problematic connection with manipulation, what sort of evidence is there about the capacity of children to distinguish commercials from television programming? According to the report, most children 'below the age of about 4–5 years exhibit low awareness of the concept of commercials'.† It is worth noting that, as children's general sophistication (not to say their media awareness) seems to be growing, the age at which they recognise

---

† American Psychological Association, *Report of the APA Task Force on Advertising and Children,* p. 6.

advertising seems to be increasing, quite without scientific explanation or justification – in the APA's November 2002 *Monitor on Psychology*, Melissa Dittmann, writing about the APA Task Force on Advertising and Children, had noted in an interview with Kunkel that 'by age 3 or 4, most children are able to differentiate an ad from a program'.[104]

Aside from the unexplained increase in the age of ad–programme differentiation, the claim has a twofold problem that relates to the report's central deficiency – its selective use of the research record to make unsubstantiated claims. First, the evidence adduced is more than 30 years old and represents but a fraction of the available literature,[105] and second, significant amounts of the literature not cited suggest that children understand the commercial–programme distinction as early as three years of age. For instance, Jaglom and Gardner argued, on the basis of a number of different testing methodologies, that the distinction between commercial and other television developed at about age three.[106] In an experiment in which videos with commercials and programmes were randomly stopped, Levin *et al.* found that children aged three to five could apply the concepts correctly about two-thirds of the time.[107] In research that did not depend on children's verbal skills (reported by Kunkel himself, but curiously not cited in this report), it was found that three-year-olds knew the difference between commercials and programmes.[108] Indeed, these and other findings suggest that the claims about the inability of young children to distinguish between advertisements and programming may be based on a confusion (due to reliance on verbal testing methodologies), in which children's inability to explain the difference between the two is assumed to be an inability to understand the difference.

Thus, the report's claim that the 'evidence indicates that most children below four to five years of age do not consistently discriminate between program and commercial content' is true if based on two 30-year-old studies,[109] but false if based on the larger research record – a record that includes the work of the report's lead author, Dale Kunkel. This bias in reporting the empirical data serves an important function in the report's ideological agenda, for it allows children's advertising literacy to be systematically discounted and children to be portrayed as more vulnerable to advertising than they really are – an argument that is vital to the case for banning advertisements.

The ability of children to distinguish advertising from programmes, while necessary to a 'mature comprehension of advertising', is not sufficient; for mature comprehension also requires an awareness, if not some degree of understanding, of what advertising is designed to do: that is, its selling intent. Unfortunately, what constitutes this awareness, and when children come to possess it, is a matter of considerable controversy. The authors of the report propose a definition of awareness that involves knowing and understanding four things: '(1) the source of the message has other perspectives and other interests than those of the receiver, (2) the source intends to persuade, (3) persuasive messages are biased, and (4) biased messages demand different interpretive strategies than do unbiased messages.' Only when a child understands all of these things, as evidenced in his 'processing of advertising messages', can he 'be said to have developed mature comprehension of the advertising process'.[110]

While the emphasis in the report's definition of advertising awareness focuses on the concept of persuasion, earlier research suggested that awareness was the ability to verbally identify the profit motive of advertising. Using this notion of mature comprehension, the researchers found that 96 per cent of 5–6-year-olds did not understand what TV commercials were about, compared to 62 per cent of 11–12-year-olds.[111] In a 1974 study, Robertson and Rossiter proposed an even more rigorous test of mature comprehension that included the abilities to understand that commercials have external sources and intended audiences, to appreciate the symbolic character of advertisement, and to distinguish between the claims of the advertisement and the reality of the product.[112] Such a criterion might count against the advertising maturity of a good many people other than children. Using this criterion,

Robertson and Rossiter found that only 43 per cent of first-grade children 'understood' advertisements – a figure that rose to 71 per cent of third-grade children and 94 per cent of fifth-grade children.

What of the other evidence? Surely there is more than this 30-year-old study with its limited scope on the crucial issue of children's understanding of persuasive intent? The report tells us that 'numerous other studies ... have produced comparable findings that age is positively correlated with an understanding of commercials' persuasive intent, with seven to eight years the approximate point that such ability typically develops'.[113] This, however, is not the case, unless, of course, 'numerous' has a different meaning at the APA. In addition to the Robertson and Rossiter study, the report mentions exactly four others, one of which is also by Rossiter and Robertson, and only one of which is more recent than 19 years. So, if we set aside Rossiter and Robertson, we are left with three other studies that tell us children do not understand what advertisements are designed to do until they are eight years old. In other words an enormously significant public policy issue is being analysed on the basis of the empirical evidence of *five* studies.[114]

There is, however, considerable other evidence, unwelcome as it may be to the APA and the IOM, that paints a substantially different picture of children's understanding of persuasive intent. For example, Gaines and Esserman, in studies in which children were required to do certain things or choose particular pictures, showed that children aged four to five were able to understand what television commercials were about.[115] In a 1988 study, Peterson and Lewis showed that children as young as six could be taught to distinguish the purely informational from the persuasive aspects of advertisements.[116] In a 1997 German study (the APA apparently failed to examine any international studies), Backe and Kommer found that 57 per cent of children aged six understood that advertising was designed to sell things,[117] a result that is sharply at odds with the APA report's claim of current research showing that 'fewer than half of 8 year olds comprehend advertising's persuasive intent'. Indeed, in the same study, 59 per cent of six-year-olds questioned the credibility of advertising at least some of the time.

Similarly, in a British survey of children's understanding of TV advertisements, when the children were asked 'What is the main reason they have advertisements on TV?', 80 per cent answered that it is because advertisers want to sell something. Less than 8 per cent of the children did not know why advertisements appeared on TV and, while there were differences in comprehension between girls and boys (with girls being more advertising literate), there was no difference in responses by age or social class.[118] When asked about the truthfulness of advertising, only 6 per cent of the children thought that advertisements always told the truth.

These sorts of findings are replicated in the extensive work on television advertising carried out by David Buckingham with British children. Arguing against the picture of children as incompetent or irrational, and hence vulnerable to persuasion, Buckingham notes that children are able 'from a very early age' to distinguish between programmes and advertisements, and that they are aware not only of what advertisements are designed to do, but, in many cases, they develop an extreme cynicism about advertising. He writes:

> In our interviews, we encountered a considerable degree of scepticism – and indeed cynicism – about television advertising. The children were clearly aware of the persuasive functions of advertising, and of the potential for deception. Many described how advertisers would attempt to 'make things look better than they are'; and many reported instances in which their experiences of products fell far short of the claims made in the advertisements. Advertising in general was rejected by many as merely a 'con' – a confidence trick. The children were also very ready to parody or mock particular advertisements, often with great hilarity. Far from admiring the glamorous role models that allegedly populate the world of advertising, the children seemed

to reject the large majority of the people featured in them as hopeless 'wallies' and 'has-beens'.[119]

In a study that suggested children's understanding of commercial intent is often underestimated because researchers rely on verbal responses, Donahue *et al.* found that, by not relying on verbal measures, children aged three to six could understand persuasive intent.[120] In a 1997 study of young children's understanding of advertising intent by Young *et al.* (apparently ignored in the APA report), children aged four to eight years were shown a series of seven commercials. They were told that the end was missing in each, and were asked to complete the advertisements by choosing one of three pictures: one that showed a promotional ending, one that showed a neutral ending, and a third that showed an entertaining ending. Almost half of the four-year-olds chose an entertaining ending, suggesting that they did not understand the promotional purpose of advertising. But in the 5–6-year-old group, over half of the children chose a promotional ending for the advertisements, leading Young and his associates to conclude that 'children understand the promotional principle in advertising as early as 5–6 years'. As Young notes, this understanding of the selling function of advertising is 'one of the central pillars of advertising literacy, and finding it at the beginnings of middle childhood can only mean that children are not as gullible and lacking in understanding as was previously thought'.[121]

Thus, the research record is much more mixed than the APA report allows: it is simply not true to claim that the 'evidence as a whole indicates that most children younger than about age 7–8 years do not typically recognize that the underlying goal of a commercial is to persuade the viewer'. While certain pieces of empirical research suggest that this is true, some other pieces – just as compelling – suggest that it is not.

Realising, perhaps, that their empirical case was so weak, the authors next turned to 'psychological theory' to defend their claim about the inability of young children to understand persuasive intent. For instance, the report claimed that 'given the complexities involved in appreciating the source's perspective in the advertising process, there is a strong theoretical basis to expect that children below age 7–8 years will have difficulty recognizing the persuasive intent underlying television advertising'. Of course, the report has never established that 'appreciating the source's perspective in the advertising process' is the necessary condition for understanding persuasive intent, so what we have is a criterion established by fiat rather than argument. Nevertheless, if we allow this notion of understanding persuasive intent, then, according to this theoretical perspective, 'children below the age of approximately 7–8' have a limited cognitive development in at least two ways: first, they 'tend toward egocentrism and have difficulty in taking the perspective of another person', and second they have not yet developed a 'coherent understanding of mental events such as beliefs, desires, and motives until at least age 6'. Egocentrism and a failure to have a 'coherent' understanding of beliefs, desires and motives means that children cannot understand an advertiser's persuasive intent.

Is this theoretical perspective in fact justified? Does cognitive psychology really hold that young children's abilities are so limited as to make it impossible for them to understand what advertising is about? We would suggest that what is happening here is another instance of the report's ideologically driven selectivity. Given that the empirical case for young children's understanding of advertising intent is so weak, the report, ignoring the fact that one study is worth a thousand theories, attempted to make its case through a highly selective account of what we know about the mental life of children. Indeed, despite its overblown claims about the strength of the empirical evidence, the report's core claim is really this theoretical picture of young children as inherently limited by their cognitive development.

What underlies this picture of cognitively limited children is a Piagetian model of childhood, in which children develop in a rigid and unvarying series of 'ages and stages' that ultimately brings them to a state of adult rationality. As James Anderson argues, this picture of children proceeds on the assumption that children suffer from cognitive deficits that render them 'incompetent' as compared to adults.[122] Commenting on Anderson, Buckingham observes that:

> [M]uch genitive research tends to regard the child as a 'deficit system' – as more or less 'incompetent' when compared with adults. Using normative developmental models, children at certain ages are defined as being unable to accomplish the 'proper' sequencing of visual images, to recall the 'essential' features of a narrative, or to identify correctly the 'messages' that are being beamed at them. This preoccupation with identifying the 'inadequacies' of children's understanding – as compared with adults – has led to a neglect of children's own perspectives.[123]

This picture, however, is open to serious question, most significantly because it ignores the revolutionary developments in our understanding of young children's cognitive development in general, and of children's understanding of mental events, that have occurred in the last 10 years. As is noted by Judy Dunn, a leading theorist on children's mental abilities, when and what children understand now 'dominates developmental psychology'.[124] It would be curious if the professional psychologists who authored the APA report were ignorant of these developments in child psychology, so it is extremely difficult to explain why they are silent about them; for silent they are. In making their theoretical case that children's cognitive abilities below the age of eight do not allow them to understand persuasion, beliefs, desires, motives and intentions, the authors rely on psychological literature almost exclusively from the 1970s. They cite six authors who support the view of the child as conceptually limited, four of whose studies were published in the 1970s, one in the 1980s, and one in 1990. With the possible exception of the 1990 study, all the studies pre-date the significant developments in understanding children's cognitive abilities that have occurred in the last 10 years.

What has emerged from these developments is a quite different picture of the capacities of young children: one that is sharply at odds with the report's 30-year-old theory that such children cannot take the 'perspective of another person' and do not have an understanding of 'beliefs, desires and motives'.

As Dunn notes, in speaking about children under the age of four, 'We now have a picture of what children understand of their own and others' mental states in the preschool years; of their growing ability to distinguish thoughts and things and to reflect on and play with hypothetical events; and of their propensity to talk about what they and other people want, feel, and see.'[125] Then, crucially, 'as they reach 4 years, their burgeoning interest in talking about thinking, knowing and remembering' is clearly documented, Dunn tells us, by a variety of researchers, including Bartsch and Wellman,[126] two authors whose recent work on child development was not cited by the report, although some of their other work was. So, the APA report's 1970s theory that young children do not understand beliefs, desires and motives is contradicted by recent empirical studies that show that young children do, in fact, understand hypothetical events, speak of what they and others want, see and feel, as well as talk about thinking and knowing.

Three sorts of interactions occur in children during their third and fourth years, providing clear evidence of the richness and sophistication of their cognitive lives, according to Dunn. First, children display 'a very early and rapidly growing curiosity about and interest in inner states':

> Over the third year, our studies showed, their questions about other people's feelings and wants, and about why they act the way they do, increase markedly in frequency ... Frequently their questions about others are focused on hurt or upset: 'Are you all right?' 'Why are you crying?' and 'What's that frighten you, Mum?'

Second, Dunn notes four studies that look at young children's abilities in what psychologists call 'joint pretend', where children jointly structure a pretend world with another child. Such pretend playing requires the young child not only to understand and develop a play line, but also to understand the other child's thoughts and intentions, so as jointly to shape the pretend world. As Dunn observes, 'The general point of importance is that these data show us that children begin to entertain multiple hypothetical realities and "decouple" reality from fantasy not as solitary cognitive enterprises but through negotiating social interactions in which these cognitive states are shared.'[127]

Dunn's research is replicated in the work of psychologist Stephen Kline's study of children at play. Commenting on a study involving 30 boys aged three to six, Kline notes:

> When one child says to another 'let's play' it is an invitation to engage in social communication with each other by using toys. But a very complex process of meaning-making underlies even the simplest acts of playfulness. A wealth of social concepts is employed regularly in playing with action toys – because play implies the active application of rules, roles, narrative structure that the player brings to the game to make play.[128]

Far from being without concepts or beliefs, these young children understand rules, roles and narratives.

A third interaction occurring during the first four years of children's lives is the telling of stories. Dunn describes both her own work and that of others as revealing young children's sophisticated 'linguistic skills – referring to inner states, sequencing events temporally and causally – when they reported events involving fear, anger or distress'. Perhaps the most compelling displays of children's linguistic and cognitive skills is found, according to Dunn, when children engage in negotiations involving disputes with others:

> A child's ability to construct her own compelling and believable account of what happened may be called on

to a greater degree in the context of a dispute than in other settings ... Our data also showed that children have multiple opportunities to learn how best to tell what happened from listening to the exchanges between older siblings and parents.[129]

Dunn's claims are supported by an impressive array of empirical evidence from such distinguished children's researchers as Meltzoff *et al.*, who note that 'preschoolers understand a great deal about perceiving, wanting, and intending'.[130] According to Meltzoff, by

18 months of age children have already adopted a fundamental aspect of folk psychology: Persons are understood within a framework involving goals and intentions ... by 36 months children can reason backwards from an emotional reaction to what the adult was striving to do ... by age 3 there is considerable evidence that children understand that our desires and intentions may differ from, and even be in conflict with, the desires of those around us.[131]

Thus, far from the report's exclusively egocentric beings, unable to understand and take the perspective of others or to understand mental events, young children early on (as early as age three, according to Howard Gardner[132]) abandon egocentrism. Indeed, as Bartsch and Wellman observe, very young children initially explain what people do in terms of feelings and desires, but it is through their social interactions that they develop the concept of belief in order to understand others' actions.[133]

In short, the claim that children below the age of eight are so limited in cognitive development that they cannot assume the perspective of another person, and do not understand mental events such as desires, intentions, motives and beliefs, is simply not supported by a reading of the post-1990 literature in the psychology of childhood development.

Setting aside the question of the young child's general cognitive abilities, there is a very specific area of the cognitive capacities of children that the report hardly touches on, and yet is crucial for a child's understanding of advertising: namely, the ideas and actions of persuasion and lying. This is a curious omission, since the report assumes, both explicitly and implicitly, that advertising is based on persuasion; and persuasion, at the very least, is founded on bias. So, rather than a discussion about what psychological theory tells us of the cognitive abilities of young children in general, what we need, on the APA report's own terms, is a much more precise account of the specific abilities of young children with respect to those skills that are needed to understand advertising: that is, persuasion and deception.

The report makes a single reference to children's abilities to persuade; but these are dismissed in younger children as being 'limited both in scope and sophistication'. This, of course, misses the point. No one would say that the persuasive abilities of young children are equal to those of older children. This is not the relevant question. The real question is whether the abilities are sufficiently developed to allow the young child to use his own experience of trying to persuade as the model for understanding a commercial's attempt to persuade him, and the report presents no evidence that this is not the case. There is a considerable body of literature concerning young children's abilities to persuade and deceive. This should not be surprising since, as Eleanor Siegel notes in the *APS Observer*, 'Nothing in life is more pervasive than persuasion. Nearly every social interaction between humans ... has a strong element of persuasion.'[134]

One of the first studies of children's use of deception was the 1928 *Studies in Deceit* by Hartshorne and May, who noted that pre-school children are already practised in deceit, and that all children, given the right circumstances, will lie and cheat.[135] More recent work by Bartsch and London,[136] and Kline and Clinton,[137] respectively, has shown that children as young as three years of age have a rich understanding of persuasion, and regularly use persuasion to influence others.

Building on the early work of Hartshorne and May, contemporary psychologists have developed a rich literature of studies on young children's understanding of deceit and persuasion.[138] For instance, Newton, in a series of studies that looked at children in natural settings, observed that children as young as three use the same types of deception as four-year-olds, though less frequently. These children used deception most often 'in situations of conflict when the child is in an emotionally charged state of opposition to parental control'. The young children had clearly mastered the concept of deception, using it most frequently to manipulate what other family members believed. Newton also noted that the young children were quite subtle in their use of deceit, as examples of 'false boasting, and bravado in the face of painful punishment demonstrated that even 3- and 4-year olds engage in impression management'.

Just as the child has learned via language to participate in a shared perspective of the world, he also quickly develops the awareness that perspective can be manipulated through concealing his intentions and his plans. With that awareness come the 'cognitive skills for tactical deception' that emerge during the first four to six years of the child's life.[139]

Summarising the cognitive abilities that young children must have in order to lie successfully, Marie Vasek writes that they must 'have knowledge of another's knowledge and beliefs, recognize the information required to sway the beliefs of the listener, and communicate such that this information, rather than information which suggests one's intent to deceive is passed on'.[140] Vasek notes that, in children six and older, this capacity for manipulation, involving the ability to assume another's perspective and understand intentionality, is developed in a sophisticated enough form to 'allow them to manipulate their opponents in complex games ... and to understand convoluted deceptions in narrative ... Children of the same age can also modify their speech to suit the informational needs of their listeners.'[141]

Alongside all the other evidence of young children's cognitive capacities, their ability to deceive suggests, contra the APA report, that they understand much about motivation, intention, beliefs and desires.

Having put aside the report's infantilist view of young children and replaced it with a contemporary understanding of young children's abilities, we can now return to the central question of whether young children are able to understand the persuasive intent of advertising. We would suggest that the answer to this question is to be found by asking what are the minimum cognitive capacities necessary for children to understand persuasive intent. This is different from the test proposed by the report, which suggests that children require a 'mature comprehension of advertising messages' and which argues that the 'younger child's limited ability to understand and manipulate complex, abstract information about relationships between message sources and receivers' means that a child cannot understand persuasive intent. Such sophistic question-begging means that young children, by definition, cannot understand advertising, since the bar of understanding is pitched unreasonably high. There is no need for a straight-faced and farcical inquiry for, if young children require mature comprehension to understand persuasive intent, then, by definition, they do not possess it. But if the question is posed differently, so that it becomes a matter of whether young children have a comprehension – a set of capacities sufficient to understand the basic intention of advertisements – then we are asking something meaningful.

What might those capacities look like? They would be, as a minimum, the capacities necessary for children to engage in persuasion and deception themselves. In other words, if young children are able to engage in actions designed to persuade (and we have seen that they are), then they are able to recognise and grasp in an essential sense what advertising is all about. In effect, Marie Vasek's inventory of the understandings and skills necessary for children to lie – knowledge of another's knowledge and beliefs, knowing the information required to convince the listener, and communicating this persuasive information while masking one's intent to deceive – can also serve as one definition of advertising itself; unflattering, of course, but one of which the APA would approve. This is not, of course, to claim that young children's understanding of advertising is complete: it is merely to claim that it is sufficient to allow them to grasp its basic intent.

For some, this view of young children as cognitively sophisticated and practised in persuasion will be unattractive, as it runs counter to a long-held and deeply ingrained perception of them as innocent and unworldly. As the historian Ludmilla Jordanova notes, children traditionally have been seen as 'tender, impressionable, vulnerable, pure, deserving of parental protection, and hence all too easily corrupted by the market-place'.[142] In a society that rightly cherishes (though perhaps too often indulges) its children, there is a tendency to dismiss the idea of children understanding and practising deceit as at once too harsh and too clinical, as if it described children from some other place and time. But the scientific view of the mental and moral lives of young children finds its counterpart in both our popular culture and our experience of the lives of our own children. The idea of a long and protected childhood, in which children are sheltered, if not screened, from the 'world', has increasingly become a polite fiction. Young children, for better or worse, increasingly interact with the adult world. As David Buckingham has observed, 'Over the past twenty or thirty years, the status of childhood and our assumptions about it have become more and more unstable. The distinctions between children and other categories – "youth" or "adults" – have become ever more difficult to sustain.'[143]

Writing about the contraction of childhood in her 2000 book *Ready or Not*, Kay Hymowitz notes:

Few Americans are unaware of the profound transformation over the last thirty years in the way children look and act ... Infants now have 'lapware' computers with education programs and work out at baby gyms. It's not uncommon to hear about soccer teams for three-year-olds and tackle football teams complete with shoulder pads and helmets for seven-year-olds. Indeed, by elementary school many children are on the fast track ... No information is off-limits for children today. Third graders recite jokes told by David Letterman the previous night ... Nor is the media their only source: kindergartners might be studying the Holocaust or AIDS in school.[144]

In a similar vein, Don Tapscott observes that one of the consequences of the expansion of the digital media is that children develop much earlier a more sceptical sense of the world, which leads them frequently to question much of what they are told.[145] As users of the Web, young children are confronted with much that is inaccurate or deceptive, and they must learn early on how to discern the fake from the authentic. As one media expert told Tapscott, 'Children today have the luxury of understanding that everything they see or hear is not necessarily true. They see a photograph and know it could be totally fabricated. Kids today are developing a higher level of self-confidence – an ability to look critically at what their parents would accept as a given.'

All of this points to a deep and central peculiarity of the APA report: while the movement of children toward adulthood is accelerating in every other aspect of their lives, when it comes to advertising it, like the report's data, is trapped in the 1970s. Regardless of how knowledgeable young children might become about everything else, they can never hope to understand what advertising – one of the most persuasive aspects of their lives – is about until age eight. Funny that.

The APA report's claim that young children lack the cognitive capacities to understand what advertisements are about is open, then, to refutation on three counts: it is inconsistent with the full range of empirical evidence about children's understanding of persuasive intent; it is contradicted by much of the recent work in cognitive psychology, itself empirically founded, and particularly by that research which has looked at children's abilities to persuade and deceive; and it is refuted by the amply documented popular accounts of curtailed or hurried childhood that are a staple of current cultural studies.

None of this is meant to suggest that young children are discriminating or sophisticated consumers: neither are many adults. The relevant question is not whether children are mature consumers or little adults, but whether they possess the skills necessary to understand what advertising is about. What this view does suggest, however, is that the sentimentalised notion of young children as so naive and malleable as to be infants until the age of eight is supported neither by the full range of psychological research and theory, nor by the picture of young children in popular culture. Stripped of its shaky claims to empirical and theoretical support, this picture of vulnerable young children emerges for what it is: an ideological, as opposed to a scientific, construct whose only purpose is to make advertising to children morally suspect.

There is, finally, one other point that is worth noting about the claim that young children are vulnerable to advertising because they do not understand its persuasive intent. It is important because of its central role in the argument against advertising. The logic of the prohibitionist case is that the failure of young children to understand the purpose of advertising makes them vulnerable to it. But the research on this issue assumes, rather than establishes, vulnerability, because it is designed to assess understanding, rather than vulnerability. The research tells us that young children do not understand what commercials are about, and from this it deduces that they are vulnerable. But actual empirical evidence of vulnerability is never adduced. If the claim were true that failure to understand the purpose of advertising equals vulnerability, then it would be a fairly straightforward matter to design an experiment involving two groups of children being shown advertisements. One group would be told what the advertisement was 'about' and the other group would not. The researchers would observe whether there were differences in their reactions. As Jeffrey Goldstein notes, 'It would be a simple matter to see whether children who are told the purpose of a commercial are less affected by it than children not so informed. To my knowledge, no study of this sort has been done.'[146] Interestingly, though, there is one study in which, as

Goldstein observes, a group of young children who did *not* understand what advertisements were about were found to be less influenced by them.[147]

THE FOUNDATION FOR A DIFFERENT STORY

Throughout this chapter we have argued that the scientific evidence, as opposed to the rhetoric, of the obesity crusaders fails to support the view that food advertising aimed at children is a cause of their diets or their weight, or that such advertising is inherently manipulative because children are unable to understand its persuasive intent. This is not to say that advertising has no effect on the purchase and consumption behaviour of children, for there is, as we have shown, substantial evidence that it does routinely affect food decisions at the brand level. Indeed, an alternative and much more evidence-based way of portraying children's food preferences and choices is as a result of multiple influences, with no single influence causing a particular choice. As we have seen, there is substantial evidence that some food choices are the result of innate preferences, while others are the result of parental, peer, cultural and commercial influences.

However, let us assume, for the moment, that this picture is fundamentally wrong, and allow that advertising might have the capacity to shape the diets of children and young people, in part because they are no match for its forceful and manipulative character. Does conceding this mean that advertising restrictions and bans are necessary to protect children and adolescents, as the critics of food advertising maintain? We would suggest not. Even if the critic of food advertising is correct in his claims about the power of advertising, his policy prescription does not follow. This is because there are at least two viable alternatives to advertising restrictions and bans – parents and programmes in advertising literacy.

First, let us consider the role of parents in terms of the supposed effects of advertising. In our adaptation of Goldstein's model, there were four steps in the causative process of advertising:

- Children see advertisements.

- Children who cannot understand the manipulative nature of the advertisements form desires for the things advertised.

- Children demand these things from their parents.

- This can result in parent–child conflict.

Consider the role of parents in the context of this model. Children, particularly those young enough to (supposedly) not understand what advertisements are about, do not routinely purchase their own food. Their access to food is through their parents. For advertisements to 'work', there must be parental acquiescence to the child's food request. As Buckingham observes, 'Ultimately, children's power as consumers is very limited: at least at this age, their earned income is generally nonexistent or minimal. Their spending power depends primarily on their ability to extract money from their parents – and in this respect, the problem of television advertising is perhaps primarily a problem for parents.'[148] In other words, one of the answers to the alleged effect of food advertising is to be found in the parent's role as food gatekeeper. Advertising can only have an effect on a child's food choices if the parent allows it to have an effect. However, as the Ofcom report showed, a majority of parents have abdicated this responsibility through their belief that healthy eating is the task of someone else.

Second, in addition to the decisive role of parents in moderating the supposed effects of advertising, there are also ways in which education in advertising literacy can counter advertising. When considering improving advertising literacy, it is important to remember that such literacy is already both widespread and significant among children. Indeed, as Buckingham observed in a 2005 British study on the media literacy of children and young people, 'Children develop media literacy even in the absence of explicit attempts to encourage and promote it. Indeed, many researchers and media producers would argue that children today are more media literate than the children of previous generations, and indeed significantly more media literate than their own parents.'[149]

Some reports, such as that of the APA, tend to be unfairly dismissive of advertising and media literacy as a solution to the supposed problems of advertising to children. As the APA notes, 'there is little evidence that media literacy interventions can effectively counteract the impact of advertising on children of any age, much less the younger ones who are most vulnerable to its influence'.[150] But this is certainly not the view of many experts in advertising literacy, or of the research literature.

For example, in a recent large-scale experimental study of the effectiveness of media literacy educational programmes, Hobbs and Frost found that a curriculum that involved children analysing various types of media messages could improve children's media literacy skills.[151] There are several studies that have examined the ways in which media literacy efforts can improve children's understanding of what advertising is and how it works, and also increase children's scepticism about it.[152] And there is considerable agreement amongst many of those who study children and the media, that children's advertising literacy can be significantly enhanced.[153]

Moreover, there is some evidence that young children – supposedly those most at risk – reap the greatest benefits from advertising literacy education. In a study that involved young children, for instance, Peterson and Lewis found that children as young as six could learn to distinguish commercials from programmes and also understand something of the selling techniques used in advertisements.[154] In an experiment involving seven- and nine-year-old children in Los Angeles, Feshbach *et al.* were able to improve children's understanding of how advertisements portray products as desirable, so that after one week children began to find advertisements less credible and the products they advertised less attractive.[155]

Nor is the role of advertising literacy education one that need be left entirely to structured programmes at school.

Singer *et al.* studied children in infant school and in their first year of primary school, and found that children who discussed advertisements at home with their parents had a better comprehension of the purpose of advertisements than their peers who did not.[156] Studies have also shown that the children who speak with their parents about advertisements and consumption have a better understanding of the consumption process, and are more discriminating, than those who do not.[157] Additionally, some work has found that parents who critically discuss commercials with their children can reduce their children's desire for an advertised product.[158]

This is particularly important when it is placed against the findings of the Ofcom report, which noted that

> few parents make any attempt to mediate the impact of television advertising on their children. Just under half of parents (44%) say they 'never' talk about advertising to their children and a further 15% say they do so 'hardly ever'. Those who do talk about them are most likely to do so only 'occasionally' and very few ever discuss the credibility of the advert or its commercial motivation.[159]

Thus, even if one were to concede that food advertising might possess the capacity to affect the diet of children, parents have the power to counter this effect, and advertising literacy education has the capacity to provide children with the knowledge and skills to understand advertising's persuasive character.

CHAPTER 4

REGULATION IS THE WRONG SOLUTION TO THE WRONG PROBLEM

> I consider it a cowardly concession to a false
> extension of the idea of democracy to make *sub rosa*
> attacks on public tastes by denouncing the people
> who serve them. It is like blaming the waiters in
> restaurants for obesity.
>
> George Stigler,
> Nobel Prize-winning economist

INTRODUCTION

The dividing line in the policy debate over obesity revolves around a single question: how much should, and can, government do to change people's behaviour? So far, only one side of this debate has resonated in policymaking circles.[1] That side insists that government must use its legislative and regulatory powers to slim down an increasingly obese nation. From such a perspective, obesity is a public health crisis. Hence, the obesity crusade necessitates a public health solution on a massive, and massively expensive, scale.

The authors of this book argue that there is another side to the debate. We do not concede that government should attempt to change the eating habits and recreational activities of its citizens. However, even if we did support this goal, as a practical matter government cannot successfully legislate either for eating less or for exercising more. The bottom line is that a person's weight, level of physical fitness, and food consumption habits and patterns are products of individual choice and personal responsibility. Neither the food industry regulators' dictates nor the obesity crusaders' enforcement mechanisms can radically alter this fact.

The preceding chapters may have convinced the reader that the 'obesity epidemic' is a manufactured, unscientific and politically expedient term that, in reality, signifies nothing more than the gentle expansion of the national waistline. However, the reader may remain convinced that obesity is a serious problem. Therefore, this chapter addresses the question of whether or not it is either necessary or feasible for the government to attempt to reduce the number of obese people in our society.

FOOD, MORALITY AND PLEASURE

The obesity crusaders' battle cry carries the implicit message that food consumption is a necessary evil. Eating is something that, regrettably, we must do in order for us to be able to do everything else in our lives. What is overlooked by some, and underappreciated by others, is the fact that, as Tim Richardson, the international confectionery historian, reminds us, 'Pleasure is a vital component of our relationship with food.'[2] The enjoyment of food is one of life's greatest pleasures, and is also of the utmost practical necessity. Stripped to its essentials, the obesity crusade is really a war on what the public health establishment conceives to be illegitimate pleasure.

The author of *Sweets: A History of Candy*,[3] Richardson discovered that 'Morality is at the center of the debate ... Since the 1960s and the counterculture whole food movement, we have absorbed the idea that healthy foods are indisputably "good" and other foods are necessarily "bad". A moral hierarchy of food has been established.' He contends that

> The entrenched moral hierarchy of food in our society is worrying ... [T]here is also the Anglo-Saxon suspicion of the concept of pleasure from food. This has dogged the nation's attitudes for at least a century, and worsened considerably after the Second World War. Where postwar generations would famously lick the platter

clean, favouring plain and sustaining food, those born later in the century have developed a pseudo-scientific, calorie-controlled attitude to diet, influenced by the way in which basic foods such as milk, eggs, sugar, meat, bread and fish have soared up and down the health league table. Just look at the way whole milk was promoted as healthy in the 1970s ... with images of healthy lads gulping down bottles of ice-cold milk – and its status now, when so many people have turned to semi-skimmed and try to consume as little milk as possible.[4]

Cornell University's Richard Klein, the author of *Eat Fat*,[5] argues that 'Not only is the British Medical Association seeking to impose on my pleasure "for my own good", it doesn't have a single good word to say about the beauty and flavour of fat. It utterly ignores the fact that, for most of human history, fat has been praised for its virtues and cele-brated for its beauty.' He is frustrated by the fact that 'At no time do our doctors, obsessed with epidemiological risk, ever consider the Epicurean principle, that health is not the aim in life, only a means to pleasure – its *sine qua non*, without which no pleasure is possible.' Klein believes that

> Our minders generally stigmatise such a view as hedonism. But hedonism has a long and respectable philosophical history. In the strictest sense, it is that system of ethical belief that considers pleasure to be inherently good ... No one objects to medical science warning us about epidemiological risks, but translating them into constraints on individual behaviour is a stark violation of our freedom to pursue happiness.[6]

An April 2006 survey conducted by the Pew Research Center found that the percentage of Americans who truly enjoy eating has fallen significantly, from 48 per cent in 1989 to 39 per cent today.[7]

THE OBESITY CRUSADE'S POLICY MENU

Three years ago, the Food Standards Agency (FSA) warned the British government that the obesity problem was a 'ticking time bomb'. If obesity actually poses a serious danger to British society, there is the troubling matter that there is a lack of substantive evidence that the significant government interventions urged to stem obesity will actually work. Furthermore, there is considerable evidence to suggest that many of these policies will be counterproductive. It is to this policy menu that we now turn our attention.

A Warning about Labels

Most food products sold throughout the European Union do not carry nutritional labelling. The fact that EU citizens manage to live their lives quite adequately without labelled food products has proved politically to be an inadequate defence of the marketplace's inherent efficiency. For the anti-free market regulators in Brussels, the overriding issue is not demonstrated results, but rather the insatiable desire to fill a regulatory void with as much red tape as possible. Hence, the European commissioner for health and consumer protection, David Byrne, pushed a directive to coerce food and beverage companies to carry labelling to support their stated health claims. On 16 May 2006, the European Parliament adopted new rules about health claims in food labelling and advertising. The rules apply to nutritional claims such as 'light', 'rich in fibre' or 'rich in calcium'. Under the new legislation, manufacturers can use health claims only if the product in question is within certain limits for quantities of two out of three food elements, namely salt, sugar and fat. Legislation to this effect is currently wending its way through the European Parliament.

With the encouragement of Brussels, the Blair government's Public Health White Paper, presented on 16 November 2004, proposed a new system of warning labels on food products. This so-called 'traffic-light' system will identify unhealthy foods in a naive attempt to encourage people to eat more healthily. High-fat, salty or sugary foods receive a red label, while healthy choices, such as fruit and vegetables, attract a green label. Nutritious but high-fat foods, such as cheese, are given an amber label.[8]

Such a scheme is typical of the 'rational thinking' that dominates policymaking in this area. Under the guise of scientific analysis, certain foods are deemed to be 'junk', while others are deemed to be 'healthy'. This approach should be challenged on its very premise. In scientific terms, the definition of certain foods as 'junk food' is contentious, to say the least. Rather than being used as a strictly scientific category, the term actually conveys a moral judgement on certain people's food preferences. The idea that a particular food is bad for you is simply outdated. In truth, a balanced, healthy diet can include almost anything, so long as moderation is the watchword. The demonising of specific foods actually runs counter to the advice of the best nutritionists, who maintain that there are no good or bad foods, only good and bad diets.[9]

For example, Professor Vincent Marks, a biochemist at the University of Surrey and co-editor of *Panic Nation: Unpicking the Myths We're Told about Food and Health*,[10] asserts that there is no such thing as junk food, full stop. 'Junk food is an oxymoron', he says. 'Food is either good, that is, it is enjoyable to eat and will sustain life, or it is good food that has gone bad, meaning that it has deteriorated and gone off. To label a food as "junk" is just another way of saying, "I disapprove of it". There are bad diets, that is, bad mixtures and quantities of food, but there are no "bad foods" except those that have become bad through contamination or deterioration.'

According to Marks, all foods – from the notorious Turkey Twizzler to the renowned freshly picked apple – are just combinations of protein, fat and carbohydrates, and our bodies will take from them what we need and get rid of the rest. 'Even hamburgers provide energy in a palatable and affordable form', asserts Marks. 'No food is "better for us" than any other; it all depends upon circumstances. For people on a limited income or in times of famine, high energy density food is best and will enable survival. For the affluent and in times of plenty ... fruit is an important part of a mixed diet.'

Marks maintains that we should focus less on individual foodstuffs and more on diet. 'There is no such thing as junk food, but there is such a thing as a "junk diet". The quantity of food consumed, over say a weekly period, is just as important as its quality.'

Labelling food products with warnings about their inherent unhealthiness is the closest we allow ourselves to come to actually labelling the consumers of these products. According to Dr Michael Fitzpatrick, a writer for the *Lancet* and author of *The Tyranny of Health: Doctors and the Regulation of Lifestyle*, eating junk food is one of the greatest social sins of our times. Observes Fitzpatrick: 'Gluttony used to be one of the seven deadly sins; now eating junk food invites moral opprobrium.'[11]

Setting aside questions of morality, one is left with the question of practicality. Is there sufficient reason to think that warning labels might work? Neither logic nor experience suggests that the traffic-light scheme will prove anything other than unworkable. Pilot programmes have already failed for a variety of reasons. For example, raspberries were labelled with an unhealthy red dot because of their sugar content. Hence, the traffic-light scheme leads to the artificial segregation of foods. The oversimplification of food choices implies that 'good' foods may be eaten with impunity, while 'bad' foods should be avoided. Such an approach can lead to unforeseen consequences, such as inadequate calcium or iron intake. This is the situation experienced by Sweden since it adopted a food labelling system several years ago.[12]

Tellingly, the American public's girth has grown somewhat, even as the information on food labels has increased over the past two decades.[13] Predictably, the bureaucratic response to such evident failure is not to rethink the entire enterprise. Instead, the public health establishment calls for a larger dose of the same medicine. Hence, US Food and Drug Administration (FDA) officials are considering placing warning labels on packages of foods deemed unhealthy by government scientists.[14] Acting FDA Commissioner Lester Crawford has said that the current system of food labelling, known as

'Nutrition Facts' (the ubiquitous boxes listing calories, fat and other dietary information on commercial food packages), may be transformed from providing information to a largely satisfied customer base into providing warnings that will serve only to unnerve and discomfit these same customers. Of course, that is the true purpose of such an otherwise indefensible scheme.

ABC-TV's John Stossel, a rare libertarian voice on American network television, has summed up the unintended consequences of further warning labels, observing:

> There are 40 warnings on a stepladder, but I don't
> think that makes us safer. In fact, ladders are a good
> example of how lawyers ... have made warning labels
> meaningless. There are so many labels on so many
> things that we don't read labels we should read. Like the
> warning label on microwave popcorn that tells you you
> could burn yourself when you open the bag. Or the label
> on some antibiotics that says it won't work if you take it
> with milk. We ought to read those, but when there's so
> much information, who reads any of it?[15]

Stossel is correct. Serious health warnings are diluted when consumers are deluged by 'warnings' about every imaginable item, ingredient and eventuality. There is already evidence from the US that consumers are confused by labelling.[16] Clearly, most of these labels should come with their own warning: 'Caution: Bureaucrats at Work'.

Bans on Fizzy Drinks and School Vending Machines

Those who constantly decry British school funding levels should note that the beverages purchased through school-based vending machines earn each school sufficient funds to cover half of a teacher's salary. Schools typically make between £13,000 and £15,000 (the total range is between £10,000 and £30,000) a year profit from vending machines, and many have come to rely on the money to pay for extra staff, new equipment and much-needed renovation.[17]

Nevertheless, banning vending machines from schools has become the cause *du jour* for obesity crusaders on both sides of the Atlantic. From September 2006, British schools were prohibited from selling junk food.[18] In America, there is a wave of regulation by school districts and state legislatures to combat reports of rising childhood obesity rates. For example, politicians in Texas, New York, Philadelphia and elsewhere removed fizzy drinks from schools. In September 2005, California enacted a law banning fizzy drinks in all government-run schools. That ban went further than the beverage association's voluntary industry guidelines, announced in August 2005, which sought to limit fizzy drink sales to no more than 50 per cent of a high-school vending machine's options.

Back in Europe, childhood obesity is also making its presence felt in France. The number of under-18s classified as overweight has doubled in France over the past decade, with one child in eight now clinically obese. Consequently, the government included in new public health legislation, passed in August 2004 and enacted in September 2005, a ban on all food-and-drink vending machines in French schools.

All of this activity, both at home and abroad, is occurring despite a lack of evidence establishing a link between fizzy drinks or vending machines and childhood obesity. In 2004, researchers from the WHO's School-Aged Children Obesity Working Group published a study involving 137,000 schoolchildren in 34 countries, including 8,904 British pupils, which looked at the alleged connection between the intake of sweets/fizzy drinks and obesity.[19] The researchers found that, in '91 percent of the countries examined, the frequency of sweets intake was lower in overweight than normal weight youth'. More importantly, they discovered that the children who ate larger amounts of so-called 'junk food' actually had less chance of being overweight. According to the WHO, 'Overweight status was not associated with the intake of ... soft drinks.'

The research confirmed several earlier studies that had also found that fizzy drinks do not cause childhood obesity. For example, a recent Harvard University study, published in the *International Journal of Obesity*, studied the eating and physical activity habits of 14,000 American schoolchildren over a three-year period.[20] It found that fizzy drinks and snack food did not lead to overweight and obesity. No matter how snack food was defined, with or without fizzy drinks, the researchers were unable to find any link between these foods and obesity. Moreover, the overweight children were not found to be eating more snack foods and fizzy drinks than the thin children.

A study presented in autumn 2005 at the North American Association for the Study of Obesity's annual meeting in Vancouver found that 'the frequency of purchases [of fizzy drinks] from school vending machines was not associated with BMI percentile or DQ [dietary quality]'.[21] Studies conducted by the Georgetown Center for Food and Nutrition Policy found no link between fizzy drink consumption and obesity in children between the ages of 12 and 18.[22] The thinnest children are often the biggest fizzy drink consumers.

New Canadian research casts additional doubt on the link between fizzy drinks and childhood obesity. The study, led by Paul Veugelers of the University of Alberta, assessed the health, nutrition and lifestyle factors of 4,299 primary schoolchildren to determine which risk factors were most important for overweight children. The study found that, in terms of the quantity of fizzy drinks consumed by children, there was no significant difference whether they attended schools that did or did not sell fizzy drinks. Children in schools that sold fizzy drinks consumed an average of four cans per week, while children at schools that did not sell fizzy drinks still consumed 3.6 cans per week. There was no relationship found between the availability of fizzy drinks at schools and the risk of children being overweight or obese, nor between the presence at schools of food vending machines and the same risk.[23] Research published last year in the *Journal of Pediatrics* also found that there was no relationship between fizzy drink consumption and BMI.[24] These findings suggest that focusing childhood obesity prevention programmes on vending machines in schools will have no significant impact on BMI.

British policymakers assume (wrongly) that schoolchildren will now spend their parents' money on unsugared, low-fat and low-salt options. According to John Dunford, the general secretary of the Secondary Heads' Association, banning the sale of junk food in school will not stop pupils eating it. Dunford predicts that, instead of buying junk food products from the school's vending machine, pupils will bring junk food to school from home or buy it in nearby shops.[25] The evidence to date suggests that Dunford's forecast will prove correct. For example, in early 2004 Queensbury School in Dunstable, Bedfordshire, was one of the first British schools to remove fizzy drinks, crisps and sweets from its vending machines. The junk food was replaced by mineral water, organic fruit juices and cereal bars. Eighteen months later, the school ended the experiment. According to the head teacher, Nigel Hill, 'We have had to remove the vending machines because students were not using them, despite the extensive programme of health education and nutrition that we introduced at the same time. The youngsters ... simply wouldn't buy the healthier food in the machines.'[26]

There are plenty of reasons to reject a fizzy drinks ban, besides the lack of a scientific foundation for such legislation. Above all, parents and teachers should be trying to educate children to make good choices. Children will never learn how to make responsible consumer choices if products are simply banned from school grounds. The 'forbidden fruit' effect is also alive and well in the experience of banning vending machines. Professor Leann Birch of Pennsylvania State University advises that 'Parents should not restrict children's access to foods they believe to be unhealthy, as this has the opposite effect. We have shown that it actually increases the child's intake of restricted food.'[27]

Advertising Bans and Restrictions

In November 2004, celebrity chef Anthony Worral Thompson spoke for the public health establishment when he informed *Independent* readers that 'The three countries with the most liberal food advertising laws are the US, Australia and the UK, and those are the three with the worst obesity problems.'[28] By contrast, the reader will recall that Chapter 3 documented the absence of a causal link between advertising and obesity. After examining the 2004 FSA report into advertising, children and obesity, Dr David Ashton, an epidemiologist at Imperial College's School of Medicine in London, said: 'I don't think the scientific evidence presented in the Food Standards Agency report supports its conclusion that ads are influencing children's diet.' He continued: 'I am not persuaded at all that there is a link. It is convenient to blame large food manufacturers. It is much easier than confronting the real issue, which is that decline in physical activity over the last few decades is to blame.'[29]

Andrew Brown, of the Advertising Association, also questions whether there is a link between childhood obesity and food advertising. He observes that 'Per capita consumption of confectionery has not gone up in ten years, and the proportion of all advertising taken up by food advertising, including fast-food advertising, is in decline. But kids are getting fatter.'[30] The proportion of food advertising within total advertising has been in decline since the late 1980s. Over the past decade, the volume of food advertisements has declined by 30 per cent. During the past six years, the number of food advertisements directed at children has also fallen by 30 per cent.[31] Yet, obesity among children aged 2–10 has risen by 25 per cent.

The 500-page report from the US National Academy of Sciences' Institute of Medicine (IOM) was billed as the most comprehensive report on obesity and food marketing to children to date.[32] Yet, the IOM report admits that current evidence is not sufficient to arrive at any finding about a causal relationship between television advertising and obesity among children and youth.[33] As Nobel Prize-winning economist Gary Becker concluded his review, 'The evidence provided by the report is weak and not persuasive.'[34] According to Becker:

> The complex report by the Institute of Medicine ... did not include any studies (presumably because none are

available) that directly look at the effects of advertising by fast food and beverage companies on the overall consumption of these goods by teenagers and younger children. Instead, virtually all the studies available to them examine the effects on children's weight of greater or lesser exposure to television ... The Institute of Medicine's report on obesity and advertising did not present any convincing evidence that television advertising oriented toward children has been responsible for the increase in children's obesity during the past quarter century.[35]

Advertising and obesity: the lack of evidence

In March 2004, more than 100 British health and consumer lobby groups called on the government to ban junk food advertising in an effort to combat obesity, which, these groups alleged, was fuelled by such advertising. Approximately 40 per cent of advertisements during children's television programmes are for food. It was asserted that most of these are for confectionery, fast food, pre-sugared breakfast cereals, savoury snacks or fizzy drinks. According to Professor Tim Lang of Thames Valley University, most of the £600 million spent on advertising food in the UK each year promotes snacks, sweets and fatty foods. Lang says children are bombarded with messages promoting unhealthy 'free' choices.[36]

This contention has carried the day in policymaking circles. Therefore, the government's autumn 2004 White Paper expressed the Orwellian wish that the large food companies 'voluntarily' agree to cut the amount of advertising of junk food aimed at children. Now, here is the regulatory rub. If the industry has not brought in satisfactory self-regulatory measures by 2007, the government has pledged to introduce legislation to force it to conform to the obesity crusaders' wishes.[37]

Such public policy flies in the face of a February 2005 report from the Social Issues Research Centre, an Oxford-based think tank. This report concluded that

We do no service to the people at risk of obesity related
morbidities in our society by 'hyping' their plight,
exaggerating their numbers or diverting limited
educational, medical and financial resources away from
where the problems really lie. Banning advertising of
'junk food' to children and similar measures may be
popular in some quarters, but they are unlikely to
impact much on the generation of people in their 50s
and 60s – those with vastly higher rates of overweight
and obesity than children and young people.[38]

The Blair government's own culture secretary opposes
banning junk food advertising on pragmatic grounds.
Questioned as to why she was not endorsing a ban on junk
food ads on television, Culture Secretary Tessa Jowell, speaking on BBC Radio 4's *Today* programme in May 2004, said
that she was sceptical about the effectiveness of such a measure. She said she doubted that banning junk food advertising
on television would help tackle the problem. Jowell argued
that individuals were responsible for their own diet and physical activity: 'The reason we have this crisis of obesity is
because too many of us are eating too much of the wrong
kind of food … and we are not exercising enough.'[39]

A leading medical journal has opined that, in the period
that the advertising of junk food remains on our screens,
celebrities should be banned from promoting it. In a November
2003 editorial, the *Lancet* suggested that celebrity endorsement
of junk food was contributing to high rates of obesity, particularly among children. It called on ministers to introduce
legislation to ban the practice: 'One of the most invidious
techniques used by junk-food advertisers is to pay sports and
pop celebrities to endorse foods – especially bizarre since sports
celebrities need a properly balanced diet to achieve fitness. Such
celebrities should be ashamed; as should others who get caught
in the web of junk-food promotion … The "British way" of
regulation is to seek voluntary agreements with manufacturers.
The time for that is past, and the junk-food industry needs to
be forced by legislation to clean up its act.'[40]

In fact, the use of celebrities in advertisements is a perfectly legitimate practice, engaged in by responsible companies. The practice of celebrity endorsement is governed by two powerful constraints, one institutional and the other sociological. In institutional terms, British food and beverage manufacturers have to abide by a strict code of practice in their advertising to children. Such a code of practice will not satisfy the fanatical obesity crusaders, for whom any advertising aimed at children is unacceptable. Reasonable people, however, recognise the constraints that those advertising to children must work within. In marketing terms, advertising has the potential to increase the sales of particular brands, but is incapable of stimulating an increase in overall food consumption.[41] As Becker explains:

> There is no doubt that McDonald's and other companies tend to increase their revenues when they raise advertising budgets – otherwise, companies would not be spending as much on advertising. But most of the increase in sales to a company when it advertises more tends to come at the expense of sales by competitors. So if Wendy's raises its advertising, sales by McDonald's and other competitors would tend to fall. To the extent that advertising mainly redistributes customers among competitors, the elimination of advertising of fast foods or sugary beverages through regulation would have relatively little effect on the overall demand for these products.[42]

Those who support an outright ban on food advertising are forced to confront the results of the only contemporary case studies in advertising bans, namely in Sweden and in the Canadian province of Quebec. Since 1980, Quebec has prohibited all food advertising to children. Yet, childhood obesity rates and the consumption of so-called 'unhealthy' foods are similar to the rest of Canada, where there is no such law.[43] The Canadian medical establishment remains either unaware of these facts or willing to overlook them for ideological reasons. How else can one explain the Ontario Medical

Association's recent report on child obesity in Ontario, Canada's most populous province? The report, *An Ounce of Prevention or a Ton of Trouble: Is There an Epidemic of Obesity in Children?*, includes the recommendation that the government introduce a ban on advertisements for high-fat foods that are targeted at children under 13 years of age.[44]

For the last decade, Sweden has also had a ban on food advertising to children. This has not resulted in significant reductions in childhood obesity or marked differences in obesity rates compared with other European countries.[45] In fact, Sweden has similar obesity rates to the UK. 'The bans have had no impact whatsoever on obesity rates', says Imperial College's Dr Ashton. 'Some people might want to say that Sweden and Quebec are not typical of the UK. That may indeed be the case. But they are the only live experiments on real people that we have and they have not shown any benefit.'[46]

The Swedish and Quebec experiments have failed, in part, as a result of an unintended, yet predictable, consequence of banning food advertising. Unable to compete with one another through conventional advertising methods, individual brands have gained a larger market share through price reductions, which have stimulated an increase in demand for that particular brand, if not the product itself. Furthermore, the removal of expensive television advertising campaigns from the budgets of food and beverage companies has enabled them to spend much larger amounts on non-broadcast marketing, thereby maximising their respective market shares via other marketing instruments.[47]

The obesity crusaders' preference for policymaking without reference to supporting scientific evidence continues apace. In the future, manufacturers who advertise sugar-rich or high-fat 'junk foods' without inserting a health warning will be liable for hefty fines, with even stricter regulations applying to products targeting children.

Healthy School Dinners

Tessa Jowell's realism is not shared by her cabinet colleagues. In September 2005, Ruth Kelly, the secretary of state for education, launched a political *jihad* against junk food. In a new government pledge to improve nutritional standards, Kelly announced that schools had until September 2006 to wipe junk food off their lunch menus. In place of the underwhelming menu exposed by celebrity chef Jamie Oliver,[48] schoolchildren will be offered healthier alternatives, such as salads, freshly cooked pasta dishes, dried fruit, etc.[49] Kelly warned that school governors who continue to allow junk food to be served after the ban comes into force could receive a criminal record. They will be 'open to the same sanctions as anyone else who breaks the law'.

Under the proposals, schoolchildren will only be able to drink water, skimmed and semi-skimmed milk, pure fruit juices, certain types of 'smoothies', and yoghurt and milk drinks made with less than 10 per cent added sugar. Colas, all other fizzy, sugary drinks, and drinks with artificial sweeteners, are to be removed from schools. Sweets, chocolate, chewing gum, cereal bars, fruit bars and chocolate-coated biscuits will also be banned. Salty snacks such as crisps and salted nuts are *verboten*, and salt will have no place on school canteen tables.

School meals, however, are a small proportion of children's food intake, and their poor standard is unlikely to affect the problem of nutrition or obesity.[50] After his or her first year at school, a child will have consumed just 5 per cent of meals in the school environment. What children eat is determined by habits acquired before they attend school and are, therefore, their parents' responsibility.[51] Mick Brookes, the general secretary of the National Association of Head Teachers, has predicted that many children will simply bring in packed lunches full of junk food.[52] David Vanstone, the head teacher at North Cestrian grammar school in Altrincham, and chair of the Independent Schools Association, was blunter than Brookes: 'I think the government should stop acting like a nanny state and realise that the young people of today know a lot more about this issue than they are given credit for.'[53]

Banning certain foods sends all the wrong signals to young people. It is an ineffective measure to combat obesity.

One of the keys to a sensible body weight is eating a balanced diet. Unfortunately, banning some foods, while encouraging the consumption of others, will not help teach our schoolchildren how to build such a balanced diet.[54]

Junk Food Tax

In 2003, the British Medical Association proposed levying a 17.5 per cent 'fat tax' on high-fat foods such as biscuits, cakes and processed meals.[55] A year later, Downing Street's Strategy Unit floated a comparable idea.[56] Last year, Britain's environmental health officers added their collective voice to the call for VAT-style taxes on unhealthy pre-prepared products.[57] Since then, the American Medical Association has come out in favour of a fat tax on fizzy drinks.[58] The public health establishment's argument is that such a tax will reduce junk food consumption, and thereby improve diets and overall public health.[59] Yet, there are many reasons to suspect that a fat tax would be at best unsuccessful, and at worst economically and socially harmful.

The latest economic research strongly suggests that a fat tax may simply prove to be a futile instrument in influencing the behaviour and habits of the overweight and the obese. Those consumers 'addicted' (to use the obesity crusaders' term) to unhealthy food will not be dissuaded from their eating habits and patterns by a tax. Those consumers who strongly prefer 'unhealthy' foods – those whom the public health establishment would label dietary 'risk takers' – will continue to eat and drink according to their individual preferences until such time as it becomes prohibitively expensive to do so.[60]

If one accepts the assumption that a fat tax would significantly alter consumer behaviour, the societal and economic consequences would be undesirable.[61] For example, the US Department of Agriculture (USDA) Economic Research Service has determined that a fat tax would be economically regressive, as a disproportionate share of the tax would be paid by low earners, who pay a higher proportion of their incomes in sales tax and also consume a disproportionate share of junk food.[62]

Medical inefficiency would result from the false 'good food' versus 'bad food' paradigm. For example, recently presented research has found that energy-dense foods like hamburgers and hot dogs, which are regularly blamed for obesity, do not appear to contribute to the problem. The researchers state that 'we found no statistically significant associations between DED [dietary energy density] and BMI, waist circumference, tricep skin folds, and subscapular skin fold. Similarly, we found no independent association between [dietary energy density] and glycosylated hemoglobin, fasting glucose, HDL ["good cholesterol"], LDL ["bad cholesterol"], total cholesterol, and triglycerides.' The study, presented at the 2005 North American Association for the Study of Obesity conference, concluded that 'DED is not significantly associated with BMI and other anthropometric measurements of obesity and adiposity. Moreover, DED is not significantly associated with the majority of common risk factors for cardiovascular disease and diabetes.'[63]

According to the Economic Research Service, another unintended consequence of a fat tax on consumer behaviour is that taxes on snack foods could lead some consumers to replace the taxed food with equally unhealthy foods.[64] Furthermore, in March 2004 the journal *Obesity Research* published an analysis that identified 'no statistically significant relationship between the percentage of calories from ice cream, baked goods, candy or chips and BMI (Body Mass Index) score' in adolescent girls.[65] According to the researchers, these 'energy dense snack foods' had no bearing on 'weight status or fatness change over the adolescent period'. Chocolate bars and crisps, often blamed for the rise in childhood obesity, are not, in fact, responsible for weight gain in children, according to research by scientists from Harvard University.[66] A leader writer for *USA Today*, a pro-regulation newspaper, disparages the WHO for encouraging fat taxes as a response to obesity. The leader argues that 'governmental Twinkie police are less effective than the marketplace in this food fight'.[67] Indeed.

Planning Restrictions

The obesity crusaders are terribly concerned about the proximity of junk food outlets to schools. Hence the call for 'food free' zones around schools. For example, officials in California's Contra Costa County, in the San Francisco area, are studying plans to restrict the number of fast-food restaurants within their jurisdiction.[68] This is a bad American idea that threatens to spread across the Atlantic.

The tendency of proponents to get their sums wrong, to add two plus two and end up with five, is again in evidence. Roger Bate, resident fellow at the American Enterprise Institute, has performed extensive research in this area. His findings indicate that the number of McDonald's restaurants in any given area has nothing to do with the prevalence of obesity. Bate writes:

> McDonald's restaurant penetration into European countries shows a negative correlation with [International Obesity Task Force] obesity data. In other words, the more McDonald's restaurants per 10,000 people, the fewer people are overweight ... fast food has little to do with overall obesity rates. If fast food were the main cause of weight gain, we would expect to see the UK and France, with high fast food penetration, being the most obese. Yet it is Greece that has the most obese population, with over 70 percent of adults clinically overweight, while the country has few McDonald's restaurants.[69]

A new study published in the *American Journal of Public Health* adds to the empirical misery of those campaigning against the proximity to schools of fast-food restaurants.[70] Researchers from the RAND Institute investigated nearly 7,000 primary schoolchildren from 59 different American cities, and found no link between childhood obesity levels and fast-food restaurant prices or the number of restaurants in a given area. They found that 'There were no significant effects for dairy or fast-food prices, nor for outlet density ... We initially expected food outlets to play an important role, but no association was found ... the absence of an effect on weight change in our data could also be an indication that density, or at least the variation in density, of food outlets has a smaller impact on diet than commonly assumed.'[71] These results corroborated a study published in the *International Journal of Obesity*, which reported that 'no relationship between availability of takeaway foods and the prevalence of obesity was found'.[72]

NATIONAL REGULATORY MODELS

In the summer of 2003, Sir Liam Donaldson, the UK's chief medical officer, declared that the country was headed for an obesity 'epidemic'. As Chapter 2 explained, there is no such thing as an obesity epidemic, either in this country or in any other developed nation. Nonetheless, for our heads-buried-in-the-empirical-sand, Leninist-minded academics, policymakers and regulators, Sir Liam's declaration raised the question, 'what is to be done?'

For the purveyors of the obesity myth, the answer is both simple and radical. According to Professor Steve Bloom of Imperial College, London, 'The answer is to stop obesity, and the way to do that is to change our society.'[73] According to Steve Webb, the Liberal Democrat health spokesman, 'Obesity is a killer and needs to be treated as such.'[74] In its seminal May 2004 report, the Commons Health Select Committee stated: 'As the main factors contributing to the rapid rises in obesity seen in recent years are societal, it is critical that obesity is tackled first and foremost at a societal rather than an individual level.'[75] Therefore, it should not surprise the reader to learn that the obesity crusaders' policy agenda is an extreme one. As R. C. Davey wrote in the *British Journal of Sports Medicine*, 'The only effective approach is for governments to implement radical policy change.'[76]

Upon closer inspection, the word 'radical' may be inadequate to capture the true nature of the changes planned to our lives by the obesity crusaders. They seek to regulate our consumption of food.[77] This will, and can only, be accomplished through state control of the food industry. In practice, this will mean advertising bans on selected produce, taxes on certain foods, and food rationing. The argument that Davey and his fellow crusaders make for a return to food rationing is based upon the empirical observation that there were very few, if any, obese or malnourished people in wartime Britain.

Do other opinion-formers have the courage of their self-anointed libertarian convictions? It would seem not. In a January 2006 speech laying out his health care policy vision, Conservative party leader David Cameron leapt upon the statist, anti-obesity bandwagon. He singled out shops, especially in train stations, that offer cut-price chocolate bars: 'As Britain faces an obesity crisis, why does W. H. Smith's promote half-price Chocolate Oranges at its checkouts instead of real oranges?' To which the executives of W. H. Smith may have replied, 'Because we conduct our business under the assumption that Britain still remotely resembles a liberal democracy.' But W. H. Smith and its retail peers have only so much to fear from any future Cameron-led government. The Conservative prime-minister-in-waiting continued, 'Of course, we cannot regulate in this regard but can point the finger, we can ask awkward questions and we can put some pressure on, and I believe politicians and others should do so.'[78]

Other members of the political class are not so patient. On the question of reducing junk food marketing to children, Charlie Powell, campaign coordinator for Sustain: The Alliance for Better Food and Farming, is alarmingly candid. He states bluntly that 'Voluntary approaches will not work.'[79]

PUBLIC HEALTH COERCION AT HOME AND ABROAD

A comparative assessment of national regulatory structures in the area of food industry regulation is a most disheartening endeavour. There is very little to recommend itself in the respective approaches to waging war on obesity. Above all, one is struck by the inability of policymakers and regulators to learn from the failures and mistakes of their peers in other countries. Consequently, each new legislative agenda in this area constitutes an exercise in reinventing the wheel. The same false assumptions are laid down as the foundation upon which the same demonstrably unworkable, even counter-productive, policies are expected to support decades-long campaigns to change the eating and drinking habits of ordinary people.

Most national governments attempt to tackle obesity by introducing an all-too-familiar menu of policies and regulatory items. The items on this policy menu include junk food advertising bans, vending machine bans, fat taxes, healthier school meals, planning restrictions and warning labels. We discuss now how such policies have been designed and implemented in the UK, the USA, France, Finland and Sweden, as well as at the supranational level in the form of the EU's own campaign against obesity.

How do you change the eating habits of tens, perhaps hundreds, of millions of people? That is the daunting problem facing each of these interventionist governments. Here is an overview of how each one is waging its own misguided obesity crusade.

The UK's New Interventionism

The central message of the May 2004 Commons Health Select Committee report was that the government, the food industry and parents had to wake up to the obesity threat. The 146-page report included stinging criticism of the government's record to date, and provided 69 recommendations on what needs to be done. These recommendations have formed the basis of what Conservative MP Boris Johnson has described as a 'jargon-laden agenda for interfering in the lives and habits of British families'.[80] To that end, on 22 August 2006, Tony Blair appointed Caroline Flint to the newly created post of 'minister for fitness' to head the British government's battle of the bulge.[81]

The select committee's report proved to be a political watershed in the fight against obesity. Above all, it calls for a more interventionist response from government. The recommendations include proposals to set up a new labelling system for food, lessons for schoolchildren on healthy eating, restrictions on food advertising, and a national campaign to try to get people to exercise more. For instance, the committee sought a new national walking strategy to encourage people to leave their cars at home.

The food and beverage industry was singled out as the major culprit in the obesity problem. The report told food manufacturers that they should implement a voluntary ban on junk food advertising targeted at children;[82] it called for an end to celebrity endorsement of less healthy foods and for super-sized products to be phased out; and it proposed that purveyors of king-size chocolate bars should be 'publicly named and shamed'. It even went so far as to recommend price changes to the industry's products to make healthier products more affordable.

The report recommended that, if the industry did not demonstrate significant improvements in product labelling and product formulation within three years, the government should step in. On 9 March 2006, the FSA recommended a traffic-light scheme that will formalise the erroneous notion of 'good' and 'bad' foods.[83] The health committee was also adamant that schools could do more to tackle obesity. Hence, its call for snack vending machines to be removed from schools. In September, the government introduced a new dietary regime for schools. When this measure was announced, the 'we-know-what's-best-for-your-child' approach extended to telling parents what to put in their children's packed lunches.[84]

In government circles, there has been no effort made to camouflage the desire for a change in the balance and the nature of food promotion. In 2006, legislation to regulate the marketing of junk food to children has been under serious consideration. As Tony Blair explained in a July 2006 health policy speech, if the government is not satisfied with the industry's response by 2007, draconian legislation will be brought in the following year.[85] The government is specifically considering whether to ban junk food advertising on television before the 9pm watershed. A ban on junk food advertising during children's television programming is a primary objective for the FSA. The broadcasting regulatory agency, Ofcom, is attempting to square the advertising circle by devising a formula that will differentiate, to nobody's satisfaction, between allegedly healthy and allegedly junk food.[86] In November 2005, a Department of Health advisory document proposed that celebrity endorsers should not be used to promote products that are high in fat, sugar or salt to children. Consequently, marketing campaigns such as the Walkers crisp advertisements featuring Gary Lineker and David Beckham may be banned.[87] Combating childhood obesity was also the focus of the government's recent decision that primary schoolchildren are to be routinely weighed and their parents told if they are obese. Ministers have decided to overrule the Children's Commissioner and their own child health officials, who fear that telling parents the test results will stigmatise some children.[88]

Sweden's Embarrassment of Fat

In Sweden, junk food advertisements are banned, but it has made no difference to levels of obesity. In February 2004, a Swedish think tank noted that 'Sweden has for a long time banned all commercials targeting children, but still Swedish children are as obese as those in comparable countries.'[89] Such an unsuccessful health policy venture is both politically and culturally embarrassing. After all, Sweden is a country that has long prided itself on its public health records. Yet, today 50 per cent of Swedish men and 33 per cent of Swedish women are overweight. Some 10 per cent are obese – almost double the numbers of the 1980s. The situation among Swedish children is regarded as particularly serious: 18 per cent of all children between six and 17 are overweight.[90]

Despite paternalistic efforts by the Swedish government to promote healthy lifestyles and to ban or tax unhealthy ones, Sweden seems to be a quite normal European country when it comes to obesity, and very much part of what the WHO calls an epidemic of obesity.[91]

The EU's Involuntary Voluntarism

A book written for a British audience cannot overlook the EU's influence on the obesity crusade's ramifications for the British consumer and taxpayer. In large part, decisions concerning the regulation of food industry advertising and labelling are made at the EU level, even if the enforcement of those decisions takes place at the local level. The very fact that the EU chose to hold an 'Obesity Summit', in Copenhagen in September 2004, did not augur well for EU policymaking in this area. It was not long before the policy rubber hit the proverbial road. According to the Dutch journalist, Joshua Livestro,

> The moment they [the health and consumer protection apparatchiks] hit upon the obesity issue, they pulled out their big guns and started shooting at anything that moved: fast-food outlets, school canteens, advertising agencies, and lately, the soft drinks industry. They issued a series of threats to ban, block or tax anything that contributed to the perceived problem. Pretty soon, Brussels will try to regulate what we can and cannot eat and drink, what we serve our children, even where we buy our meals.[92]

The EU is linking up with the food and marketing industries, consumer groups and health experts, and plans to assess national and industry efforts to counter the allegedly worsening obesity trend. It is the monitoring of the food industry's efforts that makes the EU's approach to the obesity problem 'totally novel', says Philip James, chairman of the International Obesity Task Force, a coalition of obesity scientists and research centres advising the European Union and governments around the world. 'The industry is being challenged to demonstrate, transparently, that it is going to be part of the solution', James said after the launch of the programme in Brussels.[93]

On 20 January 2005, Markos Kyprianou, the EU's health and consumer affairs commissioner, gave the European food industry until 2006 to curb its marketing of fatty and sugary products to children, to make product labels clearer, and to work with governments and health bodies to launch campaigns promoting healthy lifestyles, if the industry is to avoid continent-wide advertising bans and new labelling laws.[94] Unsurprisingly, despite the industry's conciliatory stance (critiqued in a later section of this chapter), a year later the EU Commission was preparing new anti-obesity measures.[95] Irrespective of whether the obesity crusaders themselves are situated within the EU Commission or the Parliament, or are attached via an ideological or financial umbilical cord, it is important to bear in mind their larger goal. Barbara Gallari, a food policy advisor at BEUC, a European consumer lobby group, encapsulates it thus: 'Ideally, we'd like a ban on advertising food and drink to children.'[96]

America Lets a Thousand Regulations Bloom

In America, proposals for government intervention are coming thick and fast. In 2003, for example, 150 bills regulating the food and beverage industry were introduced in state legislatures; more than double the number of the previous year, according to the National Conference of State Legislatives. In 2003, the Arkansas board of education mandated that schools send home a weight report card. Local school districts in Pennsylvania, Massachusetts, Oregon and California already require the same.[97] In state legislatures, anti-obesity advocates are pushing bills that would levy sin taxes on fizzy drinks, require calorie counts on restaurant menus and ban 'foods of minimum nutritional value' in schools. To date, 14 states have passed laws to improve either the nutritional value of school meals or to improve the food products sold in schools. Most of these new state laws include prohibitions on vending machines.

In a fiscal move illustrative of his administration's 'Big Government Conservatism' agenda, President George W. Bush's 2004 budget set aside $200 million for anti-obesity programmes. At the other end of Washington's Pennsylvania Avenue, Congress is currently considering menu-labelling laws. In June 2006, Senator Tom Harkin of Iowa, the senior Democrat on the Senate's Agriculture, Nutrition and Forestry Committee, reintroduced a bill that will require all restaurant chains with more than 20 outlets to list calories, fat and sodium on their menus and menu boards, rather than on individual products.[98] Some congressmen are calling on the Federal Trade Commission to regulate the marketing of junk food.

Many schools, required by a recent federal law to encourage students to become healthier, are drafting nutrition policies. The nutrition policies discussed in the state of Maryland, for example, are required by federal law to take effect in the 2006–07 school year. Most of the state's school systems are creating policies that follow recommendations issued by the Maryland State Board of Education in February 2005. Those recommendations forbid the sale of junk food (including sweets, chocolates and fizzy drinks) in vending machines until the end of the school day. The guidelines also throw out *à la carte* snack foods that have more than nine grams of fat, two grams of saturated fat and 15 grams of sugar.[99] In December 2005, the Institute of Medicine issued a two-year ultimatum to the food and restaurant industries to change their marketing practices 'voluntarily'.

The one ray of sunshine among these gathering legislative and regulatory clouds occurred in March 2004, when the US House of Representatives easily approved legislation to bar people from suing restaurants on the grounds that their food makes customers fat. The bill, formally known as the Personal Responsibility in Food Consumption Act (but also as the 'Cheeseburger Bill'), would have barred new cases and dismissed pending federal and state suits in which damages were being sought as compensation for medical conditions connected to weight gain or obesity that was attributed to restaurant food. To his credit, President Bush endorsed the bill, saying in a statement that 'food manufacturers and sellers should not be held liable for injury because of the person's consumption of legal, unadulterated food and a person's weight gain or obesity'.[100]

This type of legislation is extremely popular with the American people. A poll conducted in mid-2003 found 84 per cent of respondents in agreement with the statement that the government should pass laws to prevent these kinds of lawsuits.[101] Unfortunately, on this occasion, overwhelming public support did not carry the day politically. Although the House of Representatives had comfortably passed the Personal Responsibility in Food Consumption Act, and did so with the president's stamp of approval, the bill never received a vote in the Senate and therefore died a legislative death – at least temporarily. The bill was reintroduced in 2005, and on 19 October was again passed by the House by a huge margin of votes. The bill will now be sent to the Senate.

France's Futile Centralism

In the conventional view of Greg Critser, author of the influential *Fatland*,[102] in France, 'Simply put, the State regulates the excesses of modern life.'[103] Drawing upon the work of the British epidemiologist D. J. Barker, Critser argues that an interventionist French government, by focusing on prenatal care (so-called *'puericulture'*) for more than a century, has produced healthier, more metabolically efficient babies. While the French consume much more fat than the Americans, especially cheese, croissants and pastries, France's obesity rate has historically been a third that of the United States.

It is a long-standing policy of the French government to exert rigorous control over advertisements for food products aimed at children. It is particularly interesting to note, therefore, and especially noteworthy for those who purchased 2005's best-selling paean to Gallic eating habits, *French Women Don't Get Fat*,[104] that the French are also losing the battle of the bulge.[105] According to research conducted by the National Institute for Health and Medical Research, the number of clinically obese adults in France has gone up from 8 to 11 per cent in five years. In the under-15 age group, the figure doubled from 2 to 4 per cent in the same period.

This is very disappointing, especially to those scientists who have long marvelled at France's low levels of obesity.

The problem is so worrying to the French government that it is introducing a law to force food companies to put health warnings on fattening foods and beverages. Soon, food and beverage manufacturers will be forced to pay a 1.5 per cent tax on advertising, unless they display a prominent health warning approved by the health ministry. This follows a vote last year by French parliamentarians that instituted a nation-wide ban on vending machines selling sweets and fizzy drinks in schools.[106]

The French experience, replete with top-down government intervention, actually helps to make the case for less government regulation of the food and beverage industry and of our eating and drinking habits. In truth, an interfering central government cannot withstand the upward pressure being applied to the average Frenchman's weight by economic, cultural and technological trends beyond the public health establishment's control.

Finland's Illiberal Crusade

Two decades ago, Finland's obesity rate was twice that of the UK's. Since then, Britain's official obesity rate has risen significantly, while the Finnish rate has risen only modestly. This relative progress has turned Helsinki into a favourite destination for public health practitioners studying foreign regulatory structures.

The improvements in the Finnish figures stem from an assertive public education campaign to promote exercise and a healthy diet. In Finland, there is little civil libertarian sentiment. Consequently, the Finnish government had *carte blanche* to remake Finnish attitudes to weight, diet and a healthy lifestyle. Finland's social homogeneity was a blessing for the obesity crusaders, for it made the Finnish market far easier to control.[107]

Today, Finnish schoolchildren are weighed annually and the results recorded in their end-of-year reports. Each child receives a free school lunch, which must comprise one third of their calorie intake, and exercise plays a prominent part in the school day. The Finnish food and beverage industry was forced to adapt to changing consumer preferences as better-informed consumers demanded better-quality foodstuffs. Interestingly, there was no advertising ban. Instead of a mass campaign telling people what not to do, Finnish public health officials blitzed the population with positive incentives. Entire towns were set against each other in cholesterol-cutting showdowns. Local competitions were combined with sweeping nationwide changes in legislation.

Farmers were all but forced to produce low-fat milk or grow a new variety of oilseed rape, bred just for the region, that made domestic vegetable oil widely available for the first time. Privately, some claim that the Finnish public health establishment had it easier than its peers in many other nations, as Finns are happy to live in a Nanny State. In Finland, regardless of one's political views, people are largely obedient and trustful of the State.

Though Finland is widely held up by our public health establishment as an example of how to get the obesity crusade right, it is by no means a land of utopian fitness.[108] Like France, Finland faces new challenges. A huge influx of cars in the 1980s has meant fewer people now walk or cycle to work. The resulting upturn in obesity is a significant development. For example, data from the army (national service is compulsory) show that fitness on entry, as measured by a running exercise, has dropped steadily since the 1970s.[109]

THE FOOD AND BEVERAGE INDUSTRY'S NAIVE RESPONSE

There is growing pressure on food and beverage manufacturers to adjust the content, quality and marketing of their products. As the *Economist* observes, 'attacks on the industry have changed the psychological climate in which it operates, and they may yet change the legislative climate too'.[110] The policy momentum has been fuelled by the arguments presented in such books as *Consuming Kids*,[111] a critique of food marketing to children by Harvard psychologist Susan Linn; Eric Schlosser's best-selling *Fast Food Nation*,[112] which alleged that fast-food companies are guilty of contributing to America's obesity problem; and Schlosser and Charles

Wilson's *Chew on This*, which contends that fast-food companies bombard susceptible children with carefully constructed marketing and promotional campaigns.[113] The fast-food industry, in particular, was slow off the mark in taking command of the obesity issue, and this tardiness allowed special interest groups to dominate and dictate the debate.[114] In its initial response, the industry failed miserably to shift the policy spotlight to the fitness and nutrition aspects of the obesity issue.

The industry's latest, proactive response is a strategic move to pre-empt more draconian regulation of the industry.[115] The attitude of companies (particularly in Britain) is to work with, rather than to confront, the government over obesity. The strategic thinking is that cooperation is the best route to minimising regulation's negative impact on the industry. In the past couple of years, therefore, much of the industry has introduced voluntary changes in its production, advertising and labelling practices.[116] For example, PepsiCo has begun a 'Smart Spot' programme that identifies the company's more healthy products, such as orange juice, porridge, diet fizzy drinks and baked crisps. In October 2005, McDonald's introduced a nutritional labelling programme.[117] To address their critics, many other food and beverage firms have also introduced healthier products, such as reduced-sugar cereals and fruit and milk products in fast-food restaurants. In the US, PepsiCo, Coca-Cola and McDonald's all sponsor multi-million dollar children's exercise campaigns.[118] Over the past few years, 4,500 'healthier' food products have been launched.[119]

In the UK, in the autumn of 2004 chocolate manufacturers promised to scrap king-size bars. The following spring, food group Nestlé, maker of brands ranging from Kit-Kat to Nescafé, Golden Grahams and Carnation milk, announced that it was to put the calorie content of its products on the front of packs by the end of 2005, as part of a drive to make it easier for consumers to choose a healthy diet. Every bar of chocolate, packet of pasta, breakfast cereal and yoghurt produced by the world's biggest food group will carry the calorie information. The initiative, also featuring a 'nutritional compass' detailing health information on the back of packets, is part of a global plan to promote 'wellness'.

In 2004, PepsiCo initiated a policy to stop advertising its fizzy drinks to the under-12s. The following spring saw the company, whose products include Pepsi-Cola and Walkers crisps, announce that it was introducing voluntary restrictions on its advertising to children. In January 2005, Kraft, owner of Dairylea, Angel Delight and Toblerone, said it would phase out all advertising to under-12s of products that failed to meet its new nutrition criteria. In 2005, Kraft also began to cease advertising to American children. This year, it will phase out such advertising campaigns worldwide.[120]

Also in 2005, the CIAA, the confederation of food and beverage industries of the EU, agreed to introduce warning labels on its products and accepted restrictions on product advertising, especially advertising to children.[121] It was, therefore, no surprise when, on 25 January 2006, fizzy drink manufacturers in Europe agreed to the EU Commission's request to stop targeting children under the age of 12 in their advertising campaigns. Cadbury Schweppes, Coca-Cola, PepsiCo and their fellow members of the Union of European Beverages Associations (UNESDA) drew up a voluntary code of conduct that also includes commitments to end direct commercial activity in primary schools (that is, the removal of vending machines), and to offer more low-calorie beverages to consumers.[122] This announcement came as the EU Commission launched new rules to ban misleading or false claims about a product's nutritional value.[123] On the other side of the Atlantic, 2 May 2006 saw America's largest beverage companies – Cadbury Schweppes, Coca-Cola and PepsiCo – announce an agreement to end nearly all fizzy drinks sales to schools. Nearly 35 million American pupils will be affected by the deal.[124]

On 3 February 2006, Britain's largest crisp producer, Walkers, bowed to pressure from obesity crusaders and cut the amount of saturated fat in its snacks. Walkers crisps will now contain 70 per cent less saturated fat, and the salt content is also being reduced.[125] Six days later, five of Britain's largest food manufacturers (Danone, Kellogg's, Kraft, Nestlé and PepsiCo) announced an agreement to place labels on the front of all their products, telling shoppers how many calories and how much fat, saturated fat, sugar and salt a serving of each product contains.[126] The labels will also indicate how much the serving contributes to official guideline daily amounts (GDAs) for each of those nutrients.[127]

Such proactive behaviour on the part of the food and beverage industry may appear to be sensible – but only if very short-term business criteria are applied. Joshua Livestro summarises the food industry's delicate regulatory position and subsequent strategy:

> The fact that the Commission has chosen to ignore this [scientific] evidence in its quest for a new legislative agenda puts the European food and drink industry in a particularly difficult position. They certainly wouldn't want to suffer the fate of the tobacco industry, which has been demonized and marginalized and which pretty soon might be legislated out of existence altogether. By taking unilateral steps to address the issue, they hope to show that any problem – whether perceived or real – is always best tackled through self-regulation.[128]

The industry will be disappointed with the regulatory outcome. It will soon become crystal clear that the war on fat is inherently a war on the food and beverage industry itself. No pre-emptive gesture or voluntary measure will satisfy or appease the obesity crusaders. For example, the British food industry's recent announcement of a voluntary labelling scheme was immediately condemned as insufficient by spokespersons for the National Consumer Council, the Consumers' Association and the National Heart Forum.[129] Those in academia, politics and the public health establishment rallying against obesity view this war as a war of attrition. They are in this obesity campaign for the long haul. Their war-room strategy rests upon the correct assumption that the food and beverage industry has failed to learn the lessons of the tobacco industry's unsuccessful public relations campaign: that is, the industry's opponents will not be satisfied until the industry is on its financial and political knees.[130]

A recent leading article in the *Daily Telegraph* is insightful. It recognised that, regarding the manufacturers of this country's food and beverages, 'Their duty is to shareholders and customers, not to presumptuous arbiters of taste. In the name of democracy, big business should stand up to Westminster: the road to modern dictatorship runs through health and safety regulations.'[131] The food and beverage manufacturers should have confidently stood up to their self-righteous accusers; obviously, most of them did not.

Fortunately, the effort to limit our freedoms in the prosecution of the war on obesity will not fall solely upon the shoulders of the food and beverage industry. The general public is slowing waking up to the reality that preposterous policies and programmes are being enacted and planned in their name but without their consent. The following section surveys the opinions of those beyond the political class, and traces the public's truest preferences as she votes with her feet as a food and beverage shopper.

THE SOCIAL ENGINEERS WILL FAIL

What Do People Really Think about Obesity?

It is clear that those who construct and implement obesity policy either do not consult with or do not listen to the public they claim to represent, and in whose interests they claim to act. The obesity crusaders' policy agenda is replete with junk food ad bans, vending machine bans, fat taxes, warning labels and restaurant planning restrictions. This laundry list of heavy-handedness reflects the ideological and philosophical sentiments of its proponents. There is a fundamental conflict between the core democratic values of autonomy and respect and any form of social engineering. The obesity crusade's key assumption is that the State has both the right and the scientific expertise to define what constitutes healthy living.

The public health establishment does not believe that individuals are largely responsible for their own size, weight and level of fitness. It contends that the individual has an obligation to order his life according to the State's judgement about health, and that it might justifiably force him to conform if he initially demurs. However, with very few exceptions, public opinion on both sides of the Atlantic is of a decidedly more libertarian bent on questions pertaining to what government should and can do to combat obesity. Without question, the anti-fat policy agenda cannot be interpreted as a clever effort to win votes. Rather, its inability to command majority support among the public speaks of the feverish ideological commitment that, above all else, sustains the obesity crusader.

Public opinion data sympathetic to the obesity crusade are limited and largely dated. According to a poll by the Harvard School of Public Health in May 2003, half of those Americans surveyed thought that obesity was a 'private matter', while the other half said obesity was a 'public health issue that society needs to help solve'. Some 77 per cent said the government should promote exercise, and 62 per cent supported a requirement for nutritional information to appear on menus. Critically, almost every scientific poll taken in the past three years has found declining levels of support for both the philosophical underpinnings and the chosen weapons of the obesity crusade. According to a survey conducted by Lightspeed Research, almost three-quarters of Europeans blame parents for childhood obesity, compared with 13 per cent who feel that advertisers and food manufacturers are responsible.[132]

Despite the obesity crusaders' best efforts, the American public does not consider obesity to be a national health crisis.[133] Nor do Americans accept the argument that personal responsibility is not applicable in the case of obesity. Scholarly investigation into Americans' views on obesity was initiated by political scientists Eric Oliver and Taeku Lee. Their survey research has found that most Americans view obesity as a sign of individual failure, rather than stemming from environmental or genetic sources.[134] A July 2004 survey conducted by Universal McCann found that 83 per cent of Americans thought it was the responsibility of individuals to get obesity under control.[135] A 2004 poll by the *Wall Street Journal* and Harris Interactive found that 83 per cent of Americans thought the reason for an increased rate of obesity was, simply, 'People do not exercise enough.' Neither eating 'too much fast food' nor consuming 'too many calories' garnered half as much blame.

According to a November 2002 poll by the opinion research firm Planet Feedback, Americans are far less willing to blame the food and restaurant industry than they are to blame a lack of education and self-responsibility for the country's weight problem. The Universal McCann study found that only 26 per cent blamed food and beverage companies for obesity problems. Some 65 per cent of American respondents believed that advertisers were not to blame for obesity. Consequently, most Americans (56 per cent) oppose restricting advertisements for fast food on children's television programmes.[136] Some 84 per cent of those surveyed placed the primary responsibility for Americans' weight problems on 'individuals who do not exercise enough'. An Ipsos survey carried out in autumn 2005 found that parents of overweight children gave their child's lack of exercise as the principal reason for their heaviness.[137]

Closer to home, a survey conducted for the FSA suggests that most Britons think the primary responsibility for improving a child's diet rests with the child's parents (88 per cent). Schools (43 per cent) were next, followed by food manufacturers (30 per cent). In a similar vein, 83 per cent of Americans blame parents, rather than the food industry, for obesity, according to the *Wall Street Journal Online*/Harris Interactive poll. The Universal McCann study found that 42 per cent of British respondents blamed the food industry. Fifty per cent believed that food and beverage advertising was not to blame for obesity.

Recent surveys conducted by the French vending machine association Navsa have found that 67 per cent of secondary school pupils and 60 per cent of their parents thought banning junk food advertising was going too far.[138]

Only 8 per cent of Americans support a tax on junk food.[139] Neither do American consumers believe in suing restaurants and food producers for their own dietary excesses. According to a July 2003 Gallup poll, only 9 per cent were in favour of obesity lawsuits.[140] Interestingly, respondents who describe themselves as overweight are no more likely to support such litigation. Americans also overwhelmingly oppose allowing parents to sue for their children's obesity. Only 6 per cent think 'parents should be able to sue major soft-drink and snack food companies if they believe their child became obese from eating junk food and drinking soft drinks'.[141] In 2004, 56 per cent of Americans said they would not side with the plaintiff in obesity cases.[142] Meanwhile, in the UK, an opinion survey has found that most Britons think those who are obese should be charged for NHS treatment.[143]

Choosing for Ourselves – Obesity and Consumer Behaviour

As shoppers, how are people responding to the obesity crusade? Overall, it is clear that most people are paying little, if any, attention to the call for less and healthier eating. One media report has observed that consumers have responded to the government's healthy-eating message by stuffing themselves with cake, swilled down with plenty of alcohol.

In apparent defiance of warnings about obesity, cake sales rose by 5 per cent in 2004. Cake did not prove to be the only culinary vice of choice, however. According to the *Grocer* magazine's annual survey of top brands, British shoppers also spent significantly more on chocolate, biscuits and fat-laden foods in general.[144] The super-sized chocolate bar has come in for a disproportionate share of criticism for its alleged role in ruining the diet of the average Briton. Very few regular people seem to care. The latest figures confirm that king-size Mars and Snickers chocolate bars continue to sell in their millions.[145]

Britain remains a nation of snack eaters, spending more on crisps and chocolate than any other country in Europe.[146]

People are ordering larger portions of food in restaurants, according to a poll by *Caterer and Hotelkeeper* magazine.[147] New figures released in autumn 2005 found that Britons were eating more ready meals than ever before. In the 12 months prior to the report, the country spent more than £900 million on quick-fix dinners that are typically high in saturated fat, salt and sugar.[148] Some 40 per cent of British food is now eaten in restaurants, fish and chip shops, pubs and burger bars. The market in out-of-house food grew by £10 billion between 1988 and 2003.[149]

The documentation of our consumer preferences would be incomplete if we ignored the results of an experiment that could have been entitled 'Policymaker, heal thyself'. In November 2003, a week-long experiment took place in the House of Commons canteen. The plan to sell exclusively 'healthy' food did not go down a treat with the obesity crusade's legislative warriors. As the BBC reported, with characteristic understatement, the experiment failed to meet with universal approval from MPs, and many protests were registered in the customer complaint book. One dissatisfied, if pithy, member of the political class simply inquired, 'Where are the chips?'[150]

American attitudes to diet are also more relaxed than they used to be. A recent *New York Times* survey of the available data found that 'There seem to be more health unconscious consumers than anyone could have guessed.'[151] According to another survey, 'The better-for-you food pendulum that so quickly changed the look of fast food menus and that's often credited with changing consumer eating habits nationwide appears to be swinging back. Or maybe it never really swung away from indulgence in the first place.'[152] The American sales of fast-food chains grew from $6 billion in 1970 to $134 billion in 2005.[153] Additional evidence comes most recently from a survey by the NPD Group published in the journal *Rationality and Society*.[154] The article recalls that, in the late 1980s and early 1990s, American fast-food chains rushed to install salad bars. In 1989, salads as a main course peaked at 10 per cent of all restaurant meals. Today, those salad bars have declined significantly; salads now account for just 5.5 per cent of main courses.[155] At present, the fastest-growing food in American restaurants is fried chicken.[156] Sales in all fast-food categories are rising. According to *Business Week*, 'Americans are eating hamburgers, doughnuts, French fries and fried chicken like never before.'[157] During 2005, American sales of sweet baked goods rose to $12 billion; that same year, ice cream sales rose 3.1 per cent to $21.7 billion, while chocolate product sales rose 4 per cent to $17.8 billion.[158]

Far fewer Americans say that they are trying to 'avoid snacking entirely' (26 per cent in 2005, down from 45 per cent in 1985). In 2005, 53 per cent of housewives tried to avoid snacking, but that figure is down from 71 per cent in 1985.[159] Some 75 per cent of Americans said they had consumed low-fat, no-fat or reduced-fat products in the last two weeks, but that figure is down from 86 per cent in 1999, according to an NPD Group survey. The proportion of the population currently on a diet is not increasing. Twenty years ago, 25 per cent of Americans were dieting; today, it is the same.[160]

It is also true that consumer tastes are gradually changing over time. For example, the American grocery market does indicate growth in fruit and vegetable purchases for consumption at home. According to the USDA, per capita consumption of fresh fruit has increased by 30 per cent, while fresh vegetable consumption has gone up by 35 per cent.[161] However, given how cheap fresh produce is in America, it should come as no surprise that fruit and vegetable consumption has risen steadily since 1970, well before the obesity crusade became a regulatory reality.

The British experience with fruit and vegetables certainly does not inspire confidence in government programmes. Statistics recently released by the Department for Environment, Food and Rural Affairs show that Britons' daily intake of fruit and vegetables is declining, while the consumption of saturated fats and sugars is increasing.[162] Is it time for a government campaign to turn consumer habits around? The government has already gone down that particular blind alley. In 2000, it initiated a 'five-a-day' campaign to promote the consumption of fruit and vegetables – with predictably disappointing results.

Purchasing habits among non-alcoholic beverage consumers are also evolving. Fizzy drinks sales at both Coca-Cola and PepsiCo are flat in developed markets.[163] PepsiCo's position has improved relative to Coca-Cola, however, as a result of its diversification away from sugary carbonated drinks. PepsiCo was the first to realise that beverage consumers were relatively health conscious and that healthier options were increasingly in demand.[164] Hence, PepsiCo now generates 23 per cent of its worldwide profits from the fizzy drinks sector, while Coca-Cola relies on its fizzy drinks for 85 per cent of its profits.[165]

THE THREAT TO PERSONAL RESPONSIBILITY

In matters of public policy, our default position is that the State should not dictate to people how to live their lives. Citizens should be free to decide, for example, what they eat and drink. We believe these to be inviolable matters of personal freedom and taste. People do not want to be told what is good for them. They want to decide for themselves – and are perfectly capable of doing so. Our view, of course, is far from universally shared in academic, political and bureaucratic circles. Indeed, the obesity crusaders' propensity to meddle in matters best left to individual choice appears limitless.

Still, the obesity crusaders cannot have it both ways. On the one hand, the British government's November 2004 Public Health White Paper stated that it was not the role of government to force people to become healthy. The then health secretary, John Reid, observed that 'People make their own choices about health.' So far, so good. Yet Reid immediately contradicted himself with the statement that 'This government's role is to help ensure society moves in the right direction.'[166] That would not be the right direction according to individual Britons, of course, but it would be the right direction according to the government of the day and a horde of self-interested public health lobbyists. Hence the admission from the newly ensconced head of the FSA, Dame Deirdre Hutton, that 'I want the "healthy option" to be the main-stream option.'[167] Both Reid and Dame Deirdre ignore the individual Briton's right to eat, drink and exercise (or not) in whatever manner he or she desires.

Within the crusaders' tent, the logic cannot be faulted. The preference voiced by Reid and Hutton is inherently the better option. Hence, that option should and must become everyone's preference. In practice, the laws that are passed and the regulations that are enforced in the obesity crusade conspire both to restrict our choices and to make them more expensive – often prohibitively so. As the author of a Freedom Institute publication observed, 'The public health lobby ... seeks to use State coercion of various types to make us better people, at least as far as our diets are concerned.'[168] As a nation, therefore, we run the significant risk that many of the policy proposals to prevent obesity will erode further our individual liberties by enhancing the State's exclusive power to define what constitutes a good life.

Though there is a passing nod to personal responsibility in this obesity tale, generally policymakers choose to treat citizens as infantile individuals unable to cope with social problems. How do the less educated and the less well-off learn to make responsible choices for themselves if everyday decisions, such as those involving eating and drinking, are repeatedly made for them? Waldemar Ingdahl notes the paradox: 'There is something of a discrepancy in our affluent society: wealthier individuals tend to take a bigger responsibility for their health and bodies. Fortunately, such habits tend to spread throughout society over time, but not if those who need the most educating (often those of low income) are accustomed to someone else ... asserting responsibility over their bodies.'[169] Younger people are cognisant of the paradox. That is why Alex Nichols is correct. The 16-year-old student representative on the Calvert County, Maryland, school board maintains that removing vending machines from schools, for example, sends the wrong message to pupils. 'This is a big deal – huge. It's about choices', she says. 'How can we learn to make good choices if people keep making our choices for us?'[170]

All this social nannying is having an impact on the lives of ordinary people. David Lewis is a psychologist specialising in workplace health. He has noticed that:

> A lot of people think their health is someone else's concern. We drink, eat and are merry without proper consideration because we think we can just go and see a doctor and he or she will cure us. That mentality is now creeping into the workplace. If we put on weight, we sue McDonald's. Employers now fear the prospect of litigation brought against them by employees who blame their poor health on the workplace rather than high-fat, sedentary lifestyles.[171]

David Marsland, a leading sociologist, is unsurprised that the mindset of reliance on the Nanny State has moved into the workplace. After all, 'Once you have a big welfare state in place, the excuse for state nannying is infinite in scale', he says. 'This seems very dangerous as it continues the process of reducing self-reliance and handing responsibility for ourselves to external bodies.'[172]

CONCLUSION

Eating food can be, often is, and should be a pleasurable experience. However, today the pleasure of eating what we want, when we want it, and how we want it prepared, is deemed immoral by those whose received wisdom places them in the exalted position of knowing our best dietary habits. In the past few years, a moral-cum-cultural, rather than a scientific, position on overweight and obesity has metastasised into an ideological *fatwa* against those who produce, market and consume fat. The inability and unwillingness of academic, scientific, political and corporate actors to call a halt to this corruption of the scientific method and its resultant perversion of the policymaking process has confirmed the obesity crusaders' strategic wisdom. This is a strategy centred upon the expectation that those in philosophical and political opposition will prove to be their own worst enemy, presenting themselves as intellectually insecure and politically naive.

Consequently, the philosophy underpinning the obesity crusade has morphed into a policy menu riddled with pseudoscience, politically correct jargon, and intolerance of dissent and rational debate. Sadly, to date the respective British, North American and continental European experiences are uniform in their execution of doomed regulatory structures that differ only in the degree to which they have internalised and propagated the fatal conceit of a top-down, paternalistic campaign to combat obesity. This has produced a generic, statist and deeply illiberal policy framework that minimises the individual's responsibility for his own physical condition, and thereby seeks to limit his freedom to choose the dietary path and level of physical activity best suited to his own particular needs and preferences.

To the surprise of many, but not the obesity crusaders themselves, the social engineering project still gathering momentum behind closed doors in Whitehall is not taking heavy fire on the battlefield from those institutional actors whose financial self-interest is most directly threatened by the obesity crusade. Rather, it is the innate common sense of individual Britons, matched by their peers around Europe and across the Atlantic, that is providing the numerical bulwark against the obesity crusaders' siren song of a New (Thin) Man. The attitudes and the behaviour of ordinary people are the greatest threat to the obesity crusaders' attack on the principle of personal responsibility that underpins our economic and political liberties. It is to the subject of personal responsibility and the appropriate role of government that we turn in our final chapter.

CHAPTER 5

AN ALTERNATIVE PRESCRIPTION TO GOVERNMENT REGULATION

All things are poisonous and nothing is without poison. It is only the dose that makes things poisonous.

Paracelsus,
16th century pharmacologist

INTRODUCTION

In a 26 January 2006 speech at St James's Palace, Prince Charles warned the British people that they were in danger of becoming as obese as many Americans. 'We are perhaps not very far behind our American cousins in the super-sizing epidemic', said the Prince.[1] Prince Charles is, of course, completely wrong on the facts. As the preceding chapters have documented, there is no obesity epidemic, either here or in America. We do not know if Prince Charles is also aware that fat was not always considered a four-letter word. Never before in human experience has too much, rather than too little, food been considered a menace to society. Worldwide, more people (one billion) are now overfed than underfed.[2] According to the United Nations' Food and Agriculture Organization, the number of undernourished people fell from 920 million in 1980 to 799 million 20 years later, even though the world's population increased by 1.6 billion over the period.[3] Oxford University's Stanley Ulijaszek reminds us that 'In Britain, 200 years ago being fat was associated with good health. Now, being fat is not seen very positively.'[4] Early in the twentieth century, poor people were almost exclusively thin. A century later, lower-income individuals are far more likely to be overweight than the population as a whole.[5]

Social norms do not remain constant. Hence, the social pressure upon women, in particular, to be either fat or thin has fluctuated over the centuries. During certain eras, heavy women were idealised, most visibly in seventeenth-century painter Peter Paul Rubens's full-figured Rubensesque women. In other eras, society has preferred petite women with small waists. In American popular culture, there was the Gibson Girl of the 1890s; in the 1960s, British popular culture produced the supermodel, Twiggy, whose thinness set the standard for female appearance for many years.

In truth, our obsession with fat is based less on science than on morality. Politically incorrect attitudes about politics, sex, race and class are central to the focus on obesity. 'We are in a moral panic about obesity', finds Sander L. Gilman, professor of liberal arts, sciences and medicine at the University of Illinois in Chicago and the author of *Fat Boys*.[6] Gilman describes how plumpness used to be associated with affluence and the aristocracy, while today it is associated with the poor and their supposedly bad eating habits.

Social historian Peter Stearns notes the often arbitrarily shifting definitions of obesity throughout history – an arbitrariness that, as documented in an earlier chapter, continues to the present day. Stearns points out that fatness was once associated with 'good health in a time when many of the most troubling diseases were wasting diseases like tuberculosis'.[7] He traces the equation of obesity and moral deficiency to World War One. During that war, some popular magazines actually said that eating too much and gaining weight were unpatriotic, presumably because of concerns about food shortages. According to Stearns, the evolution in attitudes toward obesity constituted a moral reaction to the new abundance of food. 'I don't think we were comfortable with it because of religious legacies and hesitations', he told the *New York Times*. 'Having a target for self-control, like dieting, helped express but also reconcile moral concerns about consumer affluence', as anti-fatness became a new kind of Puritanism.[8]

THE PRODUCT OF AFFLUENCE

Two centuries ago, at the height of the Industrial Revolution, insufficient exposure to sunlight and inadequate milk consumption meant that many British children suffered from rickets, to the disgust of social reformers and public health campaigners. Today, this country's working class and its poorer citizens are no longer in danger of receiving too little sustenance; rather, it is now the concern of the self-appointed public health guardians that lower-income Britons readily consume too much food too cheaply. Vast affluence has afflicted contemporary children with obesity. Cato Institute policy analyst Radley Balko cautions us to maintain some historical perspective on the issue. He writes that

> Obesity is an affliction of prosperity. Not only has our remarkable economy managed to feed all of its citizens, our chief worry right now seems to be that our poor and middle class have *too much* to eat. That's a remarkable achievement. And in the proper historical context, it's not such a bad problem to have.[9]

Therefore, as Zoe Williams recently noted, 'Obesity ... is a function of social progress.'[10] Yet, there are many who remain decidedly uncomfortable with a definition of progress that allows for – even encourages – mass consumption of so much food at such a low cost, a circumstance unimaginable just decades ago. On both sides of the Atlantic, societies are playing out their current cultural hang-ups and expressing class-based and racial tensions through the politically correct mechanism of the obesity debate. The scientist-turned-broadcaster Vivienne Parry points out that 'Obesity is one of those areas where science meets culture full on. Science has always been used by some as a church to which they retreat for factual underpinning of their moral beliefs. Fat people are bad, fat people are lazy, fat people are symptomatic of our moral decline.'[11]

It is no secret that overweight and obesity rates are higher in minority populations. In America, for example, the obesity rate is much higher among Blacks and Hispanics than among

Anglo Whites. Legal scholar Paul Campos has studied this aspect of the obesity phenomenon and has fleshed out his concerns in *The Obesity Myth*.[12] His research has led him to the inescapable conclusion that 'Obesity is used as a socially legitimate means for the rich, who are often thinner, to express their revulsion at the poor, who tend to be fatter. By focusing on fat, it's perfectly OK for a skinny white person in an SUV to condemn a fat Guatemalan woman.'[13] Obesity in America, according to Campos, is 'primarily a cultural and political issue'. 'The war on fat', he argues, 'is unique in American history in that it represents the first concerted attempt to transform the vast majority of the nation's citizens into social pariahs, to be pitied and scorned.'[14]

Obesity is, indeed, a function of social progress. Nevertheless, as Gregg Easterbrook has suggested, obesity also epitomises the unsettled character of progress in affluent Western society.[15] Largely through implicit signals and code words, the larger debate over the relative merits of democratic capitalism versus state socialism is currently playing out through the explicit debate over the government's response to obesity. Are we responsible adults capable of rational decision-making when purchasing and consuming food and beverages for ourselves and our children? Or are we malleable, child-like creatures led hither and yonder by the siren song of advertising, a creative effort that seeks not to enrich our bodies, but to enrich the nation's food and beverage manufacturers at the expense of our health?

Today's puritanical flame is kept burning by the obesity crusaders' vocal and well-funded calls for draconian measures to halt a (manufactured) epidemic of fat people. As the previous chapter demonstrated, the obesity crusaders' legislative and regulatory weapons are blunt, crude and unsophisticated instruments destined to fail in their ultimate goal of victory on the obesity battlefield. Yet, the political momentum carrying them forward will force the rest of us to yield significant ground in the realm of our economic and civil liberties *if* the terms of the obesity debate are not recast. For the war on obesity possesses enormous potential for eroding individual liberty through employment of the engine of the State, particularly its propaganda and regulatory powers, once again to define and enforce a single vision of what constitutes a good life. The claim of State-enforced healthy living as scientifically mandated is both fundamentally fraudulent and morally illegitimate. We know that the interventionist approach will not be successful.[16] However, the call for 'something to be done' will echo around Westminster, the EU Commission in Brussels and Capitol Hill in Washington until calmer heads prevail.

In the interim, the presentation of an alternative approach to obesity control rests upon two stubborn facts. First, obesity is normally, if not exclusively, a matter of personal responsibility. Second, a variety of non-interventionist tools may be employed, at the individual rather than the political level, to arrest any growth in obesity. These measures come with a warning label of their own. They are neither politically sexy nor short-term solutions. They do constitute, however, a low-cost, positive approach to fighting obesity that has one great advantage over the current regulatory menu on offer in the UK, continental Europe and North America: they are founded upon sound science and liberal democratic principles. Collectively, they represent the potential triumph of experience over hope.

CORRUPT SCIENCE THREATENS DEMOCRATIC PUBLIC POLICY

The careful analysis of the scientific claims of the obesity epidemic provided in this book reveals a systematic disregard for the evidence about the causes, the extent and the dangers of obesity. In practice, the obesity crusaders employ a *modus operandi* that legitimises scientific misrepresentation in the service of a good cause: that is, an obesity-free society.

Is an obesity-free society sufficient justification for a public health movement founded on unsound science? Both the process of producing corrupted science and that of utilising it as the basis for public policy demand a fundamental intolerance of dissent, both scientific and otherwise.

Therefore, despite the vital role of questions, argument and dissent in science, as well as in democratic life, the process of corrupted science seeks to silence dissent in the interests not of protection of the truth, but of misrepresentation of the truth.

For all the moral problems that the use of corrupted science raises, the equally (if not far more) disturbing issue that it introduces is the implications of bad science in the public policy process. What are the consequences of introducing corrupted science into the democratic public policy process? The effects of using such science are fundamentally at odds with the character of a democratic society. The goal of democratic public policy is to minimise public harms, to the extent that this is possible within the context of such fundamental democratic values as diversity, autonomy, respect, rationality and fairness.

Both the agenda of legitimate public policy in a democracy and the process used to consider that agenda are constrained by certain non-negotiable values. What marks certain policy options and certain policy processes out as illegitimate and non-democratic is their conflict with these core non-negotiable values. Placed within this context, it is clear that the obesity crusade's use of corrupted science is a threat – not at some peripheral point, but at the very centre – to democratic values and to democratic public policy. Corrupted science and the use of corrupted science in the creation of policy threaten both the process and the values that characterise democratic public policy. This threat should be of concern to everyone, fat or thin.

THE RISKS OF DIETING

Being fit is actually more important than being fat. A burgeoning scientific literature is establishing the positive aspects of being overweight.[17] Going through life carrying excess weight may not enhance the quality of life of every overweight individual, but it is increasingly clear, from an empirical standpoint, that a healthy fat person is in better shape, so to speak, than an unhealthy thin person.

For some time, scientists have struggled to understand why soaring levels of obesity are failing to affect life expectancy. While concerns about fatness mount, the US Department of Health and Human Services has itself stressed that Americans 'are now living longer and living better than ever before'.[18] In 2004, Americans' life expectancy reached a historic high. Heart disease and cancer, the two diseases most linked to obesity, are both in decline.[19] Increasingly, therefore, researchers are challenging the conventional wisdom that there is a causal relationship between being overweight and being unhealthy. According to Steven Blair, director of research at the Cooper Institute for Aerobics Research in Dallas, the evidence suggests that fitness is more important than fatness, and being fat does not necessarily mean you are not fit. Blair studied 25,000 patients over eight years. His conclusion is that it is better to be fat and active than to be skinny and sedentary.[20]

As fatness may have received an unwarranted bad name, so dieting may not be as helpful to one's health as previously believed. In fact, research published in the journal *Public Library of Science Medicine* finds dieting may be positively harmful to one's health.[21] Finnish researchers followed 2,957 overweight or obese, but otherwise healthy, Finns for 18 years. The data showed that those who wanted to lose weight and succeeded were significantly more likely to die young than those who stayed overweight. Thorkild Sørensen, the lead researcher, observed that 'Healthy overweight or obese subjects who try to lose weight and succeed in doing so over a six-year period suffer from almost double the risk of dying during the next 18 years compared with subjects who do not try to lose weight and whose weight remains stable.'

The Finnish results replicate the findings of an earlier study by the US National Center for Chronic Disease Prevention and Health Promotion in Atlanta, Georgia.[22] This study followed 6,391 subjects and reached the same conclusion. The stress of dieting weakens the organs, decimates lean tissue, and makes people much more vulnerable to diseases far more insidious than fat.

THE IMPORTANCE OF PERSONAL RESPONSIBILITY

Two years ago, the World Health Organization (WHO) released its Global Strategy on Diet, Physical Activity and Health. Something was conspicuous by its absence from the report – any mention of personal responsibility. Fortunately, the former director of communications for the WHO's European Office, Franklin Apfel, provided ideological insight into this glaring policy omission. He later told a Dublin conference, 'we are all influenced by "hazard merchants" selling us a false view of things like … high density foodstuffs – we're given the impression that these things represent personal choice, autonomy and freedom'.[23]

Despite the WHO's best efforts, however, we cannot escape the role of personal accountability. Labelling obesity a 'disease' turns the concept of personal responsibility on its head, thereby threatening a fundamental assault on core democratic values. 'The culture of victimhood, where individuals can shunt the blame for their own actions on to someone else, has reached epic proportions', notes Dan Mindus, a senior analyst at the Washington-based Center for Consumer Freedom.[24]

In addition to one's genetic endowment, the contributors to obesity worth discussing here are those controlled by individual behaviour. These are the real 'risk factors' that may be addressed without inviting the heavy hand of the State into our supermarket trolleys.

Dietary Habits and Preferences

British eating habits have changed quite dramatically in the past generation. More people are now eating out, and people have fewer cooking skills. Our eating habits are now determined by a lifestyle of convenience. In a national study of 6,212 children and adolescents published in the journal *Pediatrics*, researchers at the US Department of Agriculture (USDA) and the Harvard Medical School found that, on a typical day, 30 per cent of the people surveyed ate fast food. The media certainly promote the message that there is a causal relationship between eating out and obesity.[25] In fact, in 2001 Britons spent an average of £7 million a day on fast food – more than any other nation in Europe.

Nevertheless, US Surgeon General Richard Carmona does not blame fast food for putting extra weight on Americans. 'Americans eat out an average of four times per week', he notes. 'That means that there are 17 meals at home per week where they are making bad choices. And even with the meals eaten out, it's still our own decision.'[26] A recent study published in the journal *Obesity Research* hypothesised that human overeating is not just a passive response to salient environmental triggers and powerful physiological drives; it is also about making choices. Eating more 'is fundamentally about making choices between short-lived and overabundant rewards in the face of a disadvantageous long-term outcome if the behavior is done in excess'. The researchers' conclusion is that 'poor decision-making skills in general lead to the food choices associated with obesity'.[27]

Whether they are eating at home or in a restaurant, the obese may simply be eating too fast. A new study by Japanese researchers suggests that slow eaters are less likely to add weight than those who quickly finish their meals. The study found a direct correlation between speed of eating and BMI. The slowest eaters showed the lowest rise in BMI from age 20, while the quickest eaters showed the greatest increase in BMI. The findings suggest that 'eating fast may lead to obesity independent of energy intake or other lifestyle factors in middle-aged, non-diabetic men and women', the research team reported at the annual meeting of the North American Association for the Study of Obesity in October 2005.[28]

Exercise

As has been detailed, contemporary weight gain is not the result of higher food consumption; rather, it reflects a reduction in physical exertion. Three years ago, then Food and Drug Administration Commissioner Dr Mark McClellan noted that actual levels of caloric intake among the young, for example, have not changed appreciably over the last 20 years.[29] Research by Professor Lisa Sutherland of the

University of North Carolina found that, while childhood obesity jumped 10 per cent between 1980 and 2000, caloric intake rose only 1 per cent. The culprit is a lack of physical activity. During the 1980s and the 1990s, physical activity declined by 13 per cent.

A study published in April 2004 in the American Medical Association's *Archives of Pediatrics and Adolescent Medicine* found that 'insufficient vigorous physical activity was the only risk factor' for overweight boys and girls.[30] A report by the UK's top medical advisor reached a similar conclusion. Rising obesity among Britons is also due to a lack of exercise.[31]

For the first time in many years, membership of British gyms is in decline.[32] Furthermore, as a survey has found, most overweight British women seeking to shed pounds choose a fashionable diet over cardiovascular exercise or lifting weights at a gym. In fact, overweight women are more likely to turn to cosmetic surgery, slimming pills or starvation to solve their problems, than to exercise.[33]

Only one American pupil in 10 walks to school; in the UK, the figure is one in two.[34] Nevertheless, nine out of 10 British schoolchildren are not doing enough exercise to ensure that they grow into healthy adults, according to a major new study. The sedentary lifestyles of many young Britons mean they are much more likely to become obese in later life.[35] Today's generation of schoolchildren spend 70 per cent less time being physically active than their parents, according to new research conducted by the polling firm IPSOS UK.[36] Children spend only three hours and 30 minutes per week being active, compared with their parents as children, who spent on average 11 hours and 35 minutes. Moreover, the parents spent five hours per week taking part in organised sporting activities outside school during their childhood, whereas today's children spend an average of only two hours. In 1971, physical recreation was by far the chief leisure activity for single people aged 15–30. Today, drinking alcohol is the chief leisure activity for people aged 15–29.[37]

Forty per cent of people use their cars to take short journeys, when perhaps they could walk.[38] More than 75 per cent of Londoners are not doing the recommended amount of weekly exercise (30 minutes of moderate activity five times a week), a YouGov poll has found.[39] Since 1960, the proportion of trips to work by walking has declined by more than 70 per cent. The typical woman who spends 14 years in a sedentary job will gain an extra 20 pounds compared to women in the least sedentary jobs, according to a study published by the National Bureau of Economic Research.[40] The Urban Institute reports that the number of American workers involved in physically demanding jobs has dropped from 20 per cent in 1950 to 8 per cent today.[41]

The situation at home has also changed considerably. Thanks to technology, we burn 20 per cent fewer calories on housework than we did a generation ago. Three decades ago, 80 per cent of American children walked or biked to school, at least occasionally. Now, more than 80 per cent never do. Today, American children are six times more likely to play a video game than ride a bike on a given day. Meanwhile, just a quarter of secondary school pupils are enrolled in PE class at any one time.[42] The number of physical education classes in American schools is declining steadily, and today Illinois is the only state that still requires daily physical education classes for pupils from infant school through secondary school. Furthermore, there is now a trend in American primary schools to ban traditional games during playtime.[43]

What do we know about the physical activity patterns of American adults? In November 2005, the Centers for Disease Control and Prevention (CDC) released a report that found that less than 50 per cent of Americans meet the government's minimum recommendations for daily physical activity, and that one American in five is completely physically inactive – that is, they do not exercise at a moderate or vigorous level for even 10 minutes per week.[44] In Washington, DC, almost four out of every 10 Hispanic adults surveyed by the Council of Latino Agencies in September 2005 did not exercise regularly.[45]

Parenting

Although the majority of parents claim that they try to make their children eat healthily, only about half of families are

255

actually doing anything about it. These were the findings of a report on childhood obesity conducted by the consumer researcher Mintel. Of the 25,000 parents surveyed, just over half claimed that they tried to limit the amount of sugar eaten by their offspring, and only 42 per cent had done anything to restrict the amount of high-fat food eaten by their youngsters. One in three families reported that they had little interest in their children's eating habits and were 'relaxed' about their diets, while one in six described themselves as 'indulgent parents' who would give their child what it wanted, whether it was healthy food or not.[46]

This indifference was confirmed in a report in autumn 2005 by the school dinner provider, Scolarest. The Scolarest Healthy Eating Report 2005 showed that nearly half of children aged 7–14 ate chocolate, cake, sweets or biscuits every day at home.[47] The study found that many parents were failing to teach children healthy eating habits, and often let them help themselves to any food they wanted. Children were more likely to survive on unhealthy snacks at home than to sit down to a freshly cooked meal. Nearly half of the 7–14-year-olds surveyed chose what they wanted to eat for breakfast, lunch or supper, and more than one third told researchers that they made their own breakfast or evening meal without supervision every day.

Sleep

Over the past 50 years, the average daily time spent in bed has dropped from more than nine hours to seven. New research published in the *International Journal of Obesity* shows that less sleep leads to increased body weight, as sleep deprivation results in reduced levels of leptin, a protein that regulates body fat, and increased levels of ghrelin, which stimulates food intake. In short, sleep restriction increases hunger and appetite.[48]

A reduction in the time people spend asleep could partly account for obesity rates, a study published in the journal *Public Library of Science Medicine* revealed. The research suggests that not only are many adults suffering chronic sleep deprivation, but children are, too. The result is hyperactive children, increased levels of stress, poor memory and obesity.[49]

Researchers at the University of Bristol have found that hormonal changes caused by lack of sleep could lead to increased appetite. According to report author Shahrad Taheri, 'Individuals who spent less than eight hours sleeping were shown to have a greater likelihood of being heavier.' This research is one of three studies published around the same time that yielded similar results: its outcomes were replicated in a second piece of research, conducted at the University of Chicago, and a third study, by Columbia University researchers, also found that people who slept four hours or less per night were 73 per cent more likely to be obese.[50] In 2004, a team from the Mailman School of Public Health and the Obesity Research Center at Columbia analysed data on 18,000 people aged between 32 and 59 who had participated in the National Health and Nutrition Examination Survey during the 1980s. They found that, even after factors such as depression, physical activity, alcohol consumption, ethnicity, level of education, age and gender had been taken into account, people were more likely to be obese the less sleep they had.[51]

Television

The latest statistics reveal that, on average, Americans spend four hours and 39 minutes watching television each day. It has been shown that television is linked to weight gain, as children are less active and eat while watching. In a study published in 2003 in the *Journal of the American Medical Association*, researchers calculated that, for every two hours a day spent watching television, there is a 23 per cent increase in obesity.[52]

A new study suggests that the amount of television children watch accurately predicts whether they will go on to become overweight. Researchers at New Zealand's University of Otago studied how much television children aged five to 15 watched. The *International Journal of Obesity* study found that the 41 per cent who were overweight or obese by the age of 26 were those who had watched the most television. Lead researcher Robert Hancock observed that 'The correlation between television viewing and BMI is stronger than reported correlations between BMI and diet or physical activity.'[53]

Yet, only 36 per cent of parents limit how much television their children watch or how much time they spend on the Internet. Consequently, the average 15-year-old now watches a screen for 53 hours a week, up from 38 hours a decade ago.[54]

Smoking

One important, if grossly underreported, catalyst for obesity has been the significant decline in smoking in most Western nations. Former smokers tend to gain weight. Appetite-suppressing cigarette usage in the UK has fallen off significantly over the past generation. In 1971, 47 per cent of adults were smokers, compared to 27 per cent in 2001.[55] According to a study by the Health and Social Care Information Centre, the proportion of men who smoked dropped from 28 per cent in 1993 to 22 per cent in 2004, while female smokers decreased more slowly – from 26 per cent to 23 per cent.[56]

Research indicates that smokers tend to weigh less than non-smokers. This is because nicotine works as an appetite suppressant. In America, CDC researchers estimate that about a quarter of the country's weight gain among men can be traced to smoking cessation.[57] Economist Michael Grossman of the City University of New York has analysed the economic causes of obesity. Grossman has calculated that, for every 10 per cent increase in the price of cigarettes, the number of obese people rises by 2 per cent. He estimates that smoking cessation has accounted for 20 per cent of the obesity increase in America.[58]

ALTERNATIVES TO GOVERNMENT REGULATION

There is no simple solution to reducing obesity, because no single factor is responsible. The nationalisation of the British diet, an extreme policy measure advocated by the obesity crusaders, would be both scientifically unsound and insufficient to address the causes. A study published recently confirms that, although primary care physicians have been advised to provide counselling on diet and exercise to their young, overweight patients, precious little reliable information is available to medical practitioners on effective anti-obesity strategies.[59]

Fundamentally, the body-weight problem is part and parcel of the way we live our lives today. University of Chicago scholars Thomas J. Philipson, an economist, and Richard A. Posner, a sitting judge and renowned legal scholar, examined whether the economic benefits and costs of obesity can be used to explain its variations across time and populations.[60] Philipson and Posner found that there are important economic factors behind the growth in obesity. Technological change has lowered the cost of calorie intake by making food cheaper, and has raised the cost of expending calories by transforming physical exercise from a vocational activity to an off-the-job leisure activity. In an agricultural or industrial society, work is strenuous; in effect, the worker is paid to exercise. Weight, then, is the result of personal choices, such as occupation, leisure-time activity or inactivity, and food consumption. As personal preferences and technology determine obesity, Philipson and Posner question the effectiveness of expanding public intervention programmes designed to reduce obesity.

Nonetheless, it is neither accurate nor helpful to argue that nothing can be done to combat obesity. Prime Minister Blair has spoken of subsidising gym memberships. Other anti-obesity campaigners recommend redesigning communities to encourage walking. Some think that planners and architects should submit 'obesity impact statements' along with their environmental impact statements. However, a cost-benefit analysis suggests that even the most attractive of these schemes offers a marginal net benefit that is too insignificant to merit serious consideration. The changes in our lifestyle over the past generation have been so significant that it is beyond the grasp, if not the reach, of government to turn the social, cultural and technological tide.[61]

Furthermore, one cannot hide from the likelihood of unintended and unwanted consequences flowing from the respective government 'solutions' to obesity. Fred Kuchler and his fellow economists caution us that 'Without evidence that food markets are failing to reflect consumer and societal preferences, food policy to curtail overweight and obesity could cause more harm than good.'[62]

As a starting point, therefore, it may be useful to revisit comments made by the renowned University of Chicago law professor, Richard Epstein.[63] Speaking at an American Enterprise Institute conference on obesity in 2004, Epstein noted that policymakers usually resort to a public health rationale when the government wants to stop an activity that can cause harm to third persons who cannot reasonably protect themselves. For example, the forcible quarantining of a person carrying a virulent disease is consistent with a public health rationale. Epstein pointed out that it is a misnomer to call the increasing number of fat people an 'epidemic', since being fat is not a communicable disease. According to Epstein, 'The broader [public health] definition ... could easily authorize interventions in economic affairs whose indirect effects are likely to reduce overall social wealth and freedom, and with it the overall health of the population.'[64]

The state of being physically fat is neither inherently good nor bad. It is, however, a physical condition that the overwhelming majority of overweight, even obese, people have the power to control. The outcome of the obesity crusade will be determined by the degree of personal responsibility exercised by currently obese and potentially obese individuals. To the extent that obesity may be a real problem, it is a problem for individuals. The taxpayers of this country should not be expected to take care of those individuals who simply refuse to take care of themselves.

Therefore, an alternative to the values-driven, empirically unsound obesity crusade consists of the following 10 non-interventionist prescriptions, which collectively petition the innate common sense and self-control of individuals.

1. An End to Corrupt Science

The most vital change we can recommend is to address the way in which the obesity crusaders misrepresent and use science and its findings to distort the policy and regulatory process. This requires a new realisation of the significant limitations of observational epidemiology as a basis both for understanding issues like population-wide obesity and for crafting policy responses to them. Integral to such a realisation will be a commitment to making evidence-based science the basis for deciding whether there is a public health problem and also what the appropriate response to that problem might be. Such a realisation will dramatically reduce the opportunities for individuals such as the obesity crusaders to pass off as genuine science a corrupted reading of what the scientific process and its results are, in order both to manufacture 'epidemics' and to hijack the policy and political processes.

2. An End to Health Promotion

Significant attention must be devoted to the public health establishment's uncritical attachment to the tenets of health promotion: most especially its beliefs, none of which is credible, that many illnesses are the result of lifestyle, that there is a scientific consensus about the one 'healthy' way to live one's life, that a major function of the public health establishment is to convince individuals to accept this consensus definition of healthy, and that coercion is justified to prevent unhealthy living. While corrupted science provides the raw materials for the obesity crusaders' claims, it is a health establishment in thrall to health promotion that provides both the environment and the institutions for launching and sustaining a war on obesity. More importantly, it is health promotion's simplistic commitment to public health over individual autonomy and respect that provides the basis for so many of the more offensive policies proposed by the obesity crusaders. If the extent of obesity is to be properly understood – and, once understood, intelligently and effectively engaged – obesity must be divorced from any association with the scientifically compromised, ineffective and offensively paternalistic practices of health promotion.

3. The Demedicalisation of Obesity

We recommend the demedicalisation of obesity. It is the medicalisation of obesity that has both allowed the obesity story to become a public 'fact', endorsed by governments at all levels, and enabled the obesity crusaders to dominate and exploit the national and international public health organisations.[65] Demedicalisation requires the exposure of the unscientific character of virtually all parts of the obesity epidemic story, but especially its claims about the extent of obesity, the connection between obesity and mortality and disease, the role of the food and beverage industry in 'creating' obesity, the advisability and possibility of significant and sustained population-wide weight loss, and the viability of government regulation as a solution to the 'obesity problem'. It will also require that the public be made aware of the conflicted and self-interested relationships that exist between certain obesity crusaders, with their assertions about obesity and science, and the weight-loss and pharmaceutical industry, certain government panels and task forces, and the wider public health establishment.

4. Focusing Resources on the Morbidly Obese

The morbidly obese, a relatively small group of people, may benefit from medical and pharmaceutical interventions of various kinds – interventions that will depend on a better biological and medical understanding of obesity. Whatever the nature of these interventions, the important point is that it is the extremely obese, and not the merely overweight and obese, that should be the focus of any obesity crusade.

5. Physical Activity

A modest programme of exercise may bring significant improvement for both adults and children. However, for children to engage in vigorous outdoor exercise, such as running or kicking a football, this country needs safer streets. Too many British streets are becoming no-go areas for increasing numbers of young children, with many too scared to play outside.[66] With both parents working outside the home, many children are often confined indoors after school for safety reasons. As a result, too many children are being 'battery reared' in their bedrooms and deprived of the freedom to play outside by worried parents.[67]

A study published recently in the *Archives of Pediatrics and Adolescent Medicine* establishes a relationship between child obesity and the lack of safe neighbourhoods.[68] The study found that children living in the least safe neighbourhoods are almost 4.5 times more likely to be overweight than children in the safest neighbourhoods. This phenomenon occurs regardless of a family's wealth. The study found that 'Measures of socioeconomic status did not eliminate the observed association between perception of neighborhood safety and overweight.' Child obesity will not be successfully tackled while schoolchildren cannot safely exercise in and around their own neighbourhoods.

6. Better Parenting

The responsibility for children's health lies with their parents. It is the duty of the parents, not of the government, to provide balanced and nutritious meals and to encourage an active lifestyle.

More mothers may choose to breast-feed their infants. This is the policy implication of research findings presented at the 2004 annual meeting of the Pediatric Academic Societies in San Francisco. According to American research, breast milk contains a protein that could reduce the risk of obesity. Researchers from the Cincinnati Children's Hospital Medical Center found high levels of a protein that affects the body's processing of fat. They believe its presence in breast milk could influence a person's 'fatness' later in life.[69] In the UK, obesity researcher Dr Ian Campbell told BBC News Online that 'We know there is a clear link between breast feeding and a reduced risk of obesity.' He said the risk appeared to be lowered further the longer a child is breast-fed. According to Campbell,

'There is an accumulative effect; the longer they are breast-fed the better it is.'[70] Parents may also directly and indirectly benefit from the knowledge that insufficient sleep is linked to changes in hormone levels that may stimulate appetite. Scientists suggest that sleeping for an extra 20 minutes each night could offer a pain-free way to lose weight.[71]

Too many parents are physically indulging their children.[72] The bottom line is that more parents need to stand up to their own children, whether in the kitchen or in the supermarket aisle.[73] If a child is obese, the solution lies within the family, not within the bureaucracy. Decisions regarding diet, exercise, television viewing and sleep habits should be solely within the parents' purview.

7. Traditional Eating Patterns

In addition to eating more slowly, those concerned with their weight may wish to revisit traditional eating patterns. Most people assume that what they eat is the cause of weight gain. How they eat is perhaps just as important, for eating behaviour is often at the root of weight problems, especially among children. Child obesity expert Frances M. Berg contends that, in normal eating (that is, eating three times a day and one or two snacks), children rely on internal signals of hunger, appetite and satiety, eating what they want and as much as they want. 'Learning how to eat well', Berg writes, 'begins by stopping all diets, meal skipping, chaotic eating, and restoring normal eating as a priority.'[74] New research suggests that the traditional practice of eating together at the table could help cut obesity among both adults and children.[75]

8. Increasing Consumer Knowledge

The best protection against obesity is a generation of informed consumers. Informed choice is what makes a non-interventionist policy feasible. However, it is the consumer's responsibility to become knowledgeable. The Dublin-based Freedom Institute argues that 'The onus is on the individual to seek out the readily available information on good nutrition. Ignorance is no excuse.'[76]

Do consumers have sufficient information to make informed choices? Such a goal is well within reach. Most consumers already know which foods, for example, will make them fat. A study by Universal McCann found that 60 per cent of American adults generally look for the nutritional labelling on food products, and that they use the information to help them decide what to buy.[77] According to the economists at the USDA's Economic Research Service,

> The sheer volume of media coverage devoted to diet and weight makes it difficult to believe that Americans are unaware of the relationship between a healthful diet and obesity. In fact, results from USDA's Diet and Health Knowledge Survey indicate that most US consumers have basic nutrition knowledge and that they can discriminate among foods on the basis of fat, fiber, and cholesterol. Most are aware of health problems related to certain nutrients.[78]

It is reasonable to assume that, in the absence of government interference and coercion, the food and beverage industry's self-interest will ensure that the amount of nutritional information provided to consumers mirrors the marketplace's collective demand for such material. Therefore, those regulatory measures introduced 'should seek to increase the amount of information in the public sphere, not restrict the capacity of consumers to make responsible choices, nor obscure the fact that they are the ones in control of their health ... Information, not restrictions, is the required prescription.'[79]

9. Less-Intrusive Government

It is a considerable irony that government policy may have encouraged obesity.[80] For example, large taxpayer-funded subsidies for sugar and beef production maintain an over-supply of these goods and commensurately cheap prices. Subsidies have proved a catalyst for both European and North American agribusiness to produce far more food than their continents' respective populations can eat. This has had the effect of reducing the cost of food.[81] According to the obesity crusaders, the cheapness of food has led restaurants to serve larger food portions, and this has significantly contributed to the obesity problem.

It is well documented that there is not a causal relationship between larger portion sizes and obesity. However, the elimination of subsidies to the sugar and beef industries is the obvious next move for the obesity crusaders' policymaking brethren. The public health establishment argues that the effect of a higher price for both sugar and beef would be a reduction in sugar and beef consumption.[82] The elimination of food subsidies will have a negative impact on European and North American food producers. However, the obesity crusaders believe that, if the elimination of subsidies proves helpful against obesity, it will constitute a win-win situation for the anti-obesity movement.

10. The Use of Discrimination

Public policy may need to discriminate against, rather than in favour of, the obese. In the American context, Balko explains that 'more and more, states are preventing private health insurers from charging overweight and obese clients higher premiums, which effectively removes any financial incentive for maintaining a healthy lifestyle'.[83] Instead of lawsuits, fat taxes and endless lists of nutritional information, Epstein suggests that we allow employers, schools, insurers and so forth to 'discriminate against any person who is obese'.[84]

First, this policy would place the costs for being overweight squarely on individuals, giving them stronger incentives to slim down. Second, since most employers want a healthy workforce, it would give them an incentive to help employees control their weight, perhaps by restricting what is served in the company canteen, or offering exercise facilities.[85] In 2002, Southwest Airlines initiated a policy of requesting that its largest passengers – those who require two seats on an aeroplane – purchase two tickets.

Such a recommendation may not prove so far fetched on this side of the Atlantic. Consider the fact that the National

Health Service has already considered refusing to treat obese people for illnesses if their lifestyle makes the treatment ineffective. In the same vein, the National Institute for Health and Clinical Excellence (NICE), the NHS's guidance body, has produced advice that raises the prospect of people who are heavy smokers or drinkers, or who are obese, being refused health care.

CONCLUSION

Contrary to the obesity crusaders' belief, we cannot overcome the obesity problem through legislation. Instead, any effort to lower body weight, if it is to prove successful, will be addressed on an individual basis, as people take personal responsibility for their own physical condition and well-being. Such an approach, however, cannot satisfy the obesity crusade's emotional needs. For this is a public health movement that verges on the religious: not in its adherence to biblical scripture, but rather in its adherence to a particular world view and belief system that cannot be argued with, or against, because its foundation is neither empirical nor scientific, but moral and cultural.

Today, science and reason are engaged in intellectual combat with a masochistic anthropological phenomenon that, in true Schumpeterian fashion, is a cultural product of the very material affluence that it finds so morally offensive and deems so physiologically dangerous. The obesity crusade's assault on affluence is so extreme that one of the greatest human accomplishments – the historically unparalleled outnumbering of those with access on a daily basis to too few calories by those with easy access to too many calories – is categorised as a disaster of epidemic proportion that requires the most radical and extreme of countermeasures. Deep moral and intense cultural pressure is subsequently applied to those who may need to, or who may simply *think* they need to, lose weight, without regard to the well-established risks of weight loss and thinness.

The obesity crusade's desire to apportion blame for obesity to an economic system that has brought us a standard of living and material well-being beyond our grandparents' wildest dreams precludes any discussion of personal responsibility, or the lack thereof, as both the cause of and the solution to the obesity issue. As a result, the obesity crusaders' 'solutions' are blunt, heavy-handed and coercive policy instruments that punish both the producers and the consumers of foods and beverages – that is, all of us: the obese, the fat, the slim and the thin – in the unscientific and unethical quest for the poisoned chalice of an obesity-free society.

In this one-sided debate, alternatives to government intervention are at best dismissed and at worst simply ignored or ridiculed. Most of these alternative prescriptions are either so obvious, so commonsensical or so politically incorrect that they cannot seriously be considered by a public health establishment that is consumed by the theoretical rather than the applied, by conjecture rather than by the rigorous testing of a measurable hypothesis.

It is unknown how long it will be before the health policy pendulum swings back in the direction of sound science, empiricism and rational debate. What is known is that there is a significant cost to the current course of treatment for an illusory disease. But the cost is not merely monetary (although that is a substantial cost). The greatest cost will consist in the sacrifice of so many of our hard-won economic and political liberties on the altar of a misguided, unwinnable crusade.

CONCLUSION

Throughout this book, we have acted as contrarians about the 'obesity epidemic' story that is continuously told to the public by the media, the public health establishment and the government. Rather than the reality of a public health disaster that threatens to overwhelm the health care system, we believe the evidence suggests that we are instead confronting the *idea* of an 'obesity epidemic': an idea that has been carefully manufactured by a group of obesity crusaders, comprising academics, public health officials and so-called public-interest science groups, many with long-standing and significant ties to the multi-billion pound weight-loss and pharmaceutical industries.

THE OBESITY EPIDEMIC'S HOUSE OF CARDS

Committed to the ideas of health promotion, and often willing to build their case for an 'obesity epidemic' on the foundation of corrupted science, the obesity crusaders have succeeded in redefining what both overweight and obesity are. At a stroke, they have created millions of new people allegedly at risk from obesity; have convinced the Centers for Disease Control and Prevention to produce studies (later discredited) purportedly showing that those who are overweight and mildly obese have significantly increased mortality risks; have skilfully used the media to disseminate the idea that thousands, if not millions, of children are at risk from obesity; and have panicked governments into bringing forward a raft of highly intrusive obesity policies, none of which has a proven track record of success.

Against this manufactured epidemic, we have shown that the scientific evidence suggests a quite different picture, namely:

● Over the same time as the supposed obesity epidemic, risk factors for many diseases have declined, as has the prevalence of many diseases, while longevity has increased.

● Overweight and modest levels of obesity are not associated with increased mortality risks.

● Rates of childhood overweight and obesity are nothing near epidemic levels, in many instances there has been no statistically significant increase in these rates, and the evidence fails to show that childhood obesity leads to greater health risks in adulthood.

● Most adults, except for the very heaviest, have gained only modest amounts of weight over the last two decades.

● The weight gain of adults and children is not convincingly linked to a diet created by the advertising of the food and beverage industry.

● There is no compelling evidence that significant long-term weight loss is either practical or confers a health benefit, and there is considerable evidence of the substantial risks attached both to dieting and to eating disorders.

● The policies proposed to resolve the 'obesity epidemic' threaten the key democratic value of individual autonomy, while at the same time offering little prospect of success.

● Alternative approaches to population-wide weight gain involving changes in diet and eating patterns, consumer knowledge, the quality of parenting, physical activity levels, sleep, and even the use of discrimination offer viable options without involving government coercion.

● The plight of the truly obese, about 3–4 per cent of the population, should be the focus of any national obesity strategy; such a strategy calls not only for a better bio-logical and medical understanding of obesity, but also quite possibly for pharmaceutical interventions of various kinds.

These conclusions and policy suggestions are much more modest than the obesity crusaders' panicked talk of an obesity epidemic and their desire for a sustained, costly and ultimately ineffective and counterproductive assault on the nation's stomach. We believe them to be far closer to what the scientific evidence shows, prudence counsels, liberty can live with, and human nature can finally tolerate.

APPENDIX

WHAT IS SCIENCE?

The claims of an obesity epidemic are supposed to be based on science, and this raises the question of what *kind* of science may underpin such claims. Are there different sciences? Indeed there are: think of political science, library science, accounting science, creation science, astrology science, social science and so on. Such sciences have diverse aims: some deal with mundane catalogue issues; others try to interpret the nuances of human nature; still others advance conjectures about historical contingencies or about presumed realities. By and large, their conclusions cannot be objectively tested to determine whether they are true and valid representations of real happenings.

It is the goal of experimental science to comprehend what actually happens in the real world. It tries to verify – in testable ways – what happens and what causes what in the physical world. This is the science we speak of in this book, and this is the science that has dramatically improved the lives and knowledge of mankind over the past few centuries, that provides abundant food, safe water, effective medicines and vaccines, and all the technologies that allow communications, transportation, space travel and much more.

Indeed, the undisputed success and power of experimental science is such that governments of modern, free societies explicitly or implicitly ensure that their public health regulations are based on testable science, while citizens implicitly expect that those norms are warranted on the basis of such science. Here, then, such an expectation raises the question of whether official claims of an obesity epidemic are indeed verifiable according to experimental science. In addressing this question it is first desirable to get briefly acquainted with the workings of science, and with the reading and interpreting of scientific reports.

TRUTH AND SCIENCE

The meaning of truth in science needs some clarification, lest it be misconstrued. What truth itself may be all about has been debated since time immemorial. The Greeks were the first to leave a written record of their speculations as to the nature of evidence, and they came to be most sceptical of human sensory perceptions, which they regarded as imperfect and deceptive. Those ancients were partial to the abstract pursuit of ideas, mathematics and geometry that allowed precise statements and conclusions – such that two plus two is four, for instance – while their interest in the physical world remained dubious, poetical and contrasting. Although not incapable of insightful natural discoveries, theirs was still a mind that mixed magic and reality. Eratosthenes, for instance, estimated the Earth's circumference and tilt, and the distance between the sun and moon, with remarkable precision, but his findings could not prevail over the misguided orthodoxy of Ptolemy's geocentric model of the cosmos, which endured for almost two millennia.

It was not until the thirteenth century, and especially from the seventeenth century onwards, in the wake of the first successful scientific experiments, that philosophers and early scientists began seriously to consider what truth there was in the empirical evidence of actual experimental tests. Perennial interlopers, philosophers were quick to note uncertainties when confronting science with logical absolutes. Hume, the Scottish sage, revived the old Greek notion that, however often observations are made, there is no guarantee of absolute agreement with the next observation. Although a conjectural truism, and a bit of sophistry, this argument has tormented philosophers of science to this very day, predictably without resolution.

Other schools of philosophers worried again that the world may not be truly observable to our imperfect and subjective senses, and that whatever theories we might construct about it are untrustworthy, leaving us mired in irresolvable scepticism. Other issues arose in the wake of Einstein's relativity, Heisenberg's uncertainty principle, the apparent paradoxes of quantum mechanics, and Gödel's demonstration that logical constructs, mathematics included, are incapable of self-justification.

Eventually, science effectively compensated for these and other uncertainties by adopting statistical and relativistic concepts that modified Newtonian concepts of exact causality. Yet a coterie of philosophers and their naive media acolytes – unschooled in science – have continued to attribute imaginary uncertainties to science, and to make it appear fatally flawed.

Other critics have also been quick to seize upon the obvious frailties of scientists, maintaining that science is the construct of cabals that end up certifying trendy hypotheses by consensus rather than by valid experiments.[1] Although more critical of the sociology than of the achievements of science, these contentions took hold in the increasingly muddled cultural climate that existed from the mid-twentieth century, which labelled as oppressive any structured form of intellectual discipline. In the end, deranged philosophers went so far as to propose cognitive anarchy as the only tenable position, putting science on an equal footing with astrology, witchcraft and prostitution – under the flag that 'anything goes'.[2]

Yet, how flawed can science be if it continues to turn out useful technologies, abundant food and effective medicines? In fact, nothing goes on in science unless it is tested and validated, so that science delivers – even to the material advantage of the most obstinate sceptics, who also drive cars and use electricity. The discrepancy lies in the fact that philosophers are obsessed with absolute and capital truth, and are generally unfamiliar with and scornful of approximations. Scientists, on the other hand, operate on the basis of the advancing discoveries and narrowing margins of measurement and error, accruing knowledge from experiments of increasing sophistication.

Absolute verification is prevented not by philosophy, but by the imperfections of observation and measurement and by the complexities of physical reality – limitations that, most often, are reduced to practical insignificance on the basis of sufficient criteria of precision, thereby reaching a point where the evidence becomes sufficiently reliable for technological applications. The other preoccupation of science is not only how to increase precision, but also how to approach objectivity – that is, to achieve results that stand proven to be what they are, irrespective of the beliefs of any observer. Thus, scientific truths are approximate, but they are also objective to the best empirical degree that experimental techniques allow.

Indeed, in their crucial function of discovering causes and effects free of judgemental interferences, experiments are the unique tools that have progressed science beyond anyone's wildest dreams. Without such a commitment to objectivity, all those technological advances that have made human life so much easier, rewarding and safe in the brief span of a few hundred years would have been unthinkable.

The whole point of science is to acquire knowledge that is reliably predictive. Knowing what the strength of steel is under different conditions eventually allows tall buildings that stand up, and reliable bridges, cars and aeroplanes to be built. Knowing how electricity moves through a transistor enables computers, televisions and CAT scans to be designed. Knowing how chemicals interact allows effective medicines and innumerable other applications.

Scientific inquiry begins with the formulation of hypotheses about possible cause-and-effect mechanisms, which are then tested experimentally to see whether they actually work, and to be validated or rejected. It is only after validation by proper experiments that causal conjectures and hypotheses can begin to be considered as credible knowledge with any degree of scientific certainty. In the words of the US National Academy of Sciences: 'An idea that has not yet been sufficiently tested is called a hypothesis. Different hypotheses are sometimes advanced to explain the same factual evidence. Rigor in the testing of hypotheses is the heart of science. If no verifiable tests can be formulated, the idea is called an ad hoc hypothesis – one that is not fruitful; such hypotheses fail to stimulate research and are unlikely to advance scientific knowledge.'[3]

Scientific practice relies on the fact that experimental conditions are planned in advance, in order to eliminate or control for the spurious corruption of results. For instance, in finding the conditions under which heat causes water to boil, it would be necessary to figure out in advance, and during the experiment, the precision of the methods for measuring temperature changes, where the measuring instruments are located, the stability of the barometric pressure, the chemical purity of the water, the shape of the vessel holding the water, how heat is applied, and other details.

Ultimately, scientific objectivity is defined by the degree of assurance that measurements are precise and that possible external corruptions have been controlled for – an assurance that is reached by observing the rules of what is known as the 'scientific method'. Again, the US National Academy: 'The task of systematizing and extending the understanding of the universe is advanced by eliminating disproved ideas and by formulating new tests of others until one emerges as the most probable explanation for any given observed phenomenon. This is called the scientific method.'

A concise statement of the scientific method is difficult to find, because philosophers have muddled its definition to the point that the US National Academy itself gives only an opaque account, despite claiming that the method is intuitive. Intuitive it ought to be, for, in order to be generally applicable, it must address the evidentiary logic of any and all experiments, regardless of the manifold complexities of their execution and the underlying theories. In fact, any scientist, regardless of the theoretical and material intricacies of an experiment, is bound to follow a set of common-sense rules aimed at the control, and possibly the elimination, of mistakes, delusions and biases that may confuse outcomes. There are three essential common-sense requirements that define a concise operational statement of the scientific method:

- A guarantee of identity and accuracy: namely, in an experiment, the thing that is being measured must be the thing that it is claimed is being measured, and it must be measured with sufficient accuracy.

- A guarantee that the effects observed are due exclusively to the causal operations studied, and not to other disturbances that interfere with an experiment's conduct and that may alter and confound the results.

- A guarantee that an experiment and its results are consistently reproducible by different experimenters.

Without the discipline of those rules, there can be no valid experiments, and no conclusions could claim scientific qualifications. No hypothesis or conjecture that does not meet these conditions could aspire to become enduring and useful knowledge with any degree of scientific objectivity, nor could it be confidently transformed into reliable technologies or reasoned policy decisions, either public or private.

At the same time, it should be obvious that the rules of the scientific method can be followed by employing a best-effort approach, using the tools and knowledge available at any given time. Factual uncertainties usually relate to the precision and specificity of measurements, and can be assessed and characterised. Possible but speculative corruptions remain non-measurable – for example, the argument that imaginary biases and confounding variables might be operating even under conditions of consistent reproducibility. Uncertainties adduce a degree of contingency to the objectivity of experimental findings, which nevertheless remain valid and useful until and unless contradicted by future findings. In other words, science proceeds by the accrual of new and improved knowledge that refines, confirms or cancels previous findings.

The US National Academy of Sciences recognises that experiments retain an essential role in science, stating that 'Truly scientific understanding cannot be attained or even pursued effectively when explanations not derived from or tested by the scientific method are accepted.'[4] With regard to the error rate, the Academy has this to say: 'The precision and accuracy of the measurements ... depend on available technology, the use of proper statistical and analytical methods, and the skills of the investigator.'[5] As for confounding variables, 'In the best experimental systems, it is common that relatively few variables have been identified and that even fewer can be controlled experimentally. Even when important variables are accounted for, the interpretation of the experimental results may be incorrect and may lead to an erroneous conclusion.'[6]

On reproducibility, the Academy has this to say: '[E]ach experiment is based on conclusions from prior studies; repeated failure of the experiment eventually calls into question those conclusions and leads to reevaluation of the measurements, generality, design, and interpretation of the earlier work ... The Investigator has a fundamental responsibility to ensure that the reported results can be replicated in his or her laboratory.'[7]

Thus, the US National Academy of Sciences acknowledges the fundamental requirements of a scientific method firmly grounded in empirical experimentation. Arguably, little more than the above triad of intuitive ground rules underpins the spectacular advances of scientific knowledge in the natural world. There is, of course, the imaginative creativity and inventiveness of scientists, but that belongs to the research phase of science, to hypotheses and knowledge in the making that still need to be tested for biases, confounders, precision and reproducibility. It is not yet knowledge that objective scientists would consider fit for validating new and reliable theories, for flying aeroplanes, producing effective and safe medicines and foods, or for informing personal decisions, public policies and court proceedings. Research scientists may work creatively with hypotheses, but only rigorous and repeatedly successful experimental validation in different hands provides an objective test of proximate truth and predictivity, albeit within the boundaries of probability. In the end, there is no science – intended as objectively usable knowledge – unless it is validated by credible and reproducible experimentation.

Are the claims of an obesity epidemic scientifically valid? Such claims are largely based on epidemiological studies, and this raises the question of what scientific validity those studies might offer.

EPIDEMIOLOGY AND SCIENTIFIC VALIDITY

Epidemiology is the study of the occurrence, distribution and temporal trends of disease and health in human populations. The primary ambition of epidemiology is to identify causes of diseases that could then be used to justify various measures of prevention and cure.

Working as it does with humans, epidemiology is constrained by ethical considerations that forbid experimentation with dangerous or infectious substances on humans. In fact, human experimentation is possible only when testing the effectiveness of vaccines and medicines that offer hope of improvement. Thus, epidemiology is denied the basic scientific opportunity of experimentation, being forced merely to observe what natural causes and effects may go on in the world of health and disease. Those causes and effects may, in fact, represent natural experiments, but each of those experiments is uniquely determined by many observable and unobservable components, and becomes impervious to clear interpretations of general validity. It might be said that epidemiology often mimics the predicament of the blind men of Hindustan, who, as they touched an elephant, attempted to figure out what it was they were confronting.

The majority of epidemiological studies are not experimental but simply observational, and are limited to observation of what may happen, with no opportunity to exert experimental control. Unable to follow the scientific method, observational studies are inevitably open to error, bias and other confounding disturbances that may be only partially controllable – if at all. With only rare exceptions, interpretations of causality from observational studies inevitably end up relying on variable judgements that cannot be objectively validated.

A tension therefore arises between judgemental epidemiology and the sensible and essential requirement for independently testable and objective evidence to be available for the formulation of public health policies. Unfortunately, observational epidemiological studies have become a principal tool of advocacy and public health claims, based on the fallacious pretence that they portray true human experiences.

Epidemiologists have long tried to portray their discipline as a science, in the hope that it will be endorsed by the popular perception that science deals with proven facts. Indeed, until some 50 years ago, epidemiology helped achieve spectacular advances in finding the causes of infectious diseases – bacteria and viruses – with the crucial assistance of laboratory and clinical studies. The removal of such causes, through sanitation, vaccination or medicine, permitted vast natural experiments, resulted in the control or eradication of the diseases in question, and confirmed unambiguously the causative roles of the bacteria and viruses. Similar success has been scored for some chronic diseases of a non-infectious nature in occupational settings, where causative factors could be specifically identified, and where their removal led to the control or disappearance of the related diseases.

As infectious diseases have waned, there has been a surge in diseases that are caused not by any single and specific agent, but that depend on a constellation of factors, and that hence are called multifactorial diseases. In general, for most such conditions, determination of causality has been elusive, and laboratory and clinical studies have proved unable to determine specific mechanisms for such diseases as cancer, cardiovascular disorders and many others, including obesity.

In an attempt to fill the gap, a set of judgemental criteria was adopted to infer causality from observational statistics of multifactorial conditions. These include the familiar criteria of consistency, strength, specificity, temporal relationship and coherence – of which more later – that were catalogued in 1965 by A. B. Hill and named after him.[8] Bereft of quantitative and qualitative benchmarks, these criteria have remained judgemental and not linked to independent experimental verification. In the words of the surgeon general's report on cigarette smoking, 'The causal significance of an association is a matter of judgment' – justifiably a prudent judgement in the case of cigarettes, owing to the exceedingly robust association between smoking and the risk of lung cancer, and the reduction of risk for those who quit smoking.[9]

Following the surgeon general, a succession of professional authorities have agreed that most causality determinations in multifactorial epidemiology have been, and continue to be, defined by sensible judgements. To mention just a few of these authorities, in a 1970 textbook McMahon and Pugh noted that 'a causal association may usefully be defined as an association between categories or events or characteristics in which an alteration in the frequency or quality of one category is followed by a change in the other'.[10] In a later textbook, Kleinbaum and associates wrote: 'In epidemiology we use a probabilistic framework to assess evidence regarding causality – or more properly to make causal inferences ... [but] we need not regard the occurrence of the disease as a random process; we employ probabilistic considerations to express our ignorance of the causal process and how to observe it.'[11]

Doll and Peto framed even more explicitly the issue of multifactorial causality when they wrote:

> [E]pidemiological observations ... have serious
> disadvantages ... [T]hey can seldom be made according
> to the strict requirements of experimental science and
> therefore may be open to a variety of interpretations.
> A particular factor may be associated with some disease
> merely because of its association with some other factor
> that causes the disease, or the association may be an
> artifact due to some systematic bias in the information
> collection ... [I]t is commonly, but mistakenly, supposed

that multiple regression, logistic regression, or various forms of standardization can routinely be used to answer the question: 'Is the correlation of exposure (E) with disease (D) due merely to a common correlation of both with some confounding factor (or factors)?' ... Moreover, it is obvious that multiple regression cannot correct for important variables that have not been recorded at all ... [T]hese disadvantages limit the value of observations in humans, but ... until we know exactly how cancer is caused and how some factors are able to modify the effects of others, the need to observe *imaginatively* what actually happens to various different categories of people will remain.[12] (emphasis added)

Parallel remarks are to be found in the 'Reference Guide on Epidemiology' of the Federal Judicial Center's *Reference Manual on Scientific Evidence*, the principal reference for instructing US courts in regard to epidemiology. The *Manual* states that 'epidemiology cannot objectively prove causation; rather, causation is a judgment for epidemiologists and others interpreting the epidemiologic data',[13] and 'the existence of some [associated] factors does not ensure that a causal relationship exists. Drawing causal inferences after finding an association and considering these factors requires judgment and searching analysis', and '[w]hile the drawing of causal inferences is informed by scientific expertise, it is not a determination that is made by using scientific methodology'.[14]

Thus, while epidemiologists insist that their discipline is a science, clearly it is not the mainstream experimental science that produces reliable causal connections to fuel new scientific discoveries and successful technological advances. More to the point, if multifactorial epidemiology does not operate in the framework of science, what guarantees of reliability can it offer? A brief inquiry into how observational studies of multifactorial epidemiology are conducted will help clarify this point.

EPIDEMIOLOGICAL STUDIES

Epidemiological studies require different structures[15] to address different survey opportunities, but, in general, risk is measured as the rate of disease incidence of exposed subjects, relative to the incidence rate of unexposed subjects, the latter usually being defined as the 'control group'. Thus, the risk of exposed subjects is called a relative risk (RR):[16]

RR = Incidence rate in exposed / Incidence rate in non-exposed

The RR ratio reflects the fact that a certain incidence of disease is observed in both non-exposed and exposed subjects, owing to multiple background causes that operate in conjunction with, or entirely separate from, the exposure under study. Therefore, risk in the exposed is said to be an increment or decrement of incidence, *relative* to the basic incidence of the non-exposed subjects.

In the above equation, if the rates are the same in exposed and non-exposed subjects, the RR is 1 and therefore there is no risk differential. If the RR is above 1 the risk is said to be increased in the exposed subjects; if the RR is below 1 the risk is said to be decreased in the exposed subjects, indicating that the exposure studied might possibly be protective.

Epidemiological studies are affected by similar difficulties of design, data collection and interpretation. Fundamental obstacles arise particularly when we attempt to reconstruct past conditions – dietary and body-weight recollections, for instance – by asking each subject to remember variable personal experiences, often over several decades of their prior life. Vague and untestable answers are obtained by interviews either in person or on the telephone, or from next of kin, thus resulting in databases that are fraught with uncertainties of unfathomable dimensions that are conveniently assumed not to exist. Reckless as this assumption is, such illusionary data are nonetheless used and subjected to statistical assessments.

Measurements, Biases and Confounders

Diseases are more prevalent at different ages, making it necessary to approximate equal age conditions when comparing dissimilar groups: a manoeuvre that requires age-standardisation procedures. Similar procedures are used in attempts to equalise different groups for socioeconomic status, education level, race, gender, housing conditions, occupation and other common variables. Useful as they may be, such standardisations remain rough approximations.

Biases are common. A selection bias occurs when the non-exposed / control subjects mismatch the exposed / case subjects in respect to characteristics that cannot be standardised for age, gender, etc. In fact, selection bias is impossible to eliminate in epidemiological studies, and its presence can only be guessed at, but not measured with any precision.

Information bias relates to inevitable inaccuracies in data collection. Recall bias is most frequent, and is of special concern in case-control studies, where cases with a disease are apt to recall more intense and longer exposures than the controls that do not have the disease. Recall bias and error may be exacerbated when exposure information is retrieved from the next of kin of deceased subjects. Exposure reconstruction from other sources may also be biased.

The variable accuracy of disease identification diagnostics and death certificates may affect the classification of subjects. A misclassification bias occurs when subjects are mistakenly assigned to a group because of inadvertently, or wilfully, wrong responses from interviewed subjects or next of kin.

Confounders are defined as hidden risk factors that could also participate in an association. For instance, bodyweight data might be confounded by the anorectic effects of cigarette smoking. Methods are used to uncover and reduce the effect of possible known confounders, but those effects can only be partially controlled for on account of the inherent uncertainties. No control is possible for hidden and unknown confounders. For instance, studies dealing with overweight and cancer should consider several risk factors as potential confounders reported in the literature, and studies of cardiovascular conditions face over 300 published accounts of risk factors as potential confounders. Without a credible control for at least all major known confounders, epidemiological studies cannot be interpreted credibly.

Statistical Error

Large as they might be, epidemiological surveys usually sample only a small fraction of a population. This raises the possibility of statistical error, the magnitude of which is inversely related to the number of subjects in a given study. Statistical error is characterised by tests of significance defined as p-values or as confidence intervals (CI). Both relate to a predefined and arbitrary level of error that is considered acceptable, the usual convention being a 5 per cent error (i.e. a 1 in 20 chance of error).[17] Detailed accounts of epidemiological methodologies for dealing with biases, confounders, standardisations and statistics can be found in textbooks.[18] Still, it would be useful to acquire a perspective on statistical significance. The conventional 1 in 20 threshold of acceptable error would be disastrous in most everyday activities. Would it be sensible to drive a car if one time in 20 the brakes failed, or it turned left when the driver attempted to steer right?

Science valid enough for reliable applications must attain much lower margins of error. Margins of error for aeroplanes need to be extremely low. A typical car engine that has run for 100,000 miles has performed without mechanical error for over 2 billion revolutions. Several million transistors on a 1 square inch chip of silicon must perform flawlessly for years. At the basis of all atomic and chemical interactions, Feynman's experimental account of quantum electrodynamics predicts accurately to some 11 decimal places, or to a level of error of less than 1 in 100 billion.[19]

Even more perplexing is that statistical elaborations presented in most epidemiological studies are based on the assumption that the original data on which statistical analyses are performed are reliable and accurate, and provide objective measurements of real conditions. In fact, this assumption is wholly unwarranted, given that the original data are obtained through manifestly unreliable individual recalls that guess compositions and amounts of lifetime diets, or levels of exposure to possible hazards. Thus, for many epidemiological studies, the inescapable conclusion is that the statistical elaborations offered are demonstrably figments of the imagination, and this holds true for studies that either may or may not support a particular issue, such as an obesity epidemic.

Combining Multiple Studies

Meta-analysis is the statistical technique used to pool results from different studies. Originally it was developed for summarising the results of homogeneous randomised clinical trials – a use that remains its legitimate application. However, using meta-analysis for pooling the results of diverse observational studies is fraught with irresolvable difficulties.

In epidemiological practice, meta-analysis gives different subjective weights to studies, and does not pool the discrete data that yielded each result, but only the final results of each study, regardless of whether they are concordant or discordant, credible or not. The procedure does not discriminate for characteristics of each study, such as design, data collection, standardisations, biases, confounders, adjustments, statistical procedures, etc. Meta-analysis, therefore, produces only a weighted average of the final numerical results of the studies, but does not standardise, relieve, or control for differential corruptions that may be present in each study. Characteristics other than study size are commonly used in weighting studies (e.g. study quality): those characteristics are likely to be discretionary, judgemental and conducive to different meta-analysis results at the hands of different analysts.

The Federal Judicial Center's 'Reference Guide on Epidemiology' warns that '[a] final problem with meta-analyses is that they generate a single estimate of risk and may lead to a false sense of security regarding the certainty of the estimate. People often tend to have an inordinate belief in the validity of findings when a single number is attached to them, and many of the difficulties that may arise in conducting a meta-analysis, especially of observational studies like epidemiologic ones, may consequently be overlooked.'[20]

Therefore, it should be manifest that meta-analysis can be used in epidemiology as a stratagem to contrive meaning from studies that have no apparent meaning. More importantly, the excerpt from the 'Reference Guide on Epidemiology' quoted above leads to a general but crucial warning in reading and interpreting epidemiological reports. Most numbers in epidemiology are metaphorical proxies for uncertain real quantities, for epidemiology rarely measures reliably, but more commonly guesses, conceives, sizes up and appraises – all within a judgemental framework.

Indeed, statistical renditions impart an undeserved sense of accuracy and credibility to a background of vagueness caused by study design deficiencies, asymmetries in data collection, statistical error, biases, confounders, limitations of adjustments and standardisations, prejudice and more. Tests of statistical significance are equally speculative, being no more than illusory summaries of metaphorical primary data. Indeed, the greater the complexity of the statistical analysis in epidemiological reports, the greater the weakness of the data is likely to be. Using the practice of 'data dredging', epidemiologists like to conjure every conceivable signal out of what is usually a confused congeries of data. How do epidemiologists approach the inherent fragility of their data?

EPIDEMIOLOGISTS AND UNCERTAINTY

Epidemiologists react to uncertainty by taking contrasting positions. A few may focus on the collection of specific and accurate data, and on controlling as best as possible for biases and confounders. This concern may be reflected further in cautious, balanced and truthful representations of epidemiological uncertainty, which generally receive less than enthusiastic attention from the media, advocates and policymakers.

The opposite happens in the case of the majority, which adheres to a long tradition of advocacy that views epidemiology as a fungible tool for promoting the financial interests of the profession, or political preferences. In fact, it would be wholly unreasonable to expect epidemiologists to lead in the criticism of epidemiology, or in waxing forthright about its shortcomings and uncertainties. Profiting from easily aroused public anxieties, academic departments and government agencies become addicted to lavish public funding, the continuation (and expansion) of which would suffer if epidemiologists were to be openly critical of their results. What happens instead is that these funding pressures often merge with personal and political views to stimulate a consuming enthusiasm for what the French would call *dirigisme*.

Not surprisingly, epidemiology may be the only discipline where the presence of several studies with contrasting outcomes is often construed as proof that a coveted hypothesis is correct. In too many instances, advocacy prevails over interpretive restraint, leading to public messages and policies that are of questionable lineage, but that the media love. Advocacy positions are typically supported on the grounds that '[d]espite philosophic injunctions concerning inductive inference, criteria have commonly been used to make such inferences. The justification offered has been that the exigencies of public health problems demand action and that despite imperfect knowledge causal inferences must be made.'[21] The circularity of such a justification is manifest, for all too often the exigencies of public health are created by epidemiologists on the basis of knowledge that is marginal, if not wholly conjectural.

Undoubtedly, advocacy has valid roles, but it should be apparent that its legitimacy is in proportion to the factual reliability of what it is maintaining. Epidemiologists are divided on this issue. A new 'paradigm' of epidemiology has been proposed: one that shows little patience with the scientific method, though it is still reluctant to be perceived as non-scientific.

Proponents claim that 'epidemiologists among others have been misled by standard interpretations of the nature of science', and therefore 'to control for confounders … strips away the essential historical and social context, as well as the multiple moderating influences that constitute true causation'.[22] For those proponents, causal agents are to 'be seen as resulting from mechanisms that are internal to the population under study and that operate dialectically, rather than involving regular associations between externally related independent objects'.[23]

A novel methodology is also proposed, where 'the solution is not to abandon scientific standards, but rather to apply them more rigorously', even though 'it is inappropriate to falsely dichotomize research methods as: quantitative vs. qualitative, hard vs. soft, deductive vs. inductive, or objective vs. subjective'. The new paradigm focuses on broader historical, cultural, socioeconomic and political determinants of health and disease because '[r]igid adherence to an arcane view of science … [is] likely to promote narrow disciplinarian sectarianism at a time when an even more multidisciplinary ecumenical approach to public health challenges is required'.[24]

Ultimately, epidemiologists are seen as 'professionals in the sense traditional to medicine, the law, and the clergy. That is, society accords them a privileged and autonomous function founded on special training.'[25]

It should be apparent that individual decisions and public policy may have serious problems with a priesthood of epidemiology that claims privileged knowledge, and that is inclined to resolve causal theories dialectically and by internal consensus. In effect, the proposed paradigm presents an alternative epidemiology, much in the spirit of alternative medicine. The alternative relies on the meek claim that nothing better is available, proposing that good intentions alone justify the imposition of creative and (usually) interested conjectures. Extreme advocacy also scorns the undeniable truth that a number of questions may have no ready answers.

The counterpoint of sober epidemiologists is that, in most advocacy positions, 'scientific principles … are … disregarded not because they are difficult to understand, but because they are difficult to carry out … [T]he customary excuse for ignoring scientific principles is the argument that they are not necessary in epidemiologic research … [and] that no additional scientific principles need be invoked because each epidemiologic procedure has its own distinctive standards …

established by a consensus of appropriate authorities.'[26] Other sensible critics of the proposed paradigm also contend that such loose thinking invites excessive reductionist assessments, which generate 'the illusory comfort of perhaps metaphorical meta-theories that appear to explain everything while accounting for nothing'.[27]

Both the conservative and the advocacy parties in epidemiology concur that causal theories are what they produce, but they differ in interpretive restraint. The distinctive characteristic of advocacy is a determination to intrude sociopolitical views into epidemiology, with the claim that this makes epidemiology 'balanced and responsible'. The claim, however, is unsustainable, for the intrusion of ideology into the evidence-gathering process negates the original element of factual truth – or approximation of such truth – that is needed for responsible and justifiable public health actions.

How is epidemiology interpreted when scientific validation remains elusive?

INTERPRETING EPIDEMIOLOGY

As has been noted, ethical considerations and the stark reality of complex multifactorial interactions preclude the possibility of controlled experiments to specify the causal responsibilities of competing hazards. In the US, the Federal Judicial Center's 'Reference Guide on Epidemiology' concurs that, in epidemiology, '[w]hile the drawing of causal inferences is informed by scientific expertise, it is not a determination that is made by using scientific methodology'.[28] In this quotation, 'scientific expertise' refers merely to the use of statistics in analysing the data.

Fact finding in epidemiology is mostly 'a matter of judgment', in the previously cited words of the US surgeon general. However, the important distinction is that, during the initial fact-finding phase, it should be a judgement of accumulated evidence and not a judgement of conditional values – the latter coming later in the context of public health policy and action, where advocacy may also find its place. Confronting uncertainty, it is common epidemiological practice to draw judgemental causal inferences on the basis of the Hill criteria mentioned above.[29]

Strength The strength of an association is a clue to causation, but a strong association is neither necessary nor sufficient to affirm causality, and a weak one is neither necessary nor sufficient to deny causality.

Consistency Consistency of results from different studies is an obvious attribute of true causal relationships. Yet false associations can also be repeatedly consistent because of a consistent correlation with different but related causes. There is no criterion to distinguish whether a consistent association is true or false in epidemiology, but epidemiological associations that are inconsistent are unlikely to be true.

Specificity Specificity requires that a cause lead to a single effect, which is seldom the case in multifactorial epidemiology. Smoking, for instance, leads to many different effects.

Temporality Effects must occur after the cause has had a chance to act. This is a valid, if self-evident and trivial, criterion of causality.

Dose-effect relationship This is a useful but not dispositive criterion of causation. An observed dose-response gradient could be due to the presence of biases and confounders, rather than to the variables in question.

Plausibility Whether an association is biologically plausible or not remains a matter of individual speculation and is far from being objective or conclusive.

Coherence Agreement with other information may be a corollary attribute of causation, but conflicting information could be erroneous.

Experimental evidence Experimental evidence in humans would indeed constitute proof of causation, but it is very rarely available for conditions that are determined by many possible hazards.

Analogy Authorities in epidemiology comment that 'whatever insight might be derived from analogy is handicapped by the inventive imagination of scientists who can find analogies everywhere'.[30] Analogy is an absolutely invalid criterion in a judgement of causation.

In their textbook of epidemiology, Rothman and Greenland summarise Hill's criteria as follows:

> As is evident, the standards of epidemiologic evidence offered by Hill are saddled with reservations and exceptions. Hill himself was ambivalent about the utility of these 'standards' (he did not use the word criteria in the paper). On the one hand, he asked, 'In what circumstances can we pass from this observed association to a verdict of causation?' Yet, despite speaking of verdicts of causation, he disagreed that any 'hard-and-fast rules of evidence' existed by which to judge causation: 'None of my nine viewpoints [criteria] can bring indisputable evidence for or against the cause-and-effect hypothesis and none can be required as a sine qua non.'[31]

Therefore, even authorities in epidemiology acknowledge that Hill's criteria have no power as primary inferential determinants of causality. Indeed, it is remarkable that epidemiologists have not seen fit to include prominently among their criteria of evidence those most important common-sense guarantees that might begin to give some measure of confidence in epidemiological studies: namely, that what has been measured is, in fact, what is said to have been measured, is of acceptable accuracy and has a stated error; that known biases and confounders have been controlled for to the best possible (and sufficient) extent; and that the results are consistently reproducible. None of the studies of overweight and obesity have met these elementary criteria of reliable evidence.

Why is epidemiology receiving such inflated attention, despite the insurmountable deficiencies? There is, of course, the usual power seeking and money grabbing by special interests in public health, academia, advocacies, government agencies, Congress and the media, but the prime reason for the attention is that epidemiological studies are expected, demanded and conducted in affluent societies that are acutely preoccupied with health and death. The results will inevitably influence public and private policies, raising a critical need for guidance in judging how deserving of attention those results might be.

As a rule of thumb, attention should be proportional to the magnitude and consistency of the risks reported. For instance, the case against cigarette smoking is built on epidemiological studies that have consistently reported lung cancer risks for smokers that are 10–20 times higher than for non-smokers. By contrast, the epidemiological risks attributed to overweight and obesity are in the order of 0.5–1 times greater than the risks run by 'normal-weight' people. Furthermore, the results are not consistent and are rendered ambiguous and questionable by a number of unaccounted confounding hazards. For instance, when mortality in relation to overweight and obesity is the issue, there are innumerable causes of death that can impinge on the results and that the studies choose to ignore. Likewise, when cardiovascular disease, cancer, hypertension and diabetes are considered in relation to overweight and obesity, hundreds of known and potential hazards that contribute to those conditions are routinely ignored by epidemiological studies. The implicit excuse given is that it would be difficult, if not impossible, to measure the impact of those extraneous hazards on the meaning of the results, but such a lame excuse simply confirms the lack of credibility of the studies. Of course, the exception is for the small fraction of people who are morbidly obese, and for whom the epidemiological signals are strong: namely high relative risks and results that are quite consistent and reproducible.

Clearly, given the scarcity of science to hand, the reasons for the unfolding worldwide campaign for body-weight control must be motivated by interests other than scientific. Here, not to be overlooked is the political pressure exerted by different constituencies and advocacies, on the basis of interests that may have little to do with objective realities, and more to do with influence, power seeking and money grabbing.

The fundamental question is whether the mounting crusade on body weight should be allowed to impose intrusive lifestyle changes on a majority of the world's population, based on pseudo-scientific factoids created by, and for the gain of, the self-appointed experts and authorities that impose such changes. All the more so, given that the health consequences of those changes could just as easily harm, rather than improve, health and longevity.

The fair answer to this question should be in the negative, but body weight is only the newest strategy of the special interests that have a long record of exploiting epidemiology for its capacity to transform collective anxieties into political concerns, and for the unique opportunities it offers for staking claims to public and private funds.

This appendix has provided a basic overview of the methods of epidemiology, and of its inherent uncertainties. A strictly rational conclusion is that it should be easier to refute than to sustain epidemiological claims that are not experimental and not scientifically justified. Lacking the immediate persuasiveness of scientific experiments, credible epidemiology requires considerable documentation, the reading of which requires a considerably sceptical mind.

NOTES

INTRODUCTION

1. Social Issues Research Centre, *Obesity and the Facts: An Analysis of Data from the Health Survey for England 2003*, February 2005.

2. K. Severson, 'Obesity a threat to U.S. Security: Surgeon General urges a cultural shift', *San Francisco Chronicle*, 7 January 2003, http://www.sfgate.com/cgi-bin/article.cgi?file=/chronicle/archive/2003/01/07/MN166871.DTL

3. N. Hellmich, 'Obesity on track as no. 1 killer', *USA Today*, 10 March 2004.

4. M. Gard and J. Wright, *The Obesity Epidemic: Science, Morality and Ideology* (London: Routledge, 2005).

5. S. Kline, 'Fast food, sluggish kids: Moral panics, risky lifestyles, and cultures of consumption', ESRC–AHRB Research Programme Working Paper No. 9, May 2004.

6. J. Eric Oliver, *Fat Politics: The Real Story Behind America's Obesity Epidemic* (New York: Oxford University Press, 2006).

7. S. Shiffman *et al.*, 'Tobacco cessation and weight loss: Trends in media coverage', *American Journal of Health Behavior* 2006 (30): 363–64.

8. K. Flegal *et al.*, 'Excess deaths associated with underweight, overweight and obesity', *Journal of the American Medical Association* 2005 (293): 1861–67; and J. Gronniger, 'A semi-parametric analysis of the body mass index's relationship to mortality', *American Journal of Public Health* 2005 (95): 1–8.

9. K. Flegal *et al.*, 'Excess deaths associated with underweight, overweight and obesity'.

10. A. Hedley *et al.*, 'Prevalence of overweight and obesity among US children, adolescents, and adults, 1999–2002', *Journal of the American Medical Association* 2004 (291): 2847–50; and C. Wright *et al.*, 'Implications of childhood obesity for adult health: Findings from thousand families cohort study', *British Medical Journal* 2001 (323): 1280–84.

11. S. Basrur, *Healthy Weights, Healthy Lives* (Toronto: Ontario Ministry of Health, 2004).

12. Hedley *et al.*, 'Prevalence of overweight and obesity among US children, adolescents, and adults, 1999–2002'.

13. R. Troiano *et al.*, 'Energy and fat intakes of children and adolescents in the United States: Data from the national health and nutrition examination surveys', *American Journal of Clinical Nutrition* 2000 (72): 1345–53.

14. *National Diet and Nutrition Survey: Young People Aged 4–18* (London: Stationery Office, 2000).

15. Friedman *et al.*, 'Trends and correlates of class 3 obesity in the United States from 1990 through 2000', *Journal of the American Medical Association* 2002 (288): 1758–61; and P. Campos, *The Obesity Myth: Why America's Obsession with Weight is Hazardous to Your Health* (New York: Gotham Books, 2004).

16. Body Mass Index is a number calculated from a person's weight and height that supposedly indicates body fatness. A person's BMI is found by taking his weight in kilograms and dividing it by the square of his height in metres (kg/m^2).

17. L. Muecke *et al.*, 'Is childhood obesity associated with high-fat foods and low physical activity?' *Journal of School Health* 1992 (62): 19–23.

18. A. Hanley *et al.*, 'Overweight among children and adolescents in a native Canadian community: Prevalence and associated factors', *American Journal of Clinical Nutrition* 2000 (71): 693–700.

19. M. Rolland-Cachera and F. Bellisle, 'Nutrition', in W. Burniat *et al.* (eds), *Child and Adolescent Obesity: Causes and Consequences, Prevention and Management* (Cambridge: Cambridge University Press, 2002).

20. R. Prentice *et al.*, 'Low-fat dietary pattern and risk of invasive breast cancer', *Journal of the American Medical Association* 2006 (295): 629–42; B. Howard *et al.*, 'Low-fat dietary pattern and risk of cardiovascular disease', *Journal of the American Medical Association* 2006 (295): 655–66; and S. Beresford *et al.*, 'Low-fat dietary pattern and risk of colorectal cancer', *Journal of the American Medical Association* 2006 (295): 643–54.

21. P. Skrabanek, 'Fat heads', *National Review*, 1 May 1995.

22. Gronniger, 'A semi-parametric analysis of the body mass index's relationship to mortality'.

23. *Ibid.*

24. UK Advertising Association, 'The advertising of food to children: A submission to the Food Standards Agency', London, 2001.

25. C. Ebbeling *et al.*, 'Childhood obesity: Public health crisis, common sense cure', *Lancet* 2002 (360): 473–82.

26. *Ibid.*

27. A. E. Field *et al.*, 'Snack food intake does not predict weight change among children and adolescents', *International Journal of Obesity* 2004 (28): 1210–16.

28. M. Duffy, 'The influence of advertising on the pattern of food consumption in the UK', *Journal of Advertising* 1999 (18): 131–68; and P. Kyle, 'The impact of advertising on markets', *Journal of Advertising* 1982 (1): 345–59.

29. J. Willms *et al.*, 'Geographical and demographic variation in the prevalence of overweight in Canadian children', *Obesity Research* 2003 (11): 668–73; and T. Lobstein and M. Frelut, 'Prevalence of overweight among children in Europe', *Obesity Review* 2003 (4): 195–200.

30. C. Hawkes, *Marketing Food to Children: The Global Regulatory Environment* (Geneva: World Health Organization, 2004).

31. M. Serdula *et al.*, 'Prevalence of attempting weight loss and strategies for controlling weight', *Journal of the American Medical Association* 1999 (282): 1353–58.

32. *Ibid.*

33. M. Serdula *et al.*, 'Weight loss counseling revisited', *Journal of the American Medical Association* 2003 (289): 1747–50; G. Foster *et al.*, 'A randomized trial of a low-carbohydrate diet for obesity', *New England Journal of Medicine* 2003 (348): 2082–90; and F. Samaha *et al.*, 'A low-carbohydrate as compared with a low-fat diet in severe obesity', *New England Journal of Medicine* 2003 (348): 2074–81.

34. Foster *et al.*, 'A randomized trial of a low-carbohydrate diet for obesity'.

35. S. Heshka, 'Weight loss with self-help compared with a structured commercial program', *Journal of the American Medical Association* 2003 (289): 1792–98.

36. P. Nilsson *et al.*, 'The enigma of increased non-cancer mortality after weight loss in healthy men who are overweight or obese', *Journal of Internal Medicine* 2002 (252): 70–78; N. Wedick *et al.*, 'The relationship between weight loss and all-cause mortality in older men and women with and without diabetes mellitus', *Journal of the American Geriatric Society* 2002 (50): 1810–15; and T. Sorenson, 'Weight loss causes increased mortality', *Obesity Review* 2003 (4): 3–7.

37. E. Pamuk *et al.*, 'Weight loss and mortality in a national cohort of adults, 1973–1987', *American Journal of Epidemiology* 1992 (136): 686–97; E. Pamuk *et al.*, 'Weight loss and subsequent death in a cohort of U.S. adults', *Annuals of Internal Medicine* 1993 (119): 744–48; and S. French *et al.*, 'Prospective study of intentional weight loss and mortality in older women: The Iowa women's health study', *American Journal of Epidemiology* 1999 (149): 504–14.

38. D. Williamson *et al.*, 'Prospective study of intentional weight loss and mortality in overweight white men aged 40–64', *American Journal of Epidemiology* 1999 (149): 491–503.

39. R. Luepker, 'Outcomes of a field trial to improve children's dietary patterns and physical activity', *Journal of the American Medical Association* 1996 (275).

40. L. Birch *et al.*, 'The variability of young children's energy intake', *New England Journal of Medicine* 1991 (324): 232–35; R. Drucker *et al.*, 'Can mothers influence their child's eating behavior', *Journal of Developmental and Behavioral Pediatrics* 1999 (20): 88–92; J. Fischer and L. Birch, 'Restricting access to foods and children's eating appetite', *Journal of Developmental and Behavioral Pediatrics* 1999 (32): 405–19; and L. Birch *et al.*, 'Learning to overeat: Maternal use of restrictive feeding practices promotes girls' eating in the absence of hunger', *American Journal of Clinical Nutrition* 2003 (78): 215–20.

41. F. Berg, *Underage and Overweight: America's Childhood Obesity Crisis – What Every Family Needs to Know* (New York: Hatherleigh Press, 2004).

42. *Ibid.*

43. R. Strauss, 'Childhood obesity and self-esteem', *Pediatrics* 2000 (11): 15.

44. N. Calonge, 'Screening and interventions for childhood obesity: Where is the evidence?' *Pediatrics* 2005 (16): 235–37.

45. Campos, *The Obesity Myth*.

46. I. Lee and R. Paffenbarger, 'How much physical activity is optimal for health? Methodological considerations', *Research Quarterly for Exercise and Sport* 1996 (67): 206–08.

47. Troiano *et al.* 'Energy and fat intakes of children and adolescents in the United States'.

48. S. Kimm *et al.* 'Relation between the changes in physical activity and body mass index during adolescence: A multicentre longitudinal study', *Lancet* 2005 (366): 301–07.

49. IFIC, 'Food and health survey: Consumer attitudes toward food, nutrition and health', 2 May 2006, http://www.ific.org/research/foodandhealthsurvey.cfm

50. 'The dietary guidance gap: Consumers know they are supposed to do something – but are fuzzy on the details', *Food Insight* Newsletter, May/June 2006.

51. Wright *et al.*, 'Implications of childhood obesity for adult health: Findings from thousand families cohort study'.

52. Gronniger, 'A semi-parametric analysis of the body mass index's relationship to mortality'.

CHAPTER 1

1. J. Sobal, 'The medicalization and demedicalization of obesity', in D. Maurer and J. Sobal (eds), *Eating Agendas: Food and Nutrition as Social Problems* (New York: Aldine De Gruyter, 1995).

2. S. Levenstein, *Revolution at the Table: The Transformation of the American Diet* (Berkeley: University of California Press, 2003).

3. Susan Bordo, *Unbearable Weight: Feminism, Western Culture, and the Body* (Berkeley: University of California Press, 1993).

4. See V. Chang and N. Christakis, 'Medical modeling of obesity: A transition from action to experience in a 20th century American medical textbook', *Sociology of Health and Illness* 2002 (24): 151–77; and P. Conrad and J. Schneider, *Deviance and Medicalization: From Badness to Sickness* (Philadelphia: Temple University Press, 1992).

5. Sobal, 'The medicalization and demedicalization of obesity'.

6. Chang and Christakis, 'Medical modeling of obesity'.

7. L. Dublin and H. Marks, 'Overweight shortens life', paper presented at the 60th annual meeting of the Association of Life Insurance Medical Directors of America, 12 October 1951, reprinted in MLIC's *Statistical Bulletin* 32: (1) and in *Postgraduate Medicine*, 10 November 1951.

8. See '1983 Metropolitan height and weight tables', *Statistical Bulletin* 1983 (64): 3.

9. For a critique of Dublin's work, see A. Stewart *et al.*, *Conceptualization and Measurement of Health Habits for Adults in the Health Insurance Study* (Santa Monica, CA: Rand Corporation, 1980); W. Bennett and J. Gurin, *The Dieter's Dilemma* (New York: Basic Books, 1982); H. Bruch, *Eating Disorders* (New York: Basic Books, 1973); and J. Mayer, *Overweight: Causes, Cost and Control* (Englewood Cliffs, NJ: Prentice Hall, 1968).

10. Roberta Seid, *Never Too Thin: Why Women Are at War with Their Bodies* (New York: Prentice Hall, 1989).

11. *Ibid.*

12. Jean Mayer, 'Overweight and obesity', *Atlantic Monthly*, August 1955.

13. R. Drake, R. Buechley and L. Breslow, 'Measuring the risk of coronary heart disease in adult population groups: An epidemiological investigation of coronary heart disease in the California health survey population', *American Journal of Public Health* 1957 (47): 43–63.

14. Sobal, 'The medicalization and demedicalization of obesity'.

15. Eric Oliver, *Fat Politics: The Real Story Behind America's Obesity Epidemic* (New York: Oxford University Press, 2006).

16. Paul Campos, *The Obesity Myth: Why America's Obsession with Weight Is Hazardous to Your Health* (New York: Gotham Books, 2004).

17. Laura Fraser, *Losing It: America's Obsession with Weight and the Industry that Feeds on It* (New York: Dutton, 1997).

18. Oliver, *Fat Politics*.

19. P. Ernsberger and R. Koletsky, 'Biomedical rationale for a wellness approach to obesity: An alternative to a focus on weight loss', *Journal of Social Issues* 1999 (55): 221–60, at p. 249.

20. *Ibid.*

21. Thomas J. Moore, *Lifespan: Who Lives Longer and Why* (New York: Simon & Schuster, 1993).

22. Oliver, *Fat Politics*.

23. Center for Consumer Freedom, *An Epidemic of Obesity Myths* (Washington, DC, 2005).

24. Quoted in Campos, *The Obesity Myth*.

25. D. Allison *et al.*, 'Annual deaths attributable to obesity in the United States', *Journal of the American Medical Association* 1999 (282): 1530–38.

26. Quoted in Center for Consumer Freedom, *An Epidemic of Obesity Myths*.

27. Denis Campbell, 'Obesity group founder in row over drug firms' cash', *Observer*, 1 January 2006.

28. Reported in *Mail on Sunday*, 6 March 2005.

29. R. Moynihan, 'Obesity task force linked to WHO takes "millions" from drug firms', *British Medical Journal* 2006 (33).

30. R. Moynihan, 'Expanding definitions of obesity may harm children', *British Medical Journal* 2006 (33).

31. Philip James, 'The worldwide obesity epidemic', *Obesity Research*, 4 November 2001.

32. 'Obesity: A report of the Royal College of Physicians', *Journal of the Royal College of Physicians* 1983 (17): 5–65.

33. A. Mokdad *et al.*, 'The spread of the obesity epidemic in the United States, 1991–1998', *Journal of the American Medical Association* 1999 (282): 1519–22.

34. U.S. Department of Health and Human Services, *The Surgeon General's Call to Action to Prevent and Decrease Overweight and Obesity*, press release and press conference statements, Rockville, MD, 2001.

35. Marion Nestle, *Food Politics: How the Food Industry Influences Nutrition and Health* (Berkeley, CA: University of California Press, 2002).

36. P. Marsh and S. Bradley, 'Sponsoring the obesity crisis', Social Issues Research Centre, 10 June 2004, http://www.sirc.org/articles/sponsoring_obesity.shtml

37. *Mail on Sunday*, 6 March 2005.

38. House of Commons Health Committee, *Obesity*, 27 May 2004, http://www.publications.parliament.uk/pa/cm200304/cmselect/cmhealth/23/23.pdf#search=%22house%20of%20commons%20health%20committee%20obesity%22, p. 7.

39. Available at http://www.who.int/gb/ebwha/pdf_files/WHA57/A57_R17-en.pdf#search= %22global%20strategy%20on%20diet%2C%20physical%20activity%20and%20health%22

40. D. Yach *et al.*, 'The World Health Organization's Framework Convention on Tobacco Control: Implications for global epidemics of food-related deaths and disease', *Journal of Public Health Policy* 2003 (24): 274–90; and D. Yach *et al.*, 'Improving diet and physical activity: 12 lessons from controlling tobacco smoking', *British Medical Journal* 2005 (330): 898–900.

41. A. Mokdad *et al.*, 'Actual causes of death in the United States, 2000', *Journal of the American Medical Association* 2004 (291): 1238–45.

42. K. Flegal *et al.*, 'Excess deaths associated with underweight, overweight, and obesity', *Journal of the American Medical Association* 2005 (293): 1861–67.

43. See John Luik, 'The fat lady ain't singing yet', TechCentralStation.com, 3 June 2004, http://www.tcsdaily.com/060305F.html+fat+lady&hl=en&ct=clnk&cd=1 &ie=UTF-8

44. E. Marshall, 'Public enemy number one: Tobacco or obesity', *Science* 2004 (304): 804.

45. K. Flegal *et al.*, 'Estimating deaths attributable to obesity in the United States', *American Journal of Public Health* 2004 (94): 1486–89.

46. For a discussion of corrupted science, see Gio B. Gori and John C. Luik, *Passive Smoke: The EPA's Betrayal of Science and Policy* (Vancouver, BC: Fraser Institute, 1999), Chapter 4.

47. Marc Lalonde, *A New Perspective on the Health of Canadians: A Working Document* (Ottawa: Government of Canada, Ministry of National Health and Welfare, 1974).

48. G. B. Gori and B. J. Richter, 'Macroeconomics of disease prevention in the United States', *Science* 1978 (200): 1124–30.

49. Daniel Callahan, *False Hopes: Why America's Quest for Perfect Health Is a Recipe for Failure* (New York: Simon and Schuster, 1998).

50. National Institutes of Health, 'Methods for voluntary weight loss and control', NIH Technological Assessment Statement, 30 March–1 April 1992, Bethesda, MD.

51. R. Kersh and J. Morone, 'The politics of obesity: Seven steps to government action', *Health Affairs* 2002 (21): 144.

52. Stephen Schneider, interview, *Discover*, October 1989.

53. P. W. Speiser *et al.*, 'Consensus statement: Childhood obesity', *Journal of Clinical Endocrinology and Metabolism* 2005 (90): 1871–87.

54. Amanda Spake, 'Rethinking weight: Hey, maybe it's not a weakness. Just maybe...it's a disease', *US News and World Report*, 9 February 2004.

55. Oliver, *Fat Politics*.

56. John Last, 'New pathways in an age of ecological and ethical concern', *International Journal of Epidemiology* 1994 (23): 1–4.

57. J. Kaplan *et al.* (eds), *Preventing Childhood Obesity: Health in the Balance* (Washington, DC: Institute of Medicine, 2005), p. xiii.

58. *Ibid.*, p. 111.

59. *Ibid.*, p. 111.

60. *Ibid.*, p. 114.

61. B. Howard *et al.*, 'Low-fat dietary pattern and risk of cardiovascular disease', *Journal of the American Medical Association*

2006 (295): 655–66; R. Prentice *et al.*, 'Low-fat dietary pattern and risk of invasive breast cancer', *Journal of the American Medical Association* 2006 (295): 629–42; S. Beresford *et al.*, 'Low-fat dietary pattern and risk of colorectal cancer', *Journal of the American Medical Association* 2006 (295): 643–54; and B. Howard *et al.*, 'Low-fat dietary pattern and weight changes over 7 years: The Women's Health Initiative Dietary Modification Trial', *Journal of the American Medical Association* 2006 (295): 629–42.

62. C. Anderson and L. Appel, 'Dietary modification and CVD prevention: A matter of fat', *Journal of the American Medical Association* 2006 (295): 693–95.

63. See, for example, Nestle, *Food Politics*; Kelly Brownell and K. Horgen, *Food Fight: The Inside Story of the Food Industry, America's Obesity Crisis, and What We Can Do About It* (Chicago: Contemporary Books, 2004); Gerard Hastings *et al.*, *Review of Research on the Effects of Food Promotion to Children* (London: Food Standards Agency, 2003), http://www.foodstandards.gov.uk/multimedia/pdfs/foodpromotiontochildren1.pdf; Susan Linn, *Consuming Kids: The Hostile Takeover of Childhood* (New York: The New Press, 2004); G. Critser, *Fat Land: How Americans Became the Fattest People in the World* (Boston: Houghton Mifflin, 2003); and S. Dalton, *Our Overweight Children* (Berkeley: University of California Press, 2004).

64. Brownell and Horgen, *Food Fight*, p. 290.

65. Nestle, *Food Politics,* p. 195.

66. For an interesting discussion of the similarities between tobacco and food, see Jacob Sullum, *Tobacco Today, Fast Food Tomorrow? The Tyranny of Public Health* (Montreal: Montreal Economic Institute, 2005).

67. Brownell and Horgen, *Food Fight.*

68. Nestle, *Food Politics.*

69. Kersh and Morone, 'The politics of obesity'.

70. Brownell and Horgan, *Food Fight*, pp. 309–13.

71. T. Marshall, 'Exploring a fiscal food policy: The case of diet and ischaemic heart disease', *British Medical Journal* 2000 (320): 301–04.

72. Quoted in M. Blanding, 'Hard on soft drinks', *Boston Globe*, 30 October 2005.

73. *New York Times*, 17 June 2006.

CHAPTER 2

1. There is no information about trends in the amount of ingested energy that is excreted and wasted in stools, although such energy wastage can be considerable, especially with diets that accelerate transit time in the digestive tract. See J. L. Murphy *et al.*, 'Variability of fecal energy content measured in healthy women', *American Journal of Clinical Nutrition* 1993 (58): 137–40; C. M. Bijleveld *et al.*, 'Wet stool weight as parameter for fecal fat and energy excretion', *Acta Paediatrica*

Scandinavica 1986 (75): 1028–29; J. G. Muir *et al.*, 'Combining wheat bran with resistant starch has more beneficial effects on fecal indexes than does wheat bran alone', *American Journal of Clinical Nutrition* 2004 (79): 1020–28; A. M. Van den Neucker *et al.*, 'Nitrogen, water and energy content of a single stool sample in healthy children and children with cystic fibrosis', *European Journal of Pediatrics* 2003 (162): 764–66; and P. L. Beyer and M. A. Flynn, 'Effects of high- and low-fiber diets on human feces', *Journal of the American Dietary Association* 1978 (72): 271–77. Surprisingly, the literature on body weight hardly mentions the significant role of wasted energy, and the possible utilisation of this opportunity in weight control measures.

2. W. D. van Marken Lichtenbelt *et al.*, 'Body composition changes in bodybuilders: A method comparison', *Medical Science Sports Exercise* 2004 (36): 490–97.

3. R. M. Siervogel *et al.*, 'Patterns of change in weight/stature from 2 to 18 years: Findings from long-term serial data for children in the Fels Longitudinal Growth Study', *International Journal of Obesity* 1991 (15): 479–85; and J. V. Freeman *et al.*, 'Weight-for-height indices of adiposity: Relationships with height in childhood and early adult life', *International Journal of Epidemiology* 1995 (24): 970–76.

4. V. P. Wickramasinghe *et al.*, 'Impact of ethnicity upon body composition assessment in Sri Lankan Australian children', *Journal of Pediatric Child Health* 2005 (41): 101–06.

5. C. Berg *et al.*, 'Trends in overweight and obesity from 1985 to 2002 in Goteborg, West Sweden', *International Journal of Obesity* 2005 (29): 916–24.

6. M. W. Plankey *et al.*, 'Prediction equations do not eliminate systematic error in self-reported body mass index', *Obesity Research* 1997 (5): 308–14.

7. E. W. Gregg *et al.*, 'Trying to lose weight, losing weight, and 9-year mortality in overweight U.S. adults with diabetes', *Diabetes Care* 2004 (27): 657–62; and V. A. Diaz, A. G. Mainous and C. J. Everett, 'The association between weight fluctuation and mortality: Results from a population-based cohort study', *Journal of Community Health* 2005 (30): 153–65.

8. D. S. Freedman *et al.*, 'Trends and correlates of class 3 obesity in the United States from 1990 through 2000', *Journal of the American Medical Association* 2002 (288): 1758–61.

9. D. B. Allison and M. S. Faith, 'On estimating the minima of BMI-mortality curves', *International Journal of Obesity* 1996 (20): 496–98.

10. R. P. Troiano and D. A. Levitsky, 'The relationship between body weight and mortality: A quantitative analysis of combined information from existing studies', *International Journal of Obesity* 1996 (20): 63–75; R. A. Durazo-Arvizu *et al.*, 'Mortality and optimal body mass index in a sample of the US population', *American Journal of*

Epidemiology 1998 (147): 739–49; and J. T. Gronniger, 'A semiparametric analysis of the relationship of body mass index to mortality', *American Journal of Public Health* 2006 (96): 173–78.

11. A. H. Mokdad *et al.*, 'Actual causes of death in the United States, 2000', *Journal of the American Medical Association* 2004 (291): 1238–45.

12. D. B. Allison *et al.*, 'Annual deaths attributable to obesity in the United States', *Journal of the American Medical Association* 1999 (282): 1530–38.

13. K. M. Flegal *et al.*, 'Excess deaths associated with underweight, overweight, and obesity', *Journal of the American Medical Association* 2005 (293): 1861–67.

14. *Ibid.*

15. *Ibid.*

16. K. M. Flegal *et al.*, 'Estimating deaths attributable to obesity in the United States', *American Journal of Public Health* 2004 (94): 1486–89; Flegal *et al.*, 'Excess deaths associated with underweight, overweight, and obesity'; and K. M. Flegal *et al.*, 'Methods of calculating deaths attributable to obesity', *American Journal of Epidemiology* 2004 (160): 331–38.

17. N. Haapanen-Niemi *et al.*, 'Body mass index, physical inactivity and low level of physical fitness as determinants of all-cause and cardiovascular disease mortality – 16 y follow-up of middle-aged and elderly men and women', *International Journal of Obesity* 200 (24): 1465–74; W. J. Strawbridge *et al.*, 'New NHLBI clinical guidelines for obesity and overweight: Will they promote health?' *American Journal of Public Health* 2000 (90): 340–43; E. E. Calle *et al.*, 'Body-mass index and mortality in a prospective cohort of U.S. adults', *New England Journal of Medicine* 1999 (341): 1097–105; S. W. Farrell *et al.*, 'The relation of body mass index, cardiorespiratory fitness, and all-cause mortality in women', *Obesity Research* 2002 (10): 417–23; A. Heiat *et al.*, 'An evidence-based assessment of federal guidelines for overweight and obesity as they apply to elderly persons', *Archives of Internal Medicine* 2001 (161): 1194–203; K. R. Fontaine *et al.*, 'Years of life lost due to obesity', *Journal of the American Medical Association* 2003 (289): 187–93; and D. L. McGee, 'Body mass index and mortality: A meta-analysis based on person-level data from twenty-six observational studies', *Annuals of Epidemiology* 2005 (15): 87–97.

18. D. M. Mark, 'Deaths attributable to obesity', *Journal of the American Medical Association* 2005 (293): 1918–19.

19. Gronniger, 'A semiparametric analysis of the relationship of body mass index to mortality'.

20. Durazo-Arvizu *et al.*, 'Mortality and optimal body mass index in a sample of the US population'; and Troiano and Levitsky, 'The relationship between body weight and mortality'.

21. For a discussion of meta-analyses, see the Appendix.

22. Troiano and Levitsky, 'The relationship between body weight and mortality'.

23. Relative risk is a measure of how much a particular risk factor (say, cigarette smoking) influences the risk of a specified outcome (say, death by age 70). For example, a relative risk of 2 associated with a risk factor means that people with that risk factor have twice the risk of having a specified outcome relative to people without that risk factor. A relative risk of 0.5 means that people with a given factor have half the risk of the specified outcome (a protective effect) relative to people without that factor. See also Appendix.

24. J. A. Manson *et al.*, 'Body weight and mortality among women', *New England Journal of Medicine* 1995 (333): 677–85.

25. M. G. Jain *et al.*, 'Body mass index and mortality in women: Follow-up of the Canadian National Breast Screening Study cohort', *International Journal of Obesity* 2005 (29): 792–97.

26. I. M. Lee *et al.*, 'Body weight and mortality. A 27-year follow-up of middle-aged men', *Journal of the American Medical Association* 1993 (270): 2823–28.

27. A. Pajak *et al.*, 'Body mass index and risk of death in middle-aged men and women in Poland. Results of POL-MONICA cohort study', *Kardiologia Polska* 2005 (62): 95–107.

28. T. L. Visscher *et al.*, 'Underweight and overweight in relation to mortality among men aged 40–59 and 50–69 years: The Seven Countries Study', *American Journal of Epidemiology* 2000 (151): 660–66.

29. M. Miyazaki *et al.*, 'Effects of low body mass index and smoking on all-cause mortality among middle-aged and elderly Japanese', *Journal of Epidemiology* 2002 (12): 40–44.

30. Haapanen-Niemi *et al.*, 'Body mass index, physical inactivity and low level of physical fitness as determinants of all-cause and cardiovascular disease mortality'.

31. R. Hayashi *et al.*, 'Body mass index and mortality in a middle-aged Japanese cohort', *Epidemiology* 2005 (15): 70–77.

32. F. Seccareccia *et al.*, 'Role of body mass index in the prediction of all cause mortality in over 62,000 men and women. The Italian RIFLE Pooling Project. Risk factor and life expectancy', *Journal of Epidemiology and Community Health* 1998 (52): 20–26.

33. Z. Wang *et al.*, 'Body mass index and mortality in aboriginal Australians in the Northern Territory', *Australian and New Zealand Journal of Public Health* 2002 (26): 305–10.

34. D. C. Grabowski and J. E. Ellis, 'High body mass index does not predict mortality in older people: Analysis of the longitudinal study of aging', *Journal of the American Geriatric Society* 2001 (49): 968–79; and D. C. Grabowski *et al.*, 'Obesity and mortality in elderly nursing home residents', *Journal of Gerontology* 2005 (60): 1184–89.

35. H. Ellekjaer *et al.*, 'Blood pressure, smoking and body mass in relation to mortality from stroke and coronary heart disease in the elderly. A 10-year follow-up in Norway', *Blood Press* 2001 (10): 156–63.

36. S. Kalmijn *et al.*, 'The association of body weight and anthropometry with mortality in elderly men: The Honolulu heart program', *International Journal of Obesity* 1999 (23): 395–402.

37. Flegal *et al.*, 'Methods of calculating deaths attributable to obesity'.

38. P. M. Nilsson *et al.*, 'The enigma of increased non-cancer mortality after weight loss in healthy men who are overweight or obese', *Journal of Internal Medicine* 2002 (252): 70–78; and M. Korkeila *et al.*, 'Weight-loss attempts and risk of major weight gain: A prospective study in Finnish adults', *American Journal of Clinical Nutrition* 1999 (70): 965–75.

39. Gronniger, 'A semiparametric analysis of the relationship of body mass index to mortality'.

40. N. M. Wedick *et al.*, 'The relationship between weight loss and all-cause mortality in older men and women with and without diabetes mellitus: The Rancho Bernardo study', *Journal of the American Geriatric Society* 2002 (50): 1810–15; J. I. Wallace *et al.*, 'Involuntary weight loss in older outpatients: Incidence and clinical significance', *Journal of the American Geriatric Society* 1995 (43): 329–37; W. B. Droyvold *et al.*, 'The Nord-Trondelag health study, weight change and mortality: The Nord-Trondelag Health Study', *Journal of Internal Medicine* 2005 (257): 338–45; S. Eilat-Adar *et al.*, 'Intentional weight loss, blood lipids and coronary morbidity and mortality', *Current Opinion in Lipidology* 2005 (16): 5–9; T. I. Sørensen *et al.*, 'Intention to lose weight, weight changes, and 18-y mortality in overweight individuals without co-morbidities', *PLoS Medicine* 2005 (2): 171; D. F. Williamson *et al.*, 'Prospective study of intentional weight loss and mortality in never-smoking overweight US white women aged 40–64 years', *American Journal of Epidemiology* 1995 (141): 1128–41; T. I. Sørensen, 'Weight loss causes increased mortality', *Obesity Review* 2003 (4): 3–7; V. A. Diaz, 'The association between weight fluctuation and mortality: Results from a population-based cohort study', *Journal of Community Health* 2005 (30): 153–65; M. W. Reynolds *et al.*, 'Weight, weight change, mortality in a random sample of older community-dwelling women', *Journal of the American Geriatric Society* 1999 (47): 1409–14; Nilsson *et al.*, 'The enigma of increased non-cancer mortality after weight loss in healthy men who are overweight or obese'; S. G. Wannamethee *et al.*, 'Characteristics of older men who lose weight intentionally or unintentionally', *American Journal of Epidemiology* 2000 (151): 667–75; A. B. Newman *et al.*, 'Cardiovascular Study Research Group. Weight change in old age and its association with mortality', *Journal of the American Geriatric Society* 2001 (49): 1309–18; D. F. Williamson, 'Weight loss and mortality in persons with type-2 diabetes

mellitus: A review of the epidemiological evidence', *Experiments in Clinical Endocrinological Diabetes* 1998 (106): 14–21; S. Yaari and U. Goldbourt, 'Voluntary and involuntary weight loss: Associations with long term mortality in 9,228 middle-aged and elderly men', *American Journal of Epidemiology* 1998 (148): 546–55; J. S. Torgerson and L. Sjostrom, 'The Swedish Obese Subjects (SOS) study – rationale and results', *International Journal of Obesity* 2001 (25): S2–4; M. T. McGuire *et al.*, 'The behavioral characteristics of individuals who lose weight unintentionally', *Obesity Research* 1999 (7): 485–90; D. F. Williamson *et al.*, 'Prospective study of intentional weight loss and mortality in overweight white men aged 40–64 years', *American Journal of Epidemiology* 1999 (149): 491–503; G. A. Gaesse, 'Thinness and weight loss: Beneficial or detrimental to longevity?' *Medical Science Sports Exercise* 1999 (31): 1118–28; and A. Heini, 'Contraindications to weight reduction', *Ther Umsch* 2000 (57): 537–41.

41. N. Chaturvedi and J. H. Fuller, 'Mortality risk by body weight and weight change in people with NIDDM', *Diabetes Care* 1995 (18): 766–74; and K. Kalantar-Zadeh *et al.*, 'Association of morbid obesity and weight change over time with cardiovascular survival in hemodialysis population', *American Journal of Kidney Disease* 2005 (46): 489–500.

42. World Health Organization, *Obesity and Overweight*, 2006, http://www.who.int/dietphysicalactivity/publications/facts/obesity/en/

43. E. W. Gregg *et al.*, 'Secular trends in cardiovascular disease risk factors according to body mass index in US adults', *Journal of the American Medical Association* 2005 (293): 1868–74.

44. Gronniger, 'A semiparametric analysis of the relationship of body mass index to mortality'.

45. W. D. Rosamond *et al.*, 'Trends in the incidence of myocardial infarction and in mortality due to coronary heart disease, 1987 to 1994', *New England Journal of Medicine* 1998 (339): 861–67; and R. Cooper, 'Trends and disparities in coronary heart disease, stroke, and other cardiovascular diseases in the United States: Findings of the national conference on cardiovascular disease prevention', *Circulation* 2000 (102): 3137–47.

46. C. D. Lee *et al.*, 'Cardiorespiratory fitness, body composition, and all-cause and cardiovascular disease mortality in men', *American Journal of Clinical Nutrition* 1999 (69): 373–80; and Farrell *et al.*, 'The relation of body mass index, cardiorespiratory fitness, and all-cause mortality in women'.

47. E. L. Eisenstein *et al.*, 'Elevated body mass index and intermediate-term clinical outcomes after acute coronary syndromes', *American Journal of Medicine* 2005 (118): 981–90.

48. F. Thomas *et al.*, 'Cardiovascular mortality in overweight subjects: The key role of associated risk factors', *Hypertension* 2005 (46): 654–59.

49. J. P. Curtis *et al.*, 'The obesity paradox: Body mass index and outcomes in patients with heart failure', *Archives of Internal Medicine* 2005 (165): 55–61.

50. L. B. Tanko and C. Christiansen, 'Can the obesity paradox be explained by the protective effects of peripheral adiposity?' *Archives of Internal Medicine* 2005 (165): 1796–97; and Kalantar-Zadeh *et al.*, 'Morbid obesity and weight change over time with cardiovascular survival in hemodialysis population'.

51. D. K. Dey *et al.*, 'Waist circumference, body mass index, and risk for stroke in older people: A 15 year longitudinal population study of 70-year-olds', *Journal of the American Geriatric Society* 2002 (50): 1510–18.

52. A. Heiat *et al.*, 'An evidence-based assessment of federal guidelines for overweight and obesity as they apply to elderly persons', *Archives of Internal Medicine* 2001 (1161): 1194–203.

53. A. Nomura *et al.*, 'Body mass index as a predictor of cancer in men', *Journal of the National Cancer Institute* 1985 (74): 319–23.

54. K. Kuulasmaa *et al.*, 'Estimation of contribution of changes in classic risk factors to trends in coronary-event rates across the WHO MONICA Project populations', *Lancet* 2000 (355): 675–87.

55. M. E. Widlansky *et al.*, 'Body mass index and total and cardiovascular mortality in men with a history of cardiovascular disease', *Archives of Internal Medicine* 2004 (164): 2326–32.

56. R. C. Kaplan *et al.*, 'Predictors of subsequent coronary events, stroke, and death among survivors of first hospitalized myocardial infarction', *Journal of Clinical Epidemiology* 2002 (55): 654–64.

57. A. R. Ness *et al.*, 'Height, body mass index, and survival in men with coronary disease: Follow up of the diet and reinfarction trial (DART)', *Journal of Epidemiology and Community Health* 2002 (56): 218–19.

58. R. Bender *et al.*, 'Assessment of excess mortality in obesity', *American Journal of Epidemiology* 1998 (147): 42–48.

59. Gronniger, 'A semiparametric analysis of the relationship of body mass index to mortality'; and Flegal *et al.*, 'Excess deaths associated with underweight, overweight, and obesity'.

60. W. N. Kernan *et al.*, 'Phenylpropanolamine and the risk of hemorrhagic stroke', *New England Journal of Medicine* 2000 (343): 1826–32; and M. H. Pittler *et al.*, 'Adverse events of herbal food supplements for body weight reduction: Systematic review', *Obesity Review* 2005 (6): 93–111.

61. B. G. Stier, 'Phenylpropanolamine and hemorrhagic stroke in the hemorrhagic stroke project: A reappraisal in the context of science, the food and drug administration, and the law', *Annuals of Epidemiology* 2006 (16): 49–52.

62. Troiano and Levitsky, 'The relationship between body weight and mortality'; Gronniger, 'A semiparametric analysis of the relationship of body mass index to mortality'; and Durazo-Arvizu *et al.*, 'Mortality and optimal body mass index in a sample of the US population'.

63. A. Lukanova *et al.*, 'Body mass index and cancer: Results from the northern Sweden health and disease cohort', *International Journal of Cancer* 2006 (118): 458–66.

64. G. Danaei *et al.*, 'Causes of cancer in the world: Comparative risk assessment of nine behavioural and environmental risk factors', *Lancet* 2005 (366): 1784–93.

65. G. D. Batty *et al.*, 'Obesity and overweight in relation to disease-specific mortality in men with and without existing coronary heart disease in London: The original Whitehall study', *Heart* 2005: 1–8.

66. M. Inoue *et al.*, 'Impact of body mass index on the risk of total cancer incidence and mortality among middle-aged Japanese: Data from a large-scale population-based cohort study – the JPHC study', *Cancer Causes Control* 2004 (15): 671–80.

67. M. K. Whiteman *et al.*, 'Body mass and mortality after breast cancer diagnosis', *Cancer Epidemiology Biomarkers Preview* 2005 (14): 2009–14.

68. L. W. Chow *et al.*, 'Association between body mass index and risk of formation of breast cancer in Chinese women', *Asian Journal of Surgery* 2005 (28): 179–84.

69. B. Tehard and F. Clavel-Chapelon, 'Several anthropometric measurements and breast cancer risk: Results of the E3N cohort study', *International Journal of Obesity* 2006 (30): 156–63.

70. Calle *et al.*, 'Body-mass index and mortality in a prospective cohort of US adults'.

71. A. Lukanova *et al.*, 'Body mass index in relation to ovarian cancer: A multi-centre nested case-control study', *International Journal of Cancer* 2002 (99): 603–08.

72. Nomura *et al.*, 'Body mass index as a predictor of cancer in men'.

73. Troiano and Levitsky, 'The relationship between body weight and mortality'; Gronniger, 'A semiparametric analysis of the relationship of body mass index to mortality'; and Durazo-Arvizu *et al.*, 'Mortality and optimal body mass index in a sample of the US population'.

74. J. H. Young *et al.*, 'Differential susceptibility to hypertension is due to selection during the out-of-Africa expansion', *PLoS Genetics* (2005), http://dx.doi.org/10.1371/journal.pgen.0010082

75. K. M. Flegal *et al.*, 'Prevalence and trends in obesity among US adults, 1999–2000', *Journal of the American Medical Association* 2002 (288): 1723–27; Berg *et al.*, 'Trends in overweight and obesity from 1985 to 2002 in Goteborg, West Sweden'; K. M. Flegal and R. P. Troiano, 'Changes in the distribution of body mass index of adults and children in the US population', *International Journal of Obesity* 2000 (24): 807–18;

J. L. Gutierrez-Fisac *et al.*, 'Increasing prevalence of overweight and obesity among Spanish adults, 1987–1997', *International Journal of Obesity* 2000 (24): 1677–82; B. L. Heitmann, 'Ten-year trends in overweight and obesity among Danish men and women aged 30–60 years', *International Journal of Obesity* 2000 (24): 1347–52; C. L. Ogden *et al.*, 'Mean body weight, height, and body mass index, United States 1960–2002', *Advance Data from Vital and Health Statistics*, No. 347, October 2004, Centers for Disease Control and Prevention, Atlanta, GA, http://www.cdc.gov/nchs/data/ad/ad347.pdf; F. Azizi *et al.*, 'Trends in overweight, obesity and central fat accumulation among Tehranian adults between 1998–1999 and 2001–2002', *Annuals of Nutrition and Metabolism* 2005 (49): 3–8; A. M. Prentice and S. A. Jebb, 'Obesity in Britain: Gluttony or sloth?' *British Medical Journal* 1995 (11): 437–39; M. Lindstrom *et al.*, 'Increasing prevalence of overweight obesity and physical inactivity: Two population-based studies 1986 and 1994', *European Journal of Public Health* 2003 (12): 306–12; and A. Evans *et al.*, 'Trends in coronary risk factors in the WHO MONICA project', *International Journal of Epidemiology* 2001 (30): 35–40.

76. R. P. Troiano *et al.*, 'Overweight prevalence and trends for children and adolescents', *Archives of Pediatric and Adolescent Medicine* 1995 (149): 1085–91; R. P. Troiano and K. M. Flegal, 'Overweight children and adolescents: Description, epidemiology, and demographics', *Pediatrics* 1998 (101): 497–504; Heitmann, 'Ten-year trends in overweight and obesity among Danish men and women aged 30–60 years'; Y. Manios *et al.*, 'Changing relationships of obesity and dyslipidemia in Greek children: 1982–2002', *Preventive Medicine* 2005 (41): 846–51; Y. Manios *et al.*, 'Implication of socio-economic status on the prevalence of overweight and obesity in Greek adults', *Health Policy* 2005 (74): 224–32; R. von Kries, 'Obesity among Bavarian children – experiences from school admittance examinations', *Gesundheitswesen* 2004 (66): 80–85; S. Kautiainen *et al.*, 'Secular trends in overweight and obesity among Finnish adolescents in 1977–1999', *International Journal of Obesity* 2002 (26): 544–52; J. D. Willms *et al.*, 'Geographic and demographic variation in the prevalence of overweight Canadian children', *Obesity Research* 2003 (11): 668–73; B. Heude *et al.*, 'Trends in height, weight, and obesity prevalence in school children from Northern France, 1992–2000', *Diabetes and Metabolism* 2003 (29): 235–40; E. M. Mathus-Vliegen, 'Overweight – prevalence and trends', *Ned Tijdschr Geneeskd* 1998 (142): 1982–89; L. Boldori and A. Marelli, 'Monitoring the trend of overweight children in Cremona', *Minerva Pediatrics* 2000 (52): 21–27; M. Romon *et al.*, 'Influence of social class on time trends in BMI distribution in 5-year-old French children from 1989 to 1999', *International Journal of Obesity* 2005 (29): 54–59; E. Stamatakis *et al.*, 'Overweight and obesity trends from 1974 to 2003 in English children: What is the role of socioeconomic factors?' *Archives of Disease in Childhood* 2005 (90): 999–1004; A. A. Hedley *et al.*,

'Prevalence of overweight and obesity among US children, adolescents, and adults, 1999–2002', *Journal of the American Medical Association* 2004 (291): 2847–50; C. Padez *et al.*, 'Prevalence of overweight and obesity in 7–9-year-old Portuguese children: Trends in body mass index from 1970–2002', *American Journal of Human Biology* 2004 (16): 670–78; K. M. Flegal, 'Overweight and obesity in the United States: Prevalence and trends, 1960–1994', *International Journal of Obesity* 1998 (22): 39–47; J. C. Seidell *et al.*, 'Prevalence and trends of obesity in the Netherlands 1987–1991', *International Journal of Obesity* 1995 (19): 924–27; L. Serra Majem *et al.*, 'Childhood and adolescent obesity in Spain', *Med Clin* 2003 (121): 725–32; C. Frye and J. Heinrich, 'Trends and predictors of overweight and obesity in East German children', *International Journal of Obesity* 2003 (27): 963–69; and C. L. Ogden *et al.*, 'Prevalence and trends in overweight among US children and adolescents, 1999–2000', *Journal of the American Medical Association* 2002 (288): 1728–32.

77. D. L. Costa *et al.*, 'Long-term trends in health, welfare, and economic growth in the United States', in R. H. Steckel and R. Floud (eds), *Health and Welfare during Industrialization* (Chicago: University of Chicago Press, 1997).

78. H. Kalies *et al.*, 'Prevalence of overweight and obesity and trends in body mass index in German pre-school children, 1982–1997', *International Journal of Obesity* 2002 (26): 1211–17; Troiano and Flegal, 'Overweight children and adolescents: Description, epidemiology, and demographics'; Kautiainen *et al.*, 'Secular trends in overweight and obesity among Finnish adolescents in 1977–1999'; Flegal, 'Overweight and obesity in the United States: Prevalence and trends, 1960–1994'; and Romon *et al.*, 'Influence of social class on time trends in BMI distribution in 5-year-old French children from 1989 to 1999'.

79. R. P. Troiano, 'Energy and fat intakes of children and adolescents in the United States: Data from the national health and nutrition examination surveys', *American Journal of Clinical Nutrition* 2000 (72): 1343S–53S; A. F. Heini and R. L. Weinsier, 'Divergent trends in obesity and fat intake patterns: The American paradox', *American Journal of Medicine* 1997 (102): 259–64; M. Kersting *et al.*, 'Nutrition of children and adolescents', *Bundesgesundheitsblatt Gesundheitsforschung Gesundheitsschutz* 2004 (47): 213–18; C. Cavadini *et al.*, 'US adolescent food intake trends from 1965 to 1996', *Archives of Disease in Childhood* 2000 (83): 18–24; S. J. Nielsen *et al.*, 'Trends in energy intake in U.S. between 1977 and 1996: Similar shifts seen across age groups', *Obesity Research* 2002 (10): 370–78; E. Kennedy and J. Goldberg, 'What are American children eating? Implications for public policy', *Nutrition Review* 1995 (53): 111–26; S. M. Jungjohann *et al.*, 'Eight-year trends in food, energy and macronutrient intake in a sample of elderly German subjects', *British Journal of Nutrition* 2005 (93):

361–78; M. F. Rolland-Cachera and F. Bellisle, 'Nutrition', in W. Burniat *et al.* (eds), *Child and Adolescence Obesity: Causes and Consequences, Prevention and Management* (Cambridge: Cambridge University Press, 2002); A. Adamson *et al.*, 'Nutritional intake, height and weight of 11–12-year-old Northumbrian children in 1990 compared with information obtained in 1980', *British Journal of Nutrition* 1992 (68): 543–63; and M. F. Rolland-Cachera *et al.*, 'Nutritional status and food intake in adolescents living in Western Europe', *European Journal of Clinical Nutrition* 2000 (54): S41–46.

80. R. A. Forshee *et al.*, 'A risk analysis model of the relationship between beverage consumption from school vending machines and risk of adolescent overweight', *Risk Analysis* 2005 (25): 1121–35.

81. J. A. Welsh *et al.*, 'Overweight among low-income preschool children associated with the consumption of sweet drinks: Missouri, 1999–2002', *Pediatrics* 2005 (115): 223–29.

82. E. Kvaavik *et al.*, 'The stability of soft drinks intake from adolescence to adult age and the association between long-term consumption of soft drinks and lifestyle factors and body weight', *Public Health Nutrition* 2005 (8): 149–57.

83. J. W. Blum *et al.*, 'Beverage consumption patterns in elementary school aged children across a two-year period', *Journal of American College of Nutrition* 2005 (24): 93–98.

84. J. D. Skinner and B. R. Carruth, 'A longitudinal study of children's juice intake and growth: The juice controversy revisited' *Journal of the American Dietary Association* 2001 (101): 432–37.

85. R. Rajeshwari *et al.*, 'Secular trends in children's sweetened-beverage consumption', *Journal of the American Dietary Association* 2005 (105): 208–14.

86. C. S. Berkey *et al.*, 'Sugar-added beverages and adolescent weight change', *Obesity Research* 2004 (12): 778–88.

87. P. K. Newby *et al.*, 'Beverage consumption is not associated with changes in weight and body mass index among low-income preschool children in North Dakota', *Journal of the American Dietary Association* 2004 (104): 1086–94.

88. A. M. Toschke *et al.*, 'Meal frequency and childhood obesity', *Obesity Research* 2005 (13): 1932–38.

89. O. M. Thompson *et al.*, 'Dietary pattern as a predictor of change in BMI z-score among girls', *International Journal of Obesity* 2006 (30): 176–82.

90. C. B. Ebbeling *et al.*, 'Compensation for energy intake from fast food among overweight and lean adolescents', *Journal of the American Medical Association* 2004 (291): 2828–33.

91. C. S. Berkey *et al.*, 'Milk, dairy fat, dietary calcium, and weight gain: A longitudinal study of adolescents', *Archives of Pediatric and Adolescent Medicine* 2005 (159): 543–50.

92. G. Barba *et al.*, 'Inverse association between body mass and frequency of milk consumption in children', *British Journal of Nutrition* 2005 (93): 15–19.

93. E. M. Taveras *et al.*, 'Association of consumption of fried food away from home with body mass index and diet quality in older children and adolescents', *Pediatrics* 2005 (116): 518–24.

94. E. M. Taveras *et al.*, 'Family dinner and adolescent overweight', *Obesity Research* 2005 (13): 900–06.

95. I. Janssen *et al.*, 'Comparison of overweight and obesity prevalence in school-aged youth from 34 countries and their relationships with physical activity and dietary patterns', *Obesity Review* 2005 (6): 123–32.

96. S. M. Phillips *et al.*, 'Energy-dense snack food intake in adolescence: Longitudinal relationship to weight and fatness', *Obesity Research* 2004 (12): 461–72.

97. A. E. Field, 'Association between fruit and vegetable intake and change in body mass index among a large sample of children and adolescents in the United States', *International Journal of Obesity* 2003 (27): 821–26.

98. J. E. Blundell *et al.*, 'Resistance and susceptibility to weight gain: Individual variability in response to a high-fat diet', *Physiology and Behavior* 2005 (86): 614–22.

99. P. J. Salsberry and P. B. Reagan, 'Dynamics of early childhood overweight', *Pediatrics* 2005 (116): 1329–38.

100. M. K. Fox, 'Relationship between portion size and energy intake among infants and toddlers: Evidence of self-regulation', *Journal of the American Dietary Association* 2006 (106): 77–83.

101. Troiano and Flegal, 'Overweight children and adolescents: Description, epidemiology, and demographics'.

102. S. J. Marshall *et al.*, 'Relationships between media use, body fatness and physical activity in children and youth: A meta-analysis', *International Journal of Obesity* 2004 (28): 1238–46.

103. T. J. Parsons *et al.*, 'Physical activity and change in body mass index from adolescence to mid-adulthood in the 1958 British cohort', *International Journal of Epidemiology* 2006 (35): 197–204.

104. S. Y. Kimm *et al.*, 'Relation between the changes in physical activity and body-mass index during adolescence: A multicentre longitudinal study', *Lancet* 2005 (366): 301–07; C. S. Berkey *et al.*, 'Activity, dietary intake, and weight changes in a longitudinal study of preadolescent and adolescent boys and girls', *Pediatrics* 2000 (105): 56; and C. S. Berkey *et al.*, 'One-year changes in activity and in inactivity among 10- to 15-year-old boys and girls: Relationship to change in body mass index', *Pediatrics* 2003 (111): 836–43.

105. H. Sugimori *et al.*, 'Analysis of factors that influence body mass index from ages 3 to 6 years', *Pediatric Int* 2004 (46): 302–10.

106. N. Stettler *et al.*, 'Electronic games and environmental factors associated with childhood obesity in Switzerland', *Obesity Research* 2004 (12): 896–903.

107. H. L. Burdette and R. C. Whitaker, 'A national study of neighborhood safety, outdoor play, television viewing, and obesity in preschool children', *Pediatrics* 2005 (116): 657–62.

108. R. M. Viner and T. J. Cole, 'Television viewing in early childhood predicts adult body mass index', *Journal of Pediatrics* 2005 (147): 429–35.

109. S. Kautiainen *et al.*, 'Use of information and communication technology and prevalence of overweight and obesity among adolescents', *International Journal of Obesity* 2005 (29): 925–33.

110. J. J. Reilly *et al.*, 'Early life risk factors for obesity in childhood: Cohort study', *British Medical Journal* 2005 (330): 1357.

111. R. Jago *et al.*, 'BMI from 3-6 y of age is predicted by TV viewing and physical activity, not diet', *International Journal of Obesity* 2005 (29): 557–64.

112. Janssen *et al.*, 'Comparison of overweight and obesity prevalence in school-aged youth from 34 countries and their relationships with physical activity and dietary patterns'.

113. R. J. Hancox and R. Poulton, 'Watching television is associated with childhood obesity: But is it clinically important?', *International Journal of Obesity* 2006 (30): 171–75.

114. A. Page *et al.*, 'Physical activity patterns in non-obese and obese children assessed using minute-by-minute accelerometry', *International Journal of Obesity* 2005 (29): 1070–76.

115. L. A. Kelly *et al.*, 'Effect of socioeconomic status on objectively measured physical activity', *Archives of Disease in Childhood* 2006 (91): 35–38; G. J. Norman *et al.*, 'Psychosocial and environmental correlates of adolescent sedentary behaviors', *Pediatrics* 2005 (116): 908–16; J. Salmon *et al.*, 'Association of family environment with children's television viewing and with low level of physical activity', *Obesity Research* 2005 (13): 1939–51; K. C. Swallen *et al.*, 'Overweight, obesity, and health-related quality of life among adolescents: The national longitudinal study of adolescent health', *Pediatrics* 2005 (115): 340–47; Manios *et al.*, 'Changing relationships of obesity and dyslipidemia in Greek children: 1982–2002'; Manios *et al.*, 'Implication of socio-economic status on the prevalence of overweight and obesity in Greek adults'; and L. N. Oliver and M. V. Hayes, 'Neighbourhood socio-economic status and the prevalence of overweight Canadian children and youth', *Canadian Journal of Public Health* 2005 (96): 415–20.

116. C. E. Flodmark, 'The happy obese child', *International Journal of Obesity* 2005 (29): 31–33; and J. Wardle and L. Cooke, 'The impact of obesity on psychological well-being', *Best Pract Res Clinical Endocrinology* 2005 (19): 421–40.

117. R. C. Klesges *et al.*, 'Smoking, body weight, and their effects on smoking behavior. A comprehensive review of the literature', *Psychological Bulletin* 1998 (106): 204–30.

118. S. Y. Chou *et al.*, 'An economic analysis of adult obesity: Results from the Behavioral Risk Factor Surveillance System', *Journal of Health Economics* 2004 (23): 565–87; C. Filozof *et al.*, 'Smoking cessation and weight gain', *Obesity Review* 2004 (5): 95–103; R. C. Klesges *et al.*, 'How much weight gain occurs following smoking cessation? A comparison of weight gain using both continuous and point prevalence abstinence', *Journal of Consulting and Clinical Psychology* 1997 (65): 286–91; and P. Froom *et al.*, 'Smoking cessation and weight gain', *Journal of Family Practise* 1998 (46): 460–64.

119. Troiano and Flegal, 'Overweight children and adolescents: Description, epidemiology, and demographics'.

120. J. Sandhu *et al.*, 'The impact of childhood body mass index on timing of puberty, adult stature and obesity', *International Journal of Obesity* 2006 (30): 14–22; and F. Greenway, 'Virus-induced obesity', *American Journal of Physiology* 2006 (290): 188–89.

121. A. E. Field *et al.*, 'Weight status in childhood as a predictor of becoming overweight or hypertensive in early adulthood', *Obesity Research* 2005 (13): 163–69; D. S. Freedman *et al.*, 'The relation of childhood BMI to adult adiposity', *Pediatrics* 2005 (115): 22–27; S. S. Guo, 'Tracking of body mass index in children in relation to overweight in adulthood', *American Journal of Clinical Nutrition* 1999 (70): 145–48; M. K. Serdula *et al.*, 'Do obese children become obese adults? A review of the literature', *Preventive Medicine* 1993 (22): 167–77; and R. Valdez *et al.*, 'Use of weight-for-height indices in children to predict adult overweight', *International Journal of Obesity* 1996 (20): 715–21.

122. P. M. Hellstrom *et al.*, 'Peripheral and central signals in the control of eating in normal, obese and binge-eating human subjects', *British Journal of Nutrition* 2004 (92): 47–57.

123. C. A. Argmann *et al.*, 'Peroxisome proliferator-activated receptor gamma: The more the merrier?', *European Journal of Clinical Investigation* 2005 (35): 82–92.

124. P. Cohen and J. M. Friedman, 'Leptin and the control of metabolism: Role for stearoyl-CoA desaturase-1 (SCD-1)', *Journal of Nutrition* 2004 (134): 2455–63; and R. V. Considine, 'Human leptin: An adipocyte hormone with weight-regulatory and endocrine functions', *Seminars in Vascular Medicine* 2005 (5): 15–24.

125. F. Greenway, 'Virus-induced obesity', *American Journal of Physiology* 2006 (290): 188–89.

126. C. F. Jan *et al.*, 'A population-based study investigating the association between metabolic syndrome and Hepatitis B/C infection', *International Journal of Obesity* 2006 (January); and X. Ye *et al.*, 'The

139H scrapie agent produces hypothalamic neurotoxicity and pancreatic islet histopathology: Electron microscopic studies', *Neurotoxicology* 1997 (18): 533–45.

127. P. W. So *et al.*, 'Adiposity induced by adenovirus 5 inoculation', *International Journal of Obesity* 2005 (29): 603–06; L. D. Whigham *et al.*, 'Adipogenic potential of multiple human adenoviruses in vivo and in vitro in animals', *American Journal of Physiology* 2006 (290): 190–94; and R. L. Atkinson *et al.*, 'Human adenovirus-36 is associated with increased body weight and paradoxical reduction of serum lipids', *International Journal of Obesity* 2005 (29): 281–86.

128. K. Clement, 'Genetics of human obesity', *Proceedings of the Nutrition Society* 2005 (64): 133–42.

129. S. G. Wilson *et al.*, 'Linkage and potential association of obesity-related phenotypes with two genes on chromosome 12q24 in a female dizygous twin cohort', *European Journal of Human Genetics* 2006 (14): 340–48; and A. Herbert *et al.*, 'A common genetic variant is associated with adult and childhood obesity', *Science* 2006 (312): 279–83.

130. Muir *et al.*, 'Combining wheat bran with resistant starch has more beneficial effects on fecal indexes than does wheat bran alone'.

CHAPTER 3

Some of the material in this chapter is taken from John C. Luik, *Ideology Masked as Scientific Truth: The Debate About Advertising and Children* (Washington, DC: Washington Legal Foundation, 2006). The authors are grateful to WLF for permission to use this material.

1. T. Philipson and R. Posner, 'The long-run growth in obesity as a function of technological change', *Perspectives in Biology and Medicine* 2003 (46): S87–107.

2. Andrew Prentice and Susan Jebb, 'Obesity in Britain: Gluttony or sloth?' *British Medical Journal* 1995 (311): 437–39.

3. R. Kersh and J. A. Morone, 'Obesity, courts, and the new politics of public health', *Journal of Health, Politics, Policy and Law* 2005 (30): 849.

4. J. McGinnis *et al.* (eds), *Food Marketing to Children and Youth: Threat or Opportunity?* (Washington, DC: Institute of Medicine National Academies Press, 2006), p. ES-4.

5. D. Freedman *et al.*, 'Trends and correlates of class 3 obesity in the United States from 1990 through 2000', *Journal of the American Medical Association* 2002 (288): 1758–61.

6. A. Hedley *et al.*, 'Prevalence of overweight and obesity among US children, adolescents, and adults 1999–2003', *Journal of the American Medical Association* 2004 (291): 2847–50.

7. Paul Campos *et al.*, 'The epidemiology of overweight and obesity: Public health crisis or moral panic?' *International Journal of Epidemiology* 2006 (35): 55–60.

8. UK Department of Health, 'Health Survey for England 2003', 17 December 2004, http://www.dh.gov.uk/PublicationsAndStatistics/ Publications/PublicationsStatistics/PublicationsStatisticsArticle/fs/en? CONTENT_ID=4098712&chk=F4kphd

9. D. Lakdawalla and T. Philipson, 'The growth of obesity and technological change: A theoretical and empirical examination', National Bureau of Economic Research Working Paper 8946, May 2004.

10. Lisa J. Harnack et al., 'Temporal trends in energy intake in the United States: An ecologic perspective', American Journal of Clinical Nutrition 2000 (71): 1478–84.

11. A. Salbe and E. Ravussin, 'The determinants of obesity', in C. Bouchard (ed.), Physical Activity and Obesity (Champaign, IL: Human Kinetics, 2000).

12. D. Dreon et al., 'Dietary fat: Carbohydrate ratio and obesity in middle-aged men', American Journal of Clinical Nutrition 1988 (47): 995–1000.

13. A. Slyper, 'The pediatric obesity epidemic: Causes and controversies', Journal of Clinical Endocrinology and Metabolism 2004 (89): 2540–47.

14. S. Kimm et al., 'Relation between the changes in physical activity and body mass index during adolescence: A multicentre longitudinal study', Lancet 2005 (366): 301–07.

15. R. Troiano et al., 'Energy and fat intakes of children and adolescents in the United States: Data from the National Health and Nutrition Examination Surveys', American Journal of Clinical Nutrition 2002 (72): 1343–53.

16. S. Jebb, 'Aetiology of obesity', British Medical Bulletin 1997 (53): 264–85.

17. P. Speiser et al., 'Consensus statement on childhood obesity', Journal of Clinical Endocrinology and Metabolism 2004 (90): 17.

18. T. Byers, 'The role of epidemiology in developing nutritional recommendations: Past, present and future', American Journal of Clinical Nutrition 1999 (69): 1304–08.

19. Ibid., p. 1304.

20. P. Skrabanek, 'Fat heads', National Review, 1 May 1995.

21. Jon Robison, 'Are there good foods and bad foods?' TechCentralStation.com, 4 February 2004, http://www.tcsdaily.com/ article.aspx?id=020404B

22. Byers, 'The role of epidemiology in developing nutritional recommendations'.

23. Multiple Risk Factor Intervention Trial Research Group, 'Multiple risk factor intervention trial: Risk factor changes and mortality results', Journal of the American Medical Association 1982 (248): 1465–77.

24. L. Hooper et al., 'Systematic review of long term effects of advice to reduce dietary salt in adults', British Medical Journal 2002 (325): 628–37.

25. L. Appel, 'Dietary patterns and blood pressure', *New England Journal of Medicine* 1997 (337): 636–38.

26. N. Graudal *et al.*, 'Effects of sodium restriction on blood pressure, renin, aldosterone, catecholamines, cholesterols, and triglyceride', *Journal of the American Medical Association* 1998 (279): 1383–91.

27. M. Townsend *et al.*, 'Low mineral intake is associated with high systolic blood pressure in the third and fourth National Health and Nutrition Examination Surveys: Could we all be right?' *American Journal of Hypertension* 2005 (18): 261–69.

28. Robison, 'Are there good foods and bad foods?'

29. David Ashton, 'Food advertising and childhood obesity', *Journal of the Royal Society of Medicine* 2004 (97): 51–52.

30. C. Ebbeling *et al.*, 'Childhood obesity: Public health crisis, common sense cure', *Lancet* 2002 (360): 473–82.

31. I. Janssen *et al.*, 'Comparison of overweight and obesity prevalence in school-aged youth from 34 countries and their relationships with physical activity and dietary patterns', *Obesity Review* 2005 (6): 123–32.

32. A. Field *et al.*, 'Snack food intake does not predict weight change among children and adolescents', *International Journal of Obesity* 2004 (28): 1210–16.

33. *Ibid.*, p. 1214.

34. P. Veugelers and A. Fitzgerald, 'Prevalence of and risk factors for childhood overweight and obesity', *Canadian Medical Association Journal* 2005 (173): 607–13.

35. B. Sherry, 'Food behaviors and other strategies to prevent and treat pediatric overweight', *International Journal of Obesity* 2005 (29): 116–26.

36. R. Forshee *et al.*, 'The role of beverage consumption, physical activity, sedentary behavior and demographics on body mass index of adolescents', *International Journal of Food Science Nutrition* 2004 (55): 463–78.

37. R. Forshee *et al.*, 'A risk analysis model of the relationship between beverage consumption from school vending machines and risk of adolescent overweight', *Risk Analysis* 2005 (25): 1121–35.

38. I. Lee and R. Paffenbarger, 'How much physical activity is optimal for health?' *Research Quarterly for Exercise and Sport* 1996 (67): 206–08.

39. House of Commons Health Committee, *Obesity*, 27 May 2004, http://www.publications.parliament.uk/pa/cm200304/cmselect/cmhealth/23/23.pdf#search=%22house%20of%20commons%20health%20committee%20obesity%22, p. 41.

40. President's Council on Physical Fitness and Sport, *Physical Activity Fact Sheet* (Washington, DC: Department of Health and Human Services, 1996).

41. Lakdawalla and Philipson, 'The growth of obesity and technological change'.

42. C. Steuerle et al., 'Can Americans work longer?', Urban Institute, 15 August 1999, http://www.urban.org/publications/309228.html

43. Jebb, 'Aetiology of obesity'.

44. Lakdawalla and Philipson, 'The growth of obesity and technological change'.

45. Ibid.

46. Troiano et al., 'Energy and fat intakes of children and adolescents in the United States'.

47. Kimm et al., 'Relation between the changes in physical activity and body mass index during adolescence'.

48. K. Patrick et al., 'Diet, physical activity and sedentary behaviors as risk factors for overweight in adolescence', Archives of Pediatrics and Adolescent Medicine 2004 (158): 385–90.

49. W. Saris et al., 'How much physical activity is enough to prevent unhealthy weight gain? Outcome of the IASO 1st Stock Conference and consensus statement', Obesity Review 2003 (4): 101–14.

50. Marion Nestle, Food Politics: How the Food Industry Influences Nutrition and Health, p. 181 (Berkeley, CA: University of California, 2002).

51. Susan Linn, Consuming Kids: The Hostile Takeover of Childhood, p. 96 (New York: The New Press, 2004).

52. Kelly Brownell and K. Horgen, Food Fight: The Inside Story of the Food Industry, America's Obesity Crisis, and What We Can Do About It, p. 116 (Chicago: Contemporary Books, 2004).

53. D. Kunkel and D. Roberts, 'Young minds and marketplace values: Issues in children's television advertising', Journal of Social Issues 1991 (47): 57–72.

54. W. Dietz and S. Gortmaker, 'Do we fatten our children at the television set? Obesity and television viewing in children and adolescents', Pediatrics 1985 (75): 807–12.

55. Gerard Hastings et al., Review of Research on the Effects of Food Promotion to Children (London: Food Standards Agency, 2003), available at http://www.foodstandards.gov.uk/multimedia/pdfs/foodpromotiontochildren1.pdf

56. J. McGinnis et al. (eds), Food Marketing to Children and Youth: Threat or Opportunity? (Washington, DC: Institute of Medicine National Academies Press, 2005).

57. C. Atkin, 'Effects of television advertising on children – survey of children's and mothers' responses to television commercials', Report no. 8, Michigan State University, East Lansing MI, 1975; and Dietz and Gortmaker, 'Do we fatten our children at the television set?' are unusual in controlling for a few of these factors.

58. World Advertising Research Center, Advertising Statistics Yearbook 2004 (22nd edn) (Henley-on-Thames: WARC, 2004).

59. T. Zwicki, 'Obesity and advertising policy', *George Mason Law Review* 2004 (12): 979–1011.

60. S. Biddle *et al.*, 'Physical activity and sedentary behaviours in youth: Issues and controversies', *Journal of the Royal Society of Health* 2004 (124): 29–33.

61. Zwicki, 'Obesity and advertising policy'.

62. R. Dickinson, 'Food and eating on television: Impacts and influences', *Nutrition and Food Science* 2000 (30): 24–29.

63. David Buckingham, *Children Talking Television: The Making of Television Literacy* (London: Falmer Press, 1993).

64. *Ibid.*, p. 251.

65. *Ibid.*, p. 257.

66. R. Bolton, 'Modeling the impact of television food advertising on children's diets', *Current Issues Research Advertising* 1983 (7): 173–99.

67. Peter Kyle, 'The impact of advertising on markets', in J. C. Luik and M. J. Waterson (eds), *Advertising & Markets: A Collection of Seminal Papers* (Oxford: NTC Publications, 1997).

68. M. Duffy, 'The influence of advertising on the pattern of food consumption in the UK', *International Journal of Advertising* 1999 (18): 131–68.

69. M. Duffy, 'Advertising and food, drink and tobacco consumption in the United Kingdom: A dynamic demand system', *Agricultural Economics* 2003 (28): 51–70.

70. H. Henry, 'Does advertising affect market size?' *Admap*, January 1996.

71. J. Yasim, 'The effects of advertising on fast-moving consumer goods markets', *International Journal of Advertising* 1995 (14): 133–47.

72. B. Eagle and T. Ambler, 'The influence of advertising on the demand for chocolate confectionery', *International Journal of Advertising* 2002 (21): 437–54.

73. Aimee Dorr, *Television and Children: A Special Medium for a Special Audience* (Beverly Hills, CA: Sage, 1986).

74. A. Huston, B. Watkins and D. Kunkel, 'Public policy and children's television', *American Psychologist* 1989 (44): 424–33.

75. Michael McGinnis, 'Actual causes of death in the United States', *Journal of the American Medical Association* 1993 (270): 2207–12.

76. A. Mokdad *et al.*, 'Actual causes of death in the United States', *Journal of the American Medical Association* 2004 (291): 1238–45.

77. J. McGinnis and W. Foege, 'The immediate vs the important', *Journal of the American Medical Association* 2004 (291): 1263–64.

78. K. Flegal *et al.*, 'Excess deaths associated with underweight, overweight and obesity', *Journal of the American Medical Association* 2005 (293): 1861–67.

79. B. Young *et al.*, *The Role of Television Advertising in Children's Food Choice* (London: MAFF, 1996).

80. Ofcom, *Childhood Obesity: Food Advertising in Context*, July 2004, http://www.ofcom.org.uk/research/tv/reports/food_ads/report.pdf

81. *Ibid.*, p. 92.

82. *Ibid.*, p. 23.

83. *Ibid.*, p. 114.

84. *Ibid.*, p. 21.

85. *Ibid.*, p. 100.

86. McGinnis *et al.* (eds), *Food Marketing to Children and Youth*, pp. 5–6.

87. American Psychological Association, *Report of the APA Task Force on Advertising and Children* (Washington, DC, 2004), at http://www.apa.org/releases/childrenads.pdf

88. G. Smith and E. Sweeney, *Children and Television Advertising: An Overview* (London: Children Research Unit, 1984).

89. American Psychological Association, *Report of the APA Task Force on Advertising and Children*, p. 1.

90. Federal Trade Commission, *Staff Report on Television Advertising to Children* (Washington, DC, 1978).

91. Jeffrey Goldstein, *Children and Advertising: Policy Implications of Scholarly Research* (London: Advertising Association, 1997).

92. A. Furnham, *Children and Advertising: The Allegations and the Evidence* (London: Social Affairs Unit, 2000).

93. American Psychological Association, *Report of the APA Task Force on Advertising and Children*, p. 5.

94. Huston *et al.*, 'Public policy and children's television'.

95. Kunkel and Roberts, 'Young minds and marketplace values: Issues in children's television advertising'.

96. Huston *et al.*, 'Public policy and children's television'.

97. W. Fletcher, *How to Capture the Advertising High Ground* (London: Century Business, 1994).

98. Stephen Bell, 'Evaluating the effects of consumer advertising on market positions over time: How to tell whether advertising ever works', Proceedings of the Marketing Science Institute Conference, Report No. 88-107, 3, 1988.

99. H. Murray, 'Advertising's effect on sales – proven or just assumed?', *International Journal of Advertising* 1986 (5): 15–36.

100. *Ibid.*, pp. 22–23.

101. IPA, *Advertising Works* case histories, NTC Publications, Henley-on-Thames, UK.

102. M. Waterson, 'Advertising, brands and markets', in J. Luik and M. Waterson (eds), *Advertising and Markets* (Henley-on-Thames: NTC, 1996), p. 23.

103. Murray, 'Advertising's effect on sales – proven or just assumed?', p. 32.

104. Melissa Dittmann, 'Selling to children', *Monitor on Psychology* 2002 (33): 37.

105. For a fuller account of the available literature, see E. Palmer, *Television and America's Children: A Crisis of Neglect* (New York: Oxford University Press, 1988); and B. Young, *Television, Advertising and Children* (Oxford: Oxford University Press, 1990).

106. L. Jaglom and H. Gardner, 'The preschool television viewer as anthropologist', in H. Kelly and H. Gardner (eds), *Viewing Children Through Television* (San Francisco: Jossey Bass, 1981).

107. S. Levin *et al.*, 'Preschoolers' awareness of television advertising', *Child Development* 1982 (53): 933–37.

108. Kunkel and Roberts, 'Young minds and marketplace values'.

109. J. Blatt *et al.*, 'A cognitive developmental study of children's reactions to television advertising', in E. Rubenstein *et al.* (eds), *Television and Social Behavior*, vol. 4, *Television in Day-to-Day Life: Patterns of Use* (Washington, DC: US Government Printing Office, 1972); S. Ward *et al.*, 'Children's perceptions, explanations and judgments of television advertising: A further exploration', in Rubenstein *et al.*, *Television and Social Behavior*.

110. American Psychological Association, *Report of the APA Task Force on Advertising and Children*, p. 6.

111. S. Ward *et al.*, *How Children Learn to Buy: The Development of Consumer Information-Processing Skills* (Beverly Hills, CA: Sage, 1977).

112. T. Robertson and J. Rossiter, 'Children and commercial persuasion: An attributional analysis', *Journal of Consumer Research* 1974 (3): 58–61.

113. American Psychological Association, *Report of the APA Task Force on Advertising and Children*, p. 8.

114. B. Blosser and D. Roberts, 'Age differences in children's perceptions of message intent', *Communication Research* 1985 (12): 455–84; Robertson and Rossiter, 'Children and commercial persuasion'; J. Rossiter and T. Robertson, 'Children's television commercials: Testing the defenses', *Journal of Communication* 1974 (24): 137–44; S. Ward and D. Wackman, 'Children's information processing of television advertising', in P. Clarke (ed.), *New Models for Mass Communication Research* (Beverly Hills, CA: Sage, 1973); and S. Ward, D. Wachman and E. Wartella, *How Children Learn to Buy* (Beverly Hills, CA: Sage, 1977).

115. L. Gaines and J. Esserman, 'A quantitative study of young children's comprehension of television programs and commercials', in J. Esserman (ed.), *Television Advertising and Children: Issues, Research and Findings* (New York: Child Research Service, 1981).

116. L. Peterson and K. Lewis, 'Preventive intervention to improve children's discrimination of the persuasive tactics in televised advertising', *Journal of Pediatric Psychology* 1988 (13): 163–70.

117. D. Backe and S. Kommer, 'Die Werbung und die Kinder', *Medien und Erziehung* 1997 (41): 228–34.

118. B. Greenberg *et al.*, *Children's Views on Advertising*, Independent Broadcasting Authority Research Report (London, 1986).

119. David Buckingham, *After the Death of Childhood: Growing Up in the Age of Electronic Media* (Cambridge: Polity Press, 2000).

120. T. Donahue *et al.*, 'Do kids know what TV commercials intend?', *Journal of Advertising Research* 1980 (20): 51–57.

121. B. Young *et al.*, 'The young child's understanding of advocacy communication', in K. Quintanilla and R. Luna (eds), *The Proceedings of the 22nd Annual Colloquium of IAREP* 1997 (2): 761–78.

122. J. Anderson, 'Research on children and television: A critique', *Journal of Broadcasting* 1981 (25): 395–400.

123. Buckingham, *After the Death of Childhood*.

124. Judy Dunn, 'Making sense of the social world: Mindreading, emotion, and relationships', in P. Zelazo *et al.* (eds), *Developing Theories of Intention: Social Understanding and Self-Control* (Mahwah, NJ: Erlbaum, 1999).

125. *Ibid.*

126. K. Bartsch and H. Wellman, *Children Talk about the Mind* (Oxford: Oxford University Press, 1995).

127. Dunn, 'Making sense of the social world: Mindreading, emotion, and relationships'.

128. Stephen Kline, 'Toys as media: The role of toy design, promotional TV and mother's reinforcement in the young males' (3–6) acquisition of pro-social play scripts for rescue hero action toys,' ITRA Conference, Halmstadt, Sweden, 18 June 1999.

129. Dunn, 'Making sense of the social world: Mindreading, emotion, and relationships'.

130. A. Meltzoff *et al.*, 'Toddlers' understanding of intentions, desires, and emotions: Explorations of the dark ages', in Zelazo *et al.* (eds), *Developing Theories of Intention: Social Understanding and Self-Control*.

131. *Ibid.*

132. Howard Gardner, *Frames of Mind: The Theory of Multiple Intelligences* (New York: Basic Books, 1983).

133. Bartsch and Wellman, *Children Talk about the Mind*.

134. Eleanor Siegel, *APS Observer*, May 1991.

135. H. Hartshorne and M. May, *Studies in Deceit* (New York: Macmillan, 1928).

136. K. Bartsch and K. London, 'Children's use of mental state information in selecting persuasive arguments', *Developmental Psychology* 2000 (36): 352–65.

137. S. Kline and B. Clinton, 'Developments in children's persuasive message practices', *Communication Education* 1998 (47): 120–35.

138. See P. La Freniere, 'The ontogeny of tactical deception in humans', in R. Byrne and A. Whiten (eds), *Machiavellian Intelligence* (Oxford: Clarendon Press, 1988); M. Vasek, 'Lying as a skill: The development of deception in children', in R. Mitchell and N. Thompson (eds), *Deception: Perspectives on Human and Nonhuman Deceit* (Albany, NY: Albany State University Press, 1986); M. Chandler *et al.*, 'Small-scale deceit: Deception as a marker of two, three and four-year olds' theories of mind', *Child Development* 1989 (60): 1263–77; P. Newton, Preschool Prevarication: An Investigation of the Cognitive Prerequisites for Deception, doctoral dissertation, University of Portsmouth, 1994; B. Sodian, 'The development of deception in children', *British Journal of Developmental Psychology* 1991 (9): 173–88; and R. Burton, 'Honesty and dishonesty', in T. Lickona (ed.), *Moral Development and Behavior* (New York: Holt, Rinehart, and Winston, 1976).

139. David Nyberg, *The Varnished Truth: Truth Telling and Deceiving in Ordinary Life* (Chicago: University of Chicago Press, 1993).

140. Vasek, 'Lying as a skill'.

141. *Ibid.*

142. Ludmilla Jordanova, 'Children in history: Concepts of nature and society', in G. Scarre (ed.), *Children, Parents and Politics* (Cambridge: Cambridge University Press, 1989).

143. Buckingham, *After the Death of Childhood.*

144. Kay Hymowitz, *Ready or Not: What Happens When We Treat Children as Small Adults* (San Francisco: Encounter Books, 2000).

145. Don Tapscott, *Growing Up Digital: The Rise of the Net Generation* (New York: McGraw Hill, 1998).

146. Goldstein, *Children and Advertising.*

147. T. Clarke, 'Situational factors affecting preschoolers' responses to advertising', *Journal of the Academy of Marketing Science* 1984 (Fall): 25–40.

148. Buckingham, *After the Death of Childhood.*

149. David Buckingham, *The Media Literacy of Children and Young People: A Review of the Research Literature on Behalf of the Ofcom Centre for the Study of Children,* http://www.ofcom.org.uk/advice/media_literacy/medlitpub/medlitpubrss/ml_children.pdf

150. American Psychological Association, *Report of the APA Task Force on Advertising and Children,* p. 21.

151. R. Hobbs and R. Frost, 'Measuring the acquisition of media literacy skills', *Reading Research Quarterly* 2003 (38): 330–56.

152. See G. Riecken and U. Yavas, 'Children's general, product and brand-specific attitudes towards television commercials', *International Journal of Advertising* 1990 (9): 136–48; D. Singer *et al.*, 'Helping elementary school children learn about TV', *Journal of Communication* 1980 (30): 84–93; W. Rapaczynski *et al.*, 'Teaching television: A

curriculum for young children', *Journal of Communication* 1982 (32): 46–55; and M. Brucks *et al.*, 'Children's use of cognitive defenses against television advertising: A cognitive response approach', *Journal of Consumer Research* 1988 (14): 471–82.

153. Riecken and Yavas, 'Children's general, product and brand-specific attitudes towards television commercials'.

154. Peterson and Lewis, 'Preventive intervention to improve children's discrimination of the persuasive tactics in televised advertising'.

155. S. Feshbach *et al.*, 'Enhancing children's discrimination in response to television advertising: The effects of psychoeducational training in two elementary school groups', *Developmental Review* 1982 (2): 3–12.

156. D. Singer *et al.*, 'Family mediation and children's cognition, aggression, and comprehension of television: A longitudinal study', *Journal of Applied Developmental Psychology* 1988 (9): 329–47.

157. G. Moschis and R. Moore, 'Consumer socialization: A theoretical and empirical analysis', *Journal of Marketing Research* 1978 (15): 599–609.

158. V. Prasad *et al.*, 'Mother vs commercial', *Journal of Communication* 1978 (28): 91–96.

159. Ofcom, *Childhood Obesity: Food Advertising in Context*, p. 18.

CHAPTER 4

1. For a rare discussion of both sides of this debate in the American context, see Kate Zernike, 'Food fight: Is obesity the responsibility of the body politic?', *New York Times*, 9 November 2003.

2. Tim Richardson, 'Let them eat sweets', *Guardian*, 6 August 2005.

3. Tim Richardson, *Sweets: A History of Candy* (New York: Bloomsbury, 2002).

4. Richardson, 'Let them eat sweets'.

5. Richard Klein, *Eat Fat* (New York: Vintage, 1996).

6. Richard Klein, 'A VAT on Fat?', BBC News Online, 18 June 2003, http://news.bbc.co.uk/go/pr/fr/-/2/hi/uk_news/2988314.stm

7. Cited in 'Eating: Now with reduced joy', Center for Consumer Freedom, 19 April 2006, http://www.consumer freedom.com.cfml?id= 3015&page=headline

8. 'Food industry slams obesity plans', BBC News Online, 15 November 2004, http://news.bbc.co.uk/go/pr/fr/-/2/hi/business/ 4013537.stm

9. See, for example, the comments by dieticians Stephanie Smith and Mary Lee Chin, reported in 'Soda scares more fizz than fact', Center for Consumer Freedom, 16 May 2002, http://www.consumerfreedom.com/ news_detail.cfm/headline/1424

10. Vincent Marks and Stanley Feldman (eds), *Panic Nation: Unpicking the Myths We're Told about Food and Health* (London: Blake, 2005).

11. Fitzpatrick, quoted in Brendan O'Neill, 'Is junk food a myth?', BBC News Online, 3 October 2005, http://news.bbc.co.uk/1/hi/magazine/4304118.stm

12. Cited in Clare Matheson, 'Food lobby weighs in on obesity debate', BBC News Online, 27 May 2004, http://news.bbc.co.uk/go/pr/fr/-/2/hi/business/3750127.stm

13. For an economic perspective on the labelling debate, see Jayachandran N. Variyam, 'Nutrition labeling in the food-away-from-home sector: An economic assessment', ERR-4, USDA Economic Research Service, April 2005.

14. Raja Mishra, 'Food warning labels on FDA's plate', *Boston Globe*, 23 April 2004, http://www.boston.com/news/nation/articles/2004/04/23/food_warning_labels_on_fdas_plate?pg=full

15. John Stossel, 'Give me a break', *20/20*, ABC-TV News, 18 July 2003.

16. See, for example, Jane Zhang, 'How much soy lecithin is in that cookie?', *Wall Street Journal*, 13 October 2005.

17. Liz Lightfoot, 'Pupils "Will still find ways to eat crisps and sweets"', *Daily Telegraph*, 29 September 2005.

18. Alexandra Blair and Tony Halpin, 'Schools to ban fizzy drinks and chocolate', *Times*, 3 March 2006.

19. I. Lissau *et al.*, 'Body mass index and overweight in adolescents in 13 European countries, Israel, and the United States', *Archives of Pediatrics and Adolescent Medicine* 2004 (158): 27–33.

20. C. S. Berkey *et al.*, 'Longitudinal study of skipping breakfast and weight change in adolescents', *International Journal of Obesity* 2003 (27): 1258–66.

21. Janet Whatley Blum *et al.*, 'Frequency of school vending machine purchases, BMI and diet quality', paper presented at the annual meeting of the North American Association for the Study of Obesity, Vancouver, 17 October 2005.

22. Georgetown Center for Food and Nutrition Policy, research presented at the Federation of American Societies for Experimental Biology annual meeting, San Diego, April 2000.

23. John Luik, 'Soda pop redux', *Western Standard*, September 2005.

24. R. A. Forshee *et al.*, 'A risk analysis model of the relationship between beverage consumption from school vending machines and risk of adolescent overweight', *Journal of Pediatrics* 2005 (25): 1121–35.

25. Lightfoot, 'Pupils "Will still find ways to eat crisps and sweets"'.

26. Quoted in Liz Lightfoot, 'Pioneering experiment fails as children reject healthy option', *Daily Telegraph*, 29 September 2005.

27. Quoted in 'Five-year-old girls "weight conscious"', BBC News Online, 7 September 2000, http://news.bbc.co.uk/1/hi/health/913435.stm

28. Anthony Worral Thompson, 'Without a bit of nannying, we'll never eat properly', *Independent*, 14 November 2004.

29. Ray Dunne, 'Should junk food ads be banned?', BBC News Online, 7 April 2004, http://news.bbc.co.uk/go/pr/fr/-/2/hi/health/3586585.stm; see also David Ashton, 'Food ads don't make kids unfit', *Guardian*, 3 March 2004.

30. Quoted in 'Child diet "is down to parents"', BBC News Online, 28 January 2004, http://news.bbc.co.uk/2/hi/health/3429999.stm

31. Cited by Jeremy Preston, director of Food Advertising Unit, Advertising Association, *Today*, BBC Radio 4, 30 January 2006, http://www.bbc.co.uk/radio/noscript.shtml?/radio/aod/radio4_aod.shtml?radio4/tip_mon

32. J. McGinnis *et al.* (eds), *Food Marketing to Children and Youth: Threat or Opportunity?* (Washington, DC: Institute of Medicine National Academies Press, 2006).

33. Institute of Medicine, http://www.nap.edu/books/0309097134/html/7.html

34. Gary Becker, 'Advertising and obesity of children', *The Becker-Posner Blog*, 11 December 2005, http://www.becker-posner-blog.com/archives/2005/12/advertising_and_1.html

35. *Ibid.*

36. 'Fighting fat: The obesity epidemic', *Breakfast News*, BBC TV, 16 July 2002.

37. 'Measures to cut obesity revealed', BBC News Online, 16 November 2004, http://news.bbc.co.uk/go/pr/fr/-/2/hi/health/4015571.stm

38. Social Issues Research Centre, *Obesity and the Facts: An Analysis of Data from the Health Survey for England 2003* (Oxford, 2005).

39. 'Food firms warned over fat crisis', BBC News Online, 29 May 2004, http://news.bbc.co.uk/go/pr/fr/-/2/hi/health/3759891.stm

40. 'Celebrity junk food ads attacked', BBC News Online, 14 November 2003, http://news.bbc.co.uk/go/pr/fr/-/2/hi/health/3266829.stm

41. See, for example, 'Sports stars blamed for obesity', BBC News Online, 13 November 2003, http://news.bbc.co.uk/go/pr/fr/-/2/hi/ uk_news/politics/3269383.stm

42. Becker, 'Advertising and obesity of children'.

43. See, for example, Margot Shields, *Measured Obesity: Overweight Canadian Children and Adolescents*, Statistics Canada, http://www.statcan.ca/english/research/82-620-MIE/2005001/pdf/cobesity.pdf

44. Ontario Medical Association, *An Ounce of Prevention or a Ton of Trouble: Is There an Epidemic of Obesity in Children?* Summary of Recommendations, http://www.oma.org/Health/Obesity/ObesitySep2805.pdf; see also Antonella Artuso, 'Obese Generation at Risk: Report', *Toronto Sun*, 2 October 2005.

45. Ashton, 'Food ads don't make kids unfit'.

46. Dunne, 'Should junk food ads be banned?'

47. See, for example, the discussion in Fred Kuchler *et al.*, 'Obesity policy and the law of unintended consequences', *Amber Waves*, June 2005.

48. Jamie Oliver's devastating Channel 4 television series in spring 2005, *Jamie's School Dinners*, on the inadequacy of school meals. Some 270,000 people signed his 'Feed Me Better' petition that he delivered to Downing Street in March. The response was a government pledge of £280 million over three years to raise the standards of school meals.

49. See, for example, Jay Rayner, 'The truth about school dinners: What happened when Jamie went home', *Observer*, 25 June 2006.

50. See, for example, the recent discussion in Lisa Belkin, 'The school lunch test', *New York Times* Magazine, 20 August 2006.

51. See, for example, John Gill, Letter, *Sunday Times*, 13 March 2005.

52. Rebecca Smithers, Felicity Lawrence and Matthew Taylor, 'Cola, crisps and sweets banned as Kelly declares war on junk food', *Guardian*, 29 September 2005.

53. *Ibid.*

54. See also the discussion in Harriet Brown, 'Well-intentioned food police may create havoc with children's diets', *New York Times*, 30 May 2006.

55. Klein, 'A VAT on fat?'.

56. Reported in 'Fat of the land', *Economist*, 4 March 2004.

57. Hugh Muir, 'Action urged on eating habits', *Guardian*, 7 September 2005.

58. Barry Wigmore, 'Doctors call for fat tax on Coca-Cola and Pepsi', *Daily Mail*, 12 June 2006.

59. See, for example, Patrick Basham, Gio Gori and John Luik, 'An analysis of the proposal to tax junk food', *Obesity Review* 2006 (7): 224, and 'Head-to-head: fat tax', BBC News Online, 6 June 2006, http://news.bbc.co.uk/1/hi/health/5051248.stm

60. Fred Kuchler, Abebayehu Tegene and J. Michael Harris, 'Taxing snack foods: Manipulating diet quality or financing information programs?' *Review of Agricultural Economics* 2005 (27): 4–20.

61. See, for example, Richard A. Epstein, 'Let the shoemaker stick to his last: A defense of the "old" public health', *Perspectives in Biology and Medicine* 2003 (46): 138–59.

62. Kuchler *et al.*, 'Obesity policy and the law of unintended consequences'. A lengthier economic analysis of fat taxes is found in Fred Kuchler *et al.*, 'Taxing snack foods: What to expect for diet and tax revenues', AIB-747-08, USDA Economic Research Service, August 2004.

63. Nancy Howarth *et al.*, 'Dietary energy density is associated with overweight status among five ethnic groups: The multiethnic cohort study', presented at the North American Association for the Study of Obesity annual meeting, Vancouver, 17 October 2005.

64. Kuchler *et al.*, 'Obesity policy and the law of unintended consequences'.

65. Sarah M. Phillips *et al.*, 'Energy-dense snack food intake in adolescence: Longitudinal relationship to weight and fatness', *Obesity Research* 2004 (12): 461–72.

66. Roger Dobson, 'Snacks not cause of obesity in children', *Independent on Sunday*, 19 September 2004.

67. 'Don't punish food companies for world's growing girth', *USA Today*, leading article, 5 February 2004.

68. Henry K. Lee, 'Supervisor wants to limit number of fast-food eateries', *San Francisco Chronicle*, 25 January 2006.

69. Roger Bate, 'Money where the mouth is', TechCentralStation.com, 15 May 2005, http://www.tcsdaily.com/ article.aspx?id=051503A

70. S. Bryn Austin *et al.*, 'Clustering of fast-food restaurants around schools: A novel application of spatial statistics to the study of food environments', *American Journal of Public Health* 2005 (95): 1575–81.

71. Roland Sturm and A. Datar, 'Body mass index in elementary school children, metropolitan area food prices and food outlet density', *Public Health* 2005 (119): 1059–68.

72. D. Simmons *et al.*, 'Choice and availability of takeaway and restaurant food is not related to the prevalence of adult obesity in rural communities in Australia', *International Journal of Obesity* 2005 (29): 703–10.

73. Quoted in 'Child diet "is down to parents"'.

74. Sarah Boseley, 'Obesity in men almost doubles in 10 years to 23.6%', *Guardian*, 17 December 2005.

75. Reported in Duncan Walker, 'Piling on the prejudice', BBC News Online, 6 September 2004, http://news.bbc.co.uk/1/hi/magazine/3622320.stm

76. R. C. Davey, 'The obesity epidemic: Too much food for thought?', *British Journal of Sports Medicine* 2004 (38): 360–63.

77. The historical precedent for such action dates to the early thirteenth century. In 1202, King John proclaimed the first food law, the Assize of Bread, which prohibited the adulteration of bread with ground peas.

78. Reported in 'Cameron attacks chocolate sellers', BBC News Online, 4 January 2006, http://news.bbc.co.uk/go/pr/fr/-/2/hi/uk_news/politics/4580778.stm; see also Matthew Tempest, 'Cameron rounds on irresponsible big business', *Guardian*, 9 May 2006.

79. 'It's high time our children stopped living la vida logo', *Guardian*, Letters, 26 October 2005.

80. Boris Johnson, 'Hewitt and her appointees are bad news for our hospitals and health', *Daily Telegraph*, 13 October 2005.

81. See 'Minister for fitness appointed', BBC News Online, 23 August 2006, http://news.bbc.co.uk/2/hi/health/5277350.stm; and 'Fat chance', *Economist*, 24 August 2006.

82. For a comprehensive overview of existing regulations governing the advertising of food products to children, see Corinna Hawkes, *Marketing Food to Children: The Global Regulatory Environment* (Geneva: World Health Organization, 2004).

83. 'Colour-coded food labelling urged', BBC News Online, 9 March 2006, http://news.bbc.co.uk/1/hi/health/4788704.stm; and Felicity Lawrence, 'Obesity crisis prompts leading food firms to add health labels', *Guardian*, 9 February 2006.

84. Richard Garner, 'Parents to be told what to put in packed lunches', *Independent*, 4 October 2005.

85. 'We cannot make health choices for people, says Blair', *Daily Telegraph*, 26 July 2006; and the *Economist*'s 'Fat chance'.

86. Valerie Elliott, 'Junk food has claimed a generation', *Times*, 24 October 2005.

87. 'Curbs on advertising proposed', *Times*, 14 November 2005.

88. Francis Elliott, 'Obesity tests: The fat police', *Independent on Sunday*, 21 May 2006; see also Francis Elliott and Megan Waitkoff, 'Fat: How the national obsession is coming into the classroom', *Independent on Sunday*, 21 May 2006.

89. Waldemar Ingdahl, 'Swedish meatballs', TechCentralStation.com, 16 February 2004, http://www.tcsdaily.com/article.aspx?id=021604D

90. *Ibid.*

91. *Ibid.*

92. Joshua Livestro, 'Thin fizzy', TechCentralStation.com, 31 January 2006, http://www.tcsdaily.com/printArticle.aspx?ID=013106H

93. 'EU leads US for men with weight problem', Associated Press report in *Guardian*, 16 March 2005.

94. See 'EU takes aim at junk food adverts', BBC News Online, 20 January 2005, http://news.bbc.co.uk/go/pr/fr/-/2/hi/business/4190313.stm; and Julia Day, 'Europe warns food firms on junk ads', *Guardian*, 20 January 2005.

95. 'Soft drink makers agree to restrict marketing aimed at children in Europe', Associated Press report, 25 January 2006.

96. Quoted in Paul Meller, 'Europe's turn to wrestle with obesity', *New York Times*, 24 November 2005.

97. Zernike, 'Food fight: Is obesity the responsibility of the body politic?'

98. See, for example, Jeremy Grant, 'Fast food outlets under pressure to put nutritional secrets higher on the menu', *Financial Times*, 25 March 2006.

99. William Wan, 'No junk food? Students shudder at nutrition plans', *Washington Post*, 8 December 2005.

100. Carl Hulse, 'Vote in House offers a shield in obesity suits', *New York Times*, 11 March 2004.

101. Survey conducted by Stony Brook University Center for Survey Research, 22 July to 12 August 2003.

102. Greg Critser, *Fatland: How Americans Became the Fattest People in the World* (Boston: Houghton Mifflin, 2003).

103. Greg Critser, 'Measuring up: New front in the battle of the bulge', *New York Times*, 18 May 2003.

104. Mireille Guiliano, *French Women Don't Get Fat: The Secret of Eating for Pleasure* (New York: Alfred A. Knopf, 2005).

105. See, for example, 'Gross national product: Contrary to popular myth, French people do get fat', *Economist*, 20 December 2005.

106. 'French fall foul of a little too much of what they fancy', *Daily Telegraph*, 18 October 2005.

107. Karen Allen, 'Fighting fat the Finnish Way', BBC News Online, 5 February 2004,
http://news.bbc.co.uk/go/pr/fr/-/2/hi/health/ 3451491.stm

108. 'EU battle of bulge expands', BBC News Online, 24 August 2006, http://www.bbc.co.uk/mediaselector/check/nolavconsole/ifs_news/hi?redirect=st.stm&news=1&bbram=1&bbwm=1&nbram=1&nbwm=1&nol_storyid=5273270

109. Ian Sample, 'Fat to fit: How Finland did it', *Guardian*, 15 January 2005.

110. 'Food firms and fat-fighters', *Economist*, 9 February 2006.

111. Susan Linn, *Consuming Kids: Protecting Our Children from the Onslaught of Marketing and Advertising* (New York: Anchor, 2005).

112. Eric Schlosser, *Fast Food Nation: The Dark Side of the All-American Meal* (New York: Harper Collins, 2001).

113. Eric Schlosser and Charles Wilson, *Chew on This: Everything You Don't Want to Know about Fast Food* (New York: Houghton Mifflin, 2006).

114. See, for example, Mark Johnson, 'Reputation management: The fast-food fight', *PR Week*, 29 October 2004.

115. See, for example, Raphael Minder and Andrew Ward, 'Soft drink makers in voluntary ban on advertising', *Financial Times*, 25 January 2006.

116. 'Food firms and fat-fighters'.

117. For a discussion of the strategic background to McDonald's move, see Jeremy Grant and Jenny Wiggins, 'McDonald's to introduce nutrition labels', *Financial Times*, 26 October 2005; Bruce Horovitz, 'You want nutrition info with that?', *USA Today*, 26 October 2005; and Melanie Warner, 'McDonald's to add facts on nutrition to packaging', *New York Times*, 26 October 2005.

118. Caroline E. Mayer, 'Work off those Cheetos!', *Washington Post*, 23 November 2005.

119. Source: American Advertising Federation, cited in 'Junior fat', *Economist*, 14 December 2005.

120. See, for example, Day, 'Europe warns food firms on junk ads'. Regarding Kraft, McDonalds and PepsiCo, see also 'Mea culpa', *Economist*, 3 July 2003; and 'Changing the menu', *Economist*, 20 May 2004.

121. Meller, 'Europe's turn to wrestle with obesity'.

122. See also Valerie Elliott, 'Obesity fears prompt child website bans', *Times*, 21 July 2006.

123. David Gow, 'Soft drink makers promise to stop targeting children', *Guardian*, 26 January 2006.

124. Samantha Gross, 'Nearly all soda sales to schools to end', *Associated Press*, 3 May 2006.

125. 'Crisp firm spends £6m cutting fat', *Daily Telegraph*, 3 February 2006.

126. 'Food firms and fat-fighters'.

127. Lawrence, 'Obesity crisis prompts leading food firms to add health labels'.

128. Livestro, 'Thin fizzy'.

129. See the comments reported in Lawrence, 'Obesity crisis prompts leading food firms to add health labels'.

130. For more on the tobacco industry analogy, see 'Can governments make people thin?', *Economist*, 11 December 2003, and 'Food firms and fat-fighters'.

131. 'Taste for meddling', *Daily Telegraph*, leading article, 7 January 2006.

132. Cited in Jennifer Whitehead, 'Most people blame parents not ads for childhood obesity', *Brand Republic*, 20 July 2006; see also Ann Widdecombe, 'Blame parents for children being fat', *Daily Express*, 22 March 2006.

133. Data provided by Harvard political scientist Taeku Lee, cited in Neil Shea, 'The party line on flab', *Harvard Magazine*, September–October 2002.

134. Taeku Lee and J. Eric Oliver, 'Public opinion and the politics of America's obesity epidemic', John F. Kennedy School of Government Faculty Research Working Papers Series, Harvard University, May 2002.

135. Reported in 'Obesity: US, UK attitudes differ', Food USA Navigator.com, 7 July 2004, http://foodnavigator-usa.com/news/printNewsBis.asp?id=53361

136. Survey conducted by Princeton Survey Research Associates International, 12 July to 13 August 2004.

137. Reported in Lauren Neergaard, 'Parents blame kids' inactivity for obesity', *Miami Herald*, 25 October 2005.

138. Jon Henley, 'Snack attack', *Guardian*, 7 September 2005.

139. Cited in 'CSPI's "9 percent" approval rating', Center for Consumer Freedom, 22 July 2003, http://www.consumerfreedom.com/news_detail.cfm/headline/2029

140. Cited in Melanie Warner, 'The food industry empire strikes back', *New York Times*, 7 July 2005.

141. Survey conducted by Stony Brook University Center for Survey Research, 22 July to 12 August 2003.

142. Kate Zernike, 'Lawyers shift focus from big tobacco to big food', *New York Times*, 8 April 2004.

143. Cited in Deborah Orr, 'The mantra of market forces blames the victims and excuses the most powerful', *Independent*, 23 November 2005.

144. Jeremy Laurance, 'Shopping habits show food advice is being ignored', *Independent*, 11 December 2004; and 'Our slow journey to healthy eating', *Independent*, 11 December 2004.

145. Martin Hickman, 'Chocolate makers eat their words on king-size snacks', *Independent*, 6 January 2006.

146. Maxine Frith, 'Unsociable hours and commuting turn Britain into nation of snackers', *Independent*, 14 January 2005.

147. Reported in 'Customers ask for bigger portions', BBC News Online, 25 March 2004, http://news.bbc.co.uk/go/pr/fr/2/hi/health/3567247.stm

148. Interview with Anushka Asthana, 'Food watchdog targets ready meals', *Observer*, 9 October 2005.

149. Cited in Patrick Wintour, 'Blame obesity on bad diets, say food chiefs', *Guardian*, 28 November 2003.

150. 'Sports stars blamed for obesity'.

151. Dan Mitchell, 'Supersize comeback for fast-food', *New York Times*, 12 November 2005.

152. Bruce Horovitz, 'Restaurant sales climb with bad-for-you food', *USA Today*, 13 to 15 May 2005.

153. Cited in 'Food firms and fat-fighters'.

154. John Cawley *et al.*, 'Size matters: The influence of adolescents' weight and height on dating and sex', *Rationality and Society* 2006 (18): 67–94.

155. According to NPD Group tracking of consumer eating habits in 2004, the 10 most popular foods consumed in American restaurants by men were: hamburger, French fries, pizza, breakfast sandwich, side salad, eggs, doughnuts, hash browns, Chinese food and main salad; the 10 most popular foods consumed by women were: French fries, hamburger, pizza, side salad, chicken sandwich, breakfast sandwich, main salad, Chinese food, chicken nuggets or strips, and rice. Cited in Horovitz, 'Restaurant sales climb with bad-for-you food'.

156. Consumer research data compiled by NPD Group, cited in Associated Press report 'Restaurants slow to drop fat menu choices', *USA Today*, 28 February 2005.

157. Pallavi Gogoi, 'Fat times for fast food', *Business Week*, 9 November 2005.

158. Cited in Bruce Horovitz, 'Foodmakers bet on sweet treats', *USA Today*, 22 December 2005.

159. NPD Group's annual eating habits report, reported in Nanci Hellmich, 'Percentage of overweight Americans stable', *USA Today*, 4 October 2005.

160. *Ibid.*

161. Cited in '127 ways Big Brother Brownell is wrong', Center for Consumer Freedom, 29 July 2004, http://www.consumerfreedom.com/news_detail.cfm/headline/2611

162. Cited in Muir, 'Action urged on eating habits'.

163. Cited in Wintour, 'Blame obesity on bad diets, say food chiefs'.

164. See, for example, Mark Paul, 'Soft drinks go in search of fizz', *Sunday Times*, 13 November 2005.

165. David Teather, 'Bubble bursts for the real thing as PepsiCo ousts Coke from top spot', *Guardian*, 27 December 2005.

166. Quoted in BBC News Online's 'Measures to cut obesity revealed'.

167. Interview with Asthana, 'Food watchdog targets ready meals'.

168. 'Obesity and personal responsibility', Freedom Institute, 27 September 2004, http://www.freedominst.org/2004/09/obesity-and-personal-responsibility.html

169. Ingdahl, 'Swedish meatballs'.

170. Quoted in Wan, 'No junk food? Students shudder at nutrition plans'.

171. Quoted in Matt Keating, 'The battle for hearts and minds', *Guardian*, 7 January 2006.

172. *Ibid.*

CHAPTER 5

1. Speech quoted in Andrew Pierce, 'Don't follow super-size Americans, says Prince', *Times*, 27 January 2006.

2. Cited in 'Battling the flab', *Economist*, 18 August 2006.

3. Cited in 'The world is too fat. Too bad', *Economist*, 11 December 2003.

4. Caroline Ryan, 'Developing world's extra burden', BBC News Online, 23 April 2004, http://news.bbc.co.uk/2/hi/in_depth/sci_tech/2002/boston_2002/1824999.stm

5. See Gregg Easterbrook, 'Wages of wealth: All this progress is killing us, bit by bite', *New York Times*, 14 March 2004; and Jonathan Bor, 'Poorer teens more apt to be fat', *Baltimore Sun*, 24 May 2006.

6. Sander L. Gilman, *Fat Boys: A Slim Book* (Lincoln, NE: University of Nebraska Press, 2004).

7. Quoted in Dinitia Smith, 'Demonizing fat in the war on weight', *New York Times*, 1 May 2004.

8. *Ibid.*

9. Radley Balko, 'Living large: We've been misled about the real threat posed by the "obesity crisis"', *Worth*, December 2005.

10. Zoe Williams, 'Fuss is a fat lot of good', *Guardian*, 11 October 2005.

11. Vivienne Parry, 'Fat versus fiction', *Guardian*, 16 June 2005.

12. Paul Campos, *The Obesity Myth: Why America's Obsession with Weight is Hazardous to Your Health* (New York: Gotham, 2004).

13. Quoted in Clare Murphy, 'Whose fat is it anyway?', BBC News Online, 27 July 2004, http://news.bbc.co.uk/go/pr/fr/-/2/hi/americas/3912711.stm

14. Quoted in Smith, 'Demonizing fat in the war on weight'.

15. Easterbrook, 'Wages of wealth'.

16. For a lengthier discussion of the inherently limited, even counterproductive, role that government can play in the campaign against obesity, see Fred Kuchler and Elise Golan, 'Is there a role for government in reducing the prevalence of overweight and obesity?', *Choices*, Fall 2004: 41–45; Radley Balko, 'Does obesity justify bigger government?', *The Freeman*, 1 October 2005; and Fred Kuchler and Nicole Ballenger, 'Societal costs of obesity: How can we assess when federal interventions will pay?', *Food Review*, USDA Economic Research Service, 25(3) December 2002: 21–27.

17. See, for example, Patrick Basham and John Luik, 'Does Fatness Kill?', *Washington Times*, 30 August 2006; see also, Sharon Kirkey, 'Simple quiz can predict your fate: Test assigns points to different risk factors for limited life expectancy', *National Post*, 15 February 2006. Researchers at the San Francisco Veterans Affairs Medical Center discovered that, in people aged 50 and over, a body mass index of 25 – the 'overweight' category – seems to be protective, so long as the person does not have diabetes. On the other hand, a body mass index under 25 was associated with a shorter life expectancy. See, too, the discussion in Jerome Burne, 'Why being fat may not be so bad for you after all', *Daily Mail*, 3 August 2006.

18. US DHHS quoted in Murphy, 'Whose fat is it anyway?'

19. Cited in Radley Balko, 'Living large'.

20. See, for example, Steven Blair, 'Fit and fat' at http://suewidemark.com/fat-fit-new.htm; Amanda Spake, 'Can you be fit and fat? Being thin isn't everything, says surprising new research', *Shape*, January 2004; and Chris Woolston, 'Fit and fat', *Consumer Health Interactive*, 14 December 2001, http://www.ahealthyme.com/topic/fitandfat

21. Thorkild I. A. Sørensen *et al.*, 'Intention to lose weight, weight changes, and 18-y mortality in overweight individuals without co-morbidities', *Public Library of Science Medicine* 2005 (2), http://medicine.plosjournals.org/perlserv/?request=get-document&doi=10.1371/journal.pmed.0020171

22. Reported in Tanya Gold, 'My life was unmanageable – and I was still fat', *Guardian*, 28 June 2005.

23. Franklin Apfel, comments to the 'Informed Patient: EU Framework for Action' conference, Dublin, 18 February 2004.

24. Quoted in Murphy, 'Whose fat is it anyway?'

25. See, for example, the discussion in John Fauber, 'Eating out linked to health risks in children', *Seattle Times*, 15 November 2005.

26. Ronald Bailey, 'Time for tubby bye bye?' *Reason Online*, 11 June 2003, http://www.reason.com/rb/rb061103.shtml

27. Caroline Davis *et al.*, 'Decision-making deficits and overeating: A risk model for obesity', *Obesity Research* 2004 (12): 929–35.

28. Reported in Sally Squires, 'Slow and steady wins the race', *Washington Post*, 27 December 2005.

29. Mark McClellan, speech, 8 May 2003, http://www.fda.gov/oc/speeches/2003/nfpc0508.html

30. Kevin Patrick *et al.*, 'Diet, physical activity, and sedentary behaviors as risk factors for overweight in adolescence', *Archives of Pediatrics and Adolescent Medicine* 2004 (158): 385–90.

31. Francis Elliott, 'Britons are the laziest fat cats of Europe', *Independent*, 28 December 2003.

32. Cited in Rachel Stevenson, 'Gym users opt to fight their debts rather than the flab', *Independent*, 27 April 2005.

33. 'Fat and happy? That's not what women say', *Independent*, 30 June 2005.

34. Paul Osborne, 'Safe routes for children: What they want and what works', *Children, Youth and Environments* 2005 (15): 234–39.

35. Denis Campbell, '90% of children set to be couch potatoes', *Observer*, 29 May 2005.

36. Gareth A. Davies, 'Latest evidence highlights children's inactivity', *Daily Telegraph*, 30 September 2005.

37. Cited in 'The fat earth society', BBC News Online, 15 February 2001, http://news.bbc.co.uk/1/hi/uk/1171806.stm

38. 'Inactivity rules among UK adults', BBC News Online, 1 April 2004, http://news.bbc.co.uk/go/pr/fr/-/2/hi/health/3590921.stm

39. 'Flabby Londoners shirk exercise', BBC News Online, 4 February 2005, http://news.bbc.co.uk/go/pr/fr/-/2/hi/uk_news/england/london/4235833.stm

40. D. Lakdawalla and T. Philipson, 'The growth of obesity and technological change: A theoretical and empirical analysis', National Bureau of Economic Research Working Paper 8946, May 2004.

41. See also David Sanderson, 'E-mail habit can make you fat', *Sunday Times*, 16 October 2005.

42. Rick Berman, 'No flabby excuses: Take responsibility', *Philadelphia Inquirer*, 30 December 2005, http://www.consumerfreedom.com/oped_detail.cfm/oped/347

43. Emily Bazar, 'Not it! More schools ban games at recess', *USA Today*, 27 July 2006.

44. Cited in Carol Glazer, 'Obesity is not just about food', *Boston Globe*, 5 December 2005.

45. *The State of Latino Health in the District of Columbia*, reported in 'Latino health risks', *Washington Post*, 17 January 2006.

46. Cited in Sarah Cassidy, 'Only half of parents encourage children to eat healthy diet', *Independent*, 29 June 2005.

47. Cited in Sarah Cassidy, 'School food provider blames parents', *Independent*, 10 October 2005.

48. Scott W. Keith *et al.*, 'Putative contributors to the secular increase in obesity: Exploring the roads less traveled', *International Journal of Obesity*, 27 June 2006, available online at http://www.nature.com/ijo/journal/vaop/ncurrent/abs/0803326a.html

49. Harriet Griffey, 'Are you dead on your feet?', *Independent*, 26 April 2004.

50. 'Obesity linked to lack of sleep', BBC News Online, 7 December 2004, http://news.bbc.co.uk/go/pr/fr/-/2/hi/health/4073897.stm

51. Reported in 'Too little sleep may make you fat', BBC News Online, 22 November 2004, http://news.bbc.co.uk/1/hi/health/4026133.stm

52. Frank B. Hu *et al.*, 'Television watching and other sedentary behaviors in relation to risk of obesity and type 2 diabetes mellitus in women', *Journal of the American Medical Association* 2003 (289): 1785–91.

53. 'Child TV hours obesity risk link', BBC News Online, 13 September 2005, http://news.bbc.co.uk/go/pr/fr/-/2/hi/health/4238386.stm

54. Cassandra Jardine, 'Cutting out TV: The toughest diet of all', *Daily Telegraph*, 13 September 2005.

55. Cited in BBC News Online's 'The fat earth society'.

56. Press Association, 'Nearly one in four UK adults obese', 16 December 2005.

57. K. M. Flegal *et al.*, 'The influence of smoking cessation on the prevalence of overweight in the United States', *New England Journal of Medicine* 1995 (333): 1165–70.

58. Reported in Gina Kolata, 'Exchanging cigarettes for bagels', *New York Times*, 19 December 2004.

59. Kevin Patrick *et al.*, 'Randomized controlled trial of a primary care and home-based intervention for physical activity and nutrition behaviors', *Archives of Pediatrics and Adolescent Medicine* 2006 (160): 128–36.

60. Thomas J. Philipson and Richard A. Posner, 'The long-run growth in obesity as a function of technological change', Working Paper Series: 99.8, Harris School, University of Chicago, 17 May 1999.

61. Berman, 'No flabby excuses'.

62. Fred Kuchler *et al.*, 'Obesity policy and the law of unintended consequences', *Amber Waves*, June 2005.

63. For a fuller explanation of his views, see Richard A. Epstein, 'Let the shoemaker stick to his last: A defense of the "old" public health', *Perspectives in Biology and Medicine* 2003 (46): 138–59.

64. Epstein, 'Let the shoemaker stick to his last'.

65. See the discussion in Jeffrey Sobal, 'The medicalization and demedicalization of obesity', in Donna Maurer and Jeffrey Sobal (eds), *Eating Agendas: Food and Nutrition as Social Problems* (New York: Aldine de Gruyter, 1995), pp. 67–90.

66. Sophie Goodchild, 'Britain's children have a bad case of outdoor play phobia', *Independent*, 23 May 2004.

67. Maxine Frith, 'Battery-reared children miss out on play', *Independent*, 22 September 2004.

68. Julie C. Lumeng *et al.*, 'Neighborhood safety and overweight status in children', *Archives of Pediatrics and Adolescent Medicine* 2006 (160): 25–31.

69. See also the discussion in Roni Rabin, 'Breast-fed babies may have a leg up in the battle against childhood obesity', *New York Times*, 13 June 2006.

70. 'Breast milk helps reduce obesity', BBC News Online, 2 May 2004, http://news.bbc.co.uk/go/pr/fr/-/2/hi/health/3673149.stm

71. Jeremy Laurance, 'How to lose weight the easy way: Go to sleep for longer', *Independent*, 11 January 2005.

72. See, for example, Elizabeth Weil, 'Heavy questions', *New York Times* Magazine, 2 January 2005.

73. See, for example, Jacob Sullum, 'Recipe for torts', *Washington Times*, 28 January 2006.

74. Frances M. Berg, *Underage and Overweight: Our Childhood Obesity Crisis – What Every Family Needs to Know* (Long Island, NY: Hatherleigh Press, 2004).

75. Sophie Goodchild and Nicholas Pyke, 'Britain regains its taste for traditional family mealtimes', *Independent*, 10 April 2005.

76. 'Obesity and personal responsibility', Freedom Institute, 27 September 2004, http://www.freedominst.org/2004/09/obesity-and-personal-responsibility.html

77. Reported in 'Obesity: US, UK attitudes differ', Food USA Navigator.com, 7 July 2004, http://foodnavigator-usa.com/news/printNewsBis.asp?id=53361

78. Kuchler *et al.*, 'Obesity policy and the law of unintended consequences'.

79. Freedom Institute, 'Obesity and personal responsibility'.

80. See, for example, James E. Tillotson, 'America's obesity: Conflicting public policies, industrial economic development, and unintended human consequences', *Annual Review of Nutrition* 2004 (24): 617–43.

81. The ability of food subsidies to distort prices is discussed at length in J. McGinnis *et al.* (eds), *Food Marketing to Children and Youth: Threat or Opportunity?* (Washington, DC: Institute of Medicine National Academies Press, 2006), pp. 6–25.

82. For an enlightening discussion of the relationship between prices and obesity, see Jayachandran N. Variyam, 'The price is right: Economics and the rise in obesity', *Amber Waves*, USDA Economic Research Service 2005 (3).

83. Radley Balko, 'Beyond personal responsibility', TechCentralStation.com, 17 May 2004. See also 'Can governments make people thin?', *Economist*, 11 December 2003; and 'The world is too fat. Too bad', 11 December 2003.

84. Epstein, speech to the American Enterprise Institute, Washington, DC, 10 June 2003, as reported in Bailey, 'Time for tubby bye bye?'

85. *Ibid.*

APPENDIX

1. T. S. Kuhn, *The Structure of Scientific Revolutions* (Chicago: University of Chicago Press, 1970); and I. Lakatos (ed.), *The Problem of Inductive Logic* (Amsterdam: North Holland, 1969), p. 397.

2. Paul Feyerabend, 'Science and the anarchist', *Science* 1979 (206): 534–37; Feyerabend, *Against Method: Outline of an Anarchistic Theory of Knowledge* (London: New Left Books, 1975); and L. A. Kelly *et al.*, 'Effect of socioeconomic status on objectively measured physical activity', *Archives of Disease in Childhood* 2006 (91): 35–38.

3. National Academy of Sciences, *Responsible Science: Ensuring the Integrity of the Research Process* (Washington, DC: National Academy Press, 1992), vol. 1, p. 38.

4. *Ibid.*, vol. 1, p. 39.

5. *Ibid.*, vol. 1, p. 56.

6. *Ibid.*, vol. 1, p. 57.

7. *Ibid.*, vol. 1, p. 58.

8. A. B. Hill, 'The environment and disease: Association or causation?', *Proceedings of the Royal Society of Medicine* 1965 (58): 295–300.

9. US Surgeon General, 'Smoking and Health', Report of the Advisory Committee to the Surgeon General of the Public Health Service, 1964, p. 354; US Department of Health, Education, and Welfare, *Public Health Service*, No. 1103, Washington, DC, p. 19.

10. B. McMahon and T. F. Pugh, *Epidemiology: Principles and Methods* (Boston: Little Brown, 1970).

11. D. G. Kleinbaum *et al.*, *Epidemiologic Research* (London: Wadsworth, 1982).

12. R. Doll and R. Peto, 'The causes of cancer', *Journal of the National Cancer Institute* 1981 (66): 1192–312.

13. M. D. Green *et al.*, 'Reference guide on epidemiology', in *Reference Manual on Scientific Evidence* (Washington, DC: Federal Judicial Center, 2000), p. 374.

14. *Ibid.*

15. For exhaustive information, consult K. J. Rothman and S. Greenland, *Modern Epidemiology* (Philadelphia: Lippincott, Williams & Wilkins, 1998). Cohort studies are utilised to observe differences of disease frequency in groups (cohorts) of people exposed or not exposed to possible hazards. Cohort studies can follow a group of subjects over time (longitudinal studies) or simply at a particular moment in time (cross-sectional studies). Case-control studies are utilised when it is only feasible to observe differences of exposure to postulated hazards in groups of people with or without disease. Cohort studies can be prospective or retrospective. The former identify groups of subjects exposed or not exposed to potential hazards, and follow them over time – often years – to record the disease experience of each group. The latter identify groups of subjects with different incidences of diseases, and attempt to reconstruct the past exposures of these groups to possible hazards. Both prospective and retrospective studies may identify different levels of exposure, where higher incidences in relation to higher exposures are interpreted as increasing estimates of risk. Risk reduction or protection is assumed if incidence decreases at increasing exposure levels. Case-control studies are necessarily retrospective, as they compare past experiences in groups with or without a specific disease. Because disease incidence is 0 per cent in the controls and 100 per cent in the cases, a key understanding is that, in case-control studies, risks are inferred as differentials of exposure, and not actually estimated as differentials of incidence. Increased risk is inferred but not directly estimated if exposure is found to be higher among cases, and protection is inferred but not directly estimated if exposure is found to be higher among controls. Other distinctions of studies are made. Of interest here, ecological studies do not compile statistics from individual members of a group, but rather compare overall statistical data of populations against generic characteristics of the same, such as dietary habits, genetic traits, geographic and environmental conditions, and the like. In general, ecological studies produce weaker clues that may call for more specific cohort or case-control studies.

16. Relative risk (RR) is a very common index in epidemiology, along with several indexes not here illustrated, such as odds ratios (OD), hazard ratios (HR), Standard Mortality Ratios (SMR), and others.

17. Under such a consensus definition the threshold of statistical significance is $p=0.05$, that is a 1/20 value. Thus, a relative risk or odds ratio of 1.6 with a $p=0.03$ is said to be statistically significant at the 95 per cent level, whereas a relative risk of 2.3 with a $p=0.07$ is not. The confidence interval (CI) is more informative than p-values, although based on the same concepts. In standard format it gives a range of values within which the value of a relative risk or odds ratio may be located

with a probability of 95 per cent. In interpreting a confidence interval, it is important to recall how risk or odds ratios are calculated. For both indexes a value of 1 means no change in risk because incidence is the same in non-exposed and exposed, or because exposure is the same in cases and controls. Values below 1 imply risk reduction or protection and values above 1 imply increased risk. Therefore: RR=1.9 (95 per cent CI 1.2–4.6) means that the best estimate of the risk may be 1.9, but that its true value could be between 1.2 and 4.6, with a probability of 95 per cent. It also means that, within that range, all values are statistically significant at the 95 per cent level, because all would mean an increase of risk, the lowest value still being >1. RR=1.9 (95 per cent CI 0.7–2.3) means that the best estimate of the risk may be 1.9, but that its true value could be between 0.7 and 2.3, with a probability of 95 per cent. It also means that some values could be <1 and could mean protection, others could be >1 and could mean risk. As a consequence, the result is said to be equivocal and not statistically significant. RR=0.7 (95 per cent CI 0.2–0.9) means that the best estimate of the risk may be 0.7, but that its true value could be between 0.2 and 0.9, with a probability of 95 per cent. It also means that, within that range, all values are statistically significant at the 95 per cent level, because all would mean a reduction of risk, the highest value still being <1. RR=0.7 (95 per cent CI 0.3–1.9) means that the best estimate of the risk may be 0.7, but its true value could be between 0.3 and 1.9, with a probability of 95 per cent. It also means that some values could be <1 and could mean protection, others could be >1 and could mean risk. As a consequence the result is said to be equivocal and not statistically significant.

18. Rothman and Greenland, *Modern Epidemiology*.

19. R. Feynman, *QED* (Princeton, NJ: Princeton University Press, 1985).

20. Green *et al.*, 'Reference guide on epidemiology', p. 381.

21. K. J. Rothman, *Modern Epidemiology* (Boston: Little Brown & Co., 1986).

22. M. Susser and E. Susser, 'Choosing a future for epidemiology: From black box to Chinese boxes and eco-epidemiology', *American Journal of Public Health* 1996 (86): 674–77.

23. N. Pearce, 'Traditional epidemiology, modern epidemiology, and public health', *American Journal of Public Health* 1996 (86): 678–83.

24. N. Pearce and J. B. McKinlay, 'Back to the future in epidemiology and public health: Response to Dr. Gori', *Journal of Clinical Epidemiology* 1998 (51): 643–46.

25. Susser and Susser, 'Choosing a future for epidemiology'.

26. A. R. Feinstein, 'Epidemiologic analyses of causation: The unlearned scientific lessons of randomized trials', *Journal of Clinical Epidemiology* 1989 (42): 481–89.

27. G. Davey Smith, 'Learning to live with complexity: Ethnicity, socioeconomic position, and health in Britain and the United States', *American Journal of Public Health* 2000 (90): 1694–98.

28. Green *et al.*, 'Reference guide on epidemiology', p. 375.

29. Hill, 'The environment and disease: Association or causation?'.

30. Rothman and Greenland, *Modern Epidemiology*, p. 27.

31. *Ibid.*